CASE REVIEW
Gastrointestinal Imaging

Series Editor

David M. Yousem, MD, MBA
Professor of Radiology
Director of Neuroradiology
Russell H. Morgan Department of Radiology and Radiological Science
The Johns Hopkins Medical Institutions
Baltimore, Maryland

Other Volumes in the CASE REVIEW Series

- Brain Imaging
- Breast Imaging
- Cardiac Imaging
- General and Vascular Ultrasound, Second Edition
- Genitourinary Imaging, Second Edition
- Head and Neck Imaging, Second Edition
- Musculoskeletal Imaging, Second Edition
- Nuclear Medicine
- Obstetric and Gynecologic Ultrasound, Second Edition
- Pediatric Imaging
- Spine Imaging, Second Edition
- Thoracic Imaging
- Vascular and Interventional Imaging

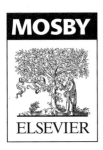

MOSBY
ELSEVIER

Robert D. Halpert, MD, FACR
Professor of Radiology
Department of Radiology
University of Mississippi Medical Center
Jackson, Mississippi

CASE REVIEW

Gastrointestinal Imaging

SECOND EDITION

CASE REVIEW SERIES

1600 John F. Kennedy Blvd.
Suite 1800
Philadelphia, PA 19103-2899

GASTROINTESTINAL IMAGING:
CASE REVIEW, Second Edition
Copyright © 2008, 2000 by Mosby, Inc.

ISBN-13: 978-0-323-04094-5

NOTICE

Knowledge and best practice in this field are constantly changing. As new research and experience broaden our knowledge, changes in practice, treatment and drug therapy may become necessary or appropriate. Readers are advised to check the most current information provided (i) on procedures featured or (ii) by the manufacturer of each product to be administered, to verify the recommended dose or formula, the method and duration of administration, and contraindications. It is the responsibility of the practitioner, relying on their own experience and knowledge of the patient, to make diagnoses, to determine dosages and the best treatment for each individual patient, and to take all appropriate safety precautions. To the fullest extent of the law, neither the Publisher nor the Author assumes any liability for any injury and/or damage to persons or property arising out of or related to any use of the material contained in this book.

Library of Congress Cataloging-in-Publication Data

Halpert, Robert D., M.D.
    Gastrointestinal imaging : case review / Robert D. Halpert. — 2nd ed.
      p. ; cm. — (Case review series)
    Rev. ed. of: Gastrointestinal imaging / Peter J. Feczko, Robert D. Halpert. c2000.
    Includes bibliographical references and index.
    ISBN 978-0-323-04094-5
    1. Gastrointestinal system—Imaging—Case studies. I. Feczko, Peter J. Gastrointestinal imaging.
    II. Title. III. Series.
    [DNLM: 1. Gastrointestinal Diseases—diagnosis—Examination Questions.
  2. Diagnostic Imaging—methods—Examination Questions. WI 18.2 H195g 2008]
  RC804.D52F43 2008
  616.3'30754—dc22

2007010332

Acquisitions Editor: Maria Lorusso
Developmental Editor: Colleen McGonigal
Project Manager: Bryan Hayward
Design Direction: Steven Stave

Printed in the United States of America.

Last digit is the print number: 9 8 7 6 5 4 3 2 1

The book is dedicated to the memory of Cecil H. Greenhow and to my father-in-law, John W. Jenkins, who at 92 years of age is still diligently occupied and busy on a daily basis with the work he loves. From the many hundreds, and perhaps thousands, of people whose lives were influenced by these men, please accept our gratitude and thanks.

I have been very gratified by the popularity and positive feedback that the authors of the Case Review Series have received on publication of the first edition volumes. Reviews in journals and word-of-mouth comments have been uniformly favorable. The authors have done an outstanding job in filling the niche of an affordable, easy-to-read, case-based learning tool that supplements the material in *THE REQUISITES* series.

While some students learn best in a noninteractive study-book mode, others need the anxiety or excitement of being quizzed, being put on the hot seat. The format that was selected for the Case Review Series simulates the Boards by showing a limited number of images needed to construct a differential diagnosis and asking a few clinical and imaging questions (the only difference is that the Case Review books give you the correct answer and immediate feedback!). Cases are scaled from relatively easy to very difficult to test the limit of the reader's knowledge. In addition, a brief author's commentary and a cross-reference to *THE REQUISITES* volume are provided for each case.

Because of the success of the series, we have begun to roll out the second editions of the Case Review volumes. The expectation is that the second editions will bring the material to the state-of-the-art, introduce new modalities and new techniques, and provide new and even more graphic examples of pathology.

This volume of the Case Review Series, *Gastrointestinal Imaging* by Dr. Robert D. Halpert, is the latest of the second editions. Dr. Halpert has updated his edition with new and improved cases, discussions, and techniques. *Gastrointestinal Imaging* encompasses far more than just fluoroscopic images of yesteryear. This is a multi-modality specialty that is inclusive of CT, MRI, ultrasound, and now molecular imaging. Perfusion imaging, three-dimensional processing, spectroscopy, and various enhancement techniques make this a rich field indeed. Fortunately, this one volume includes cases that provide residents with the knowledge they will need to feel comfortable interpreting clinical cases. Dr. Halpert's success in the first edition is revisited here, and residents preparing for the oral Boards will find here a treasure-trove of quality material that will serve them well in Louisville (or wherever Boards will be held in the future).

I am pleased to present for your viewing pleasure the latest volume of the second editions of the Case Review Series, joining the previous second editions of *Head and Neck Imaging* by David M. Yousem and Carol da Motta; *Genitourinary Imaging* by Ronald J. Zagoria, William W. Mayo-Smith, and Julia R. Fielding; *Obstetric and Gynecologic Ultrasound* by Karen L. Reuter and T. Kemi Babagbemi; *General and Vascular Ultrasound* by William D. Middleton; *Spine Imaging* by Brian Bowen, Alfonso Rivera, and Efrat Saraf-Lavi; and *Musculoskeletal Imaging* by Joseph Yu.

David M. Yousem, MD

This second edition of *Gastrointestinal Imaging: Case Review* is an attempt to further the goals put forth with such diligence by Dr. Peter Feczko in the first edition. Its intended use is to supplement *THE REQUISITES* series with self-evaluation and practical applications as well as the enjoyment of being challenged in the area of Gastrointestinal Imaging. You will note the smaller number of plain images and barium studies in this edition and the increased emphasis on MDCT imaging. This is a true reflection of the nature of the practice as we enter the 21st century. Indeed the sharp drop in the number of barium studies performed over the past five years is not transient, and it is safe to say that the barium examination will soon follow the pneumoencephalogram. Although barium studies are still justified in a small niche of cases, there will continue to be fewer and fewer such cases, and the number of radiologists with sufficient expertise in this area will continue to diminish. The boundaries of our specialty are inexact, and we must constantly adapt to these changes. But the good news is that while we might lose some territory on one front, on another we are presenting the profession, general public, and third-party payers with examinations and therapeutic procedures that are viable, less invasive, less expensive, and less risky than before. Even the name of our specialty, "Diagnostic Radiology," needs to be reconsidered as we undertake more and more therapeutic procedures in our departments. From my perspective, it is an exciting time to be embarking on a career in imaging.

Once again I would like to thank and acknowledge the efforts of Renea Hays in the preparation of the manuscript and illustrations. I must also mention and acknowledge my faculty colleague Dr. Tom Cole and the several enthusiastic radiology residents at the University of Mississippi Medical Center who were interested in and helpful in the development of this project.

Robert D. Halpert, MD

Opening Round

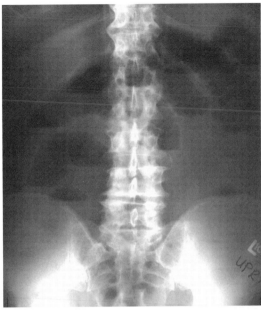

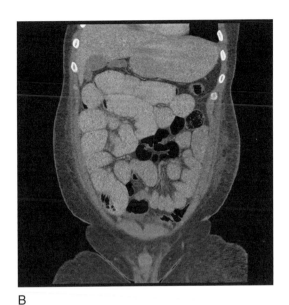

A   B

1. Which of the following statements are true? This patient presents with abdominal pain, distention, and cramps.

2. The patient very likely has a history of abdominal surgery.

3. A barium enema would most likely reveal no colonic abnormalities.

4. All of the above may be correct.

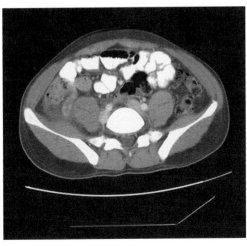

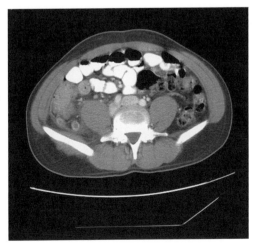

A   B

1. What is the most common cause of acute abdominal emergencies seen in the Western world?

2. The classic surface anatomy of the appendix was first described by whom?

3. The normal width of the appendix on CT is 10 to 12 mm. True or false?

4. The commonest finding for acute appendicitis on plain film is an acute focal ileus. True or false?

Small Bowel Obstruction

1. The upright plain film of the abdomen demonstrates a classic small bowel obstruction. All of these symptoms might apply.

2. The vast majority of patients presenting with small bowel obstruction have had previous abdominal surgery. Without the history of prior surgery, small bowel obstruction becomes more ominous.

3. In cases of small bowel obstruction, a barium enema would probably be of little benefit. However, if the terminal ileum can be refluxed and the terminal ileum demonstrated to be collapsed or of normal caliber, it is presumptive evidence of small bowel obstruction.

4. All of the above are correct.

Cross-Reference
Gastrointestinal Imaging: THE REQUISITES, ed 3, p 107.

Comment
The routine plain films of the abdomen are upright and supine images when possible. It is true that, increasingly, CT of the abdomen is being done for any abdominal complaint. However, CT is an expensive route for screening the nonsurgical abdomen and in such cases is not recommended. Plain films of the abdomen should be the first step if bowel obstruction is suspected. When CT is used, the findings are dilated loops of small bowel. A transition zone can sometimes be identified and occasionally the cause is demonstrated (if it is other than an adhesion, which is rarely seen on CT).

The classic differential air-fluid levels seen in the first 48 to 72 hours of a small bowel obstruction are almost pathognomonic of a mechanical SBO. The only exception occurs in rare cases of appendicitis in which the inflammatory phlegmon acts as an obstruction process. It is important to clearly understand what constitutes a differential air-fluid level. It represents two different air-fluid levels in the *same* loop of bowel. Air-fluid levels, in themselves, are nonspecific and can be seen in any number of conditions apart from mechanical obstruction. However, in mechanical obstruction, the motility of the bowel is exaggerated as it forcefully tries to push intestinal content past the narrowed segment, resulting in a to-and-fro movement of fluid. As a result there is an uneven distribution of fluid when the patient is raised to the upright position. Hence, differential air-fluid levels are seen in the same loop of bowel. With an ileus, on the other hand, the bowel movement is diminished or absent, and water distribution is equalized throughout the bowel, and as a result, differential air-fluid levels are not seen.

Notes

Acute Appendicitis

1. Acute appendicitis is the most common acute abdominal emergency in industrialized countries. Its incidence is approximately 10 to 11 per 10,000 but has been slowly declining over the last 30 years.

2. The surface anatomy of the appendix was first described by McBurney in the 19th century, giving rise to the well-known "McBurney's point" in the right lower quadrant.

3. False. The normal width of the appendix is about 4 mm. Anything wider is suspect.

4. False.

Cross-Reference
Gastrointestinal Imaging: THE REQUISITES, ed 3, p 317.

Comment
Acute appendicitis is a common abdominal emergency condition. Although there has been much discussion about the merits of various imaging modalities in the diagnosis, it is now clear that MDCT is the imaging tool of choice. It is able to not only see the appendix easier than other methods but can also provide other crucial information regarding complications, etc. Findings on MDCT include, in simple uncomplicated acute appendicitis, thickening of the appendix beyond 6 mm, appendiceal enhancement (vascular congestion), periappendiceal stranding, and occasionally small amounts of fluid around the appendix or in the cul-de-sac.

Plain film evaluation of acute appendicitis is usually not helpful. If a calcified appendolith is seen in a patient with appropriate clinical symptoms, it is pathognomonic. However, this is unusual. Occasionally one might see a focal ileus effect in the right lower quadrant, but by far the most common plain film finding is normal. Medical students and residents should discipline themselves to find the appendix on every abdominal CT case they encounter. Sometimes finding an unusually located appendix can be a chore. The more you do, the better you get at it.

Notes

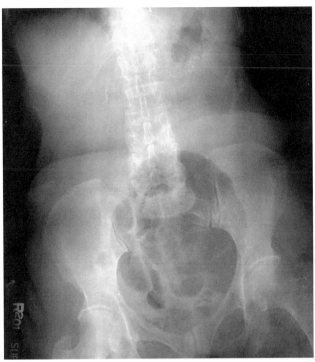

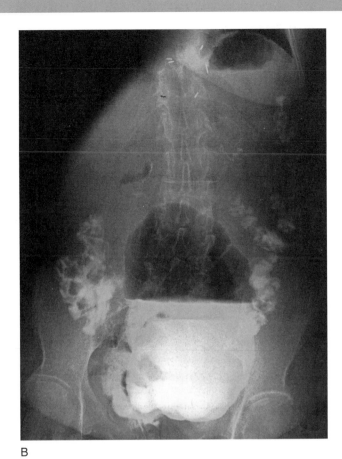

A

B

1. What is the most common type of torsion abnormality of the bowel?

2. A cecal volvulus tends to result in a dilated cecum crossing the midline and directed toward the spleen. True or false?

3. What other condition can mimic a sigmoid volvulus?

4. What are the complications of volvulus of the bowel?

Cecal Bascule

1. Sigmoid volvulus.

2. True.

3. Severe colonic ileus, often postoperative; occasionally redundant distended but unobstructive sigmoid megacolon in a patient with neuromuscular disease or on certain medications.

4. Obstruction; compromise of the vascular pedicle and bowel necrosis.

Cross-Reference

Gastrointestinal Imaging: THE REQUISITES, ed 3, p 310.

Comments

A volvulus is the twisting or torsion of a segment of bowel. The degree of severity and possibility of complications depend on the tightness of the twist and lack of spontaneous untwisting of the bowel. The number of volvuli that occur and spontaneously resolve is probably much higher than most radiologists appreciate.

The most common volvulus occurs in the sigmoid colon (50–75% of cases). The cecum is the next most common site, seen in 20% to 40% of cases. Much less common are volvuli of the transverse colon and, rarely, the splenic flexure.

There are two types of cecal volvulus: the common torsion type and the much less common cecal bascule (about 10% of all cecal volvuli are bascules, as shown in this case). The more common cecal volvulus twists around its lumen axis. The torsion acts as an obstruction of the ascending colon. If the ileocecal valve is competent (allows only unidirectional flow) the luminal axis of the air-distended cecum will be directed across the abdomen toward the spleen. Obviously, at a certain point, a greatly dilated thin-walled cecum will burst, resulting in perforation, spillage of colon content, and peritonitis. If the ileocecal value is not competent, the findings can be less clear.

In the case of a bascule, the cecum does not twist about its luminal axis, but instead flips up and over an adhesion across the ascending colon, and the dilated cecum is seen clearly as a right-sided or midline subhepatic air-filled structure with a vertical luminal axis. The cause of the adhesion or band, over which the cecum flips, is unknown. It may be congenital.

Notes

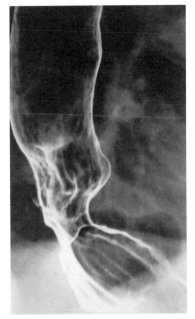

A

B

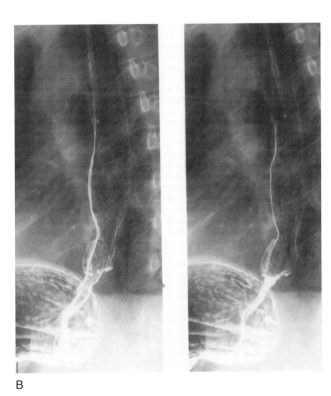

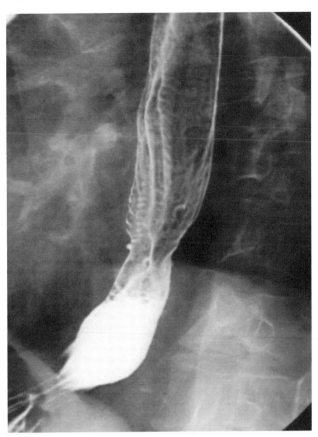

C

Indicate whether the following statements are true or false:

1. There is almost a 25% prevalence of gastroesophageal reflux disease (GERD) in the population.

2. The radiologic findings of Barrett's metaplasia have been well described in the radiologic literature.

3. A manifestation of chronic GERD is episodic insomnia.

4. The proximal esophagus is not spared in GERD.

Reflux Esophagitis

1. False. The prevalence of GERD in the general population is thought to be somewhere between 50% and 75%.

2. False. Radiologic findings associated with Barrett's metaplasia have been reported. However, there are no specific radiologic findings for the condition.

3. True. Many patients report symptoms that wake them up at night. Some can be severe with coughing fits and asthma-like symptoms. Rolling to the right side from a supine position seems to induce symptoms in many patients.

4. False. Almost universally, the symptoms and endoscopic and radiologic findings involve the distal esophagus.

Cross-Reference
Gastrointestinal Imaging: THE REQUISITES, ed 3, p 16.

Comments
Radiologically, the findings of GERD are seen in the chronic phase. Radiographs are not yet able to identify the red mucosal coloring of early or acute disease. When seen in chronic disease, findings include fold thickening, granular appearance of the mucosa, superficial ulcerations, and developing luminal narrowing. Occasionally one may encounter a "feline" esophagus (as in the image shown here) in which symmetrically arranged furrows are seen in the esophagus and are though to be a response to gastric acid on the mucosa. However, recently the endoscopic literature has described a surprising similar finding in young patients with eosinophilic esophagitis. The presence of spontaneous GE reflux and the manner in which the esophagus handles it are most important. Is the gastric content cleared quickly from the esophagus by secondary wave activity? CT evaluation is less specific and may disclose some mild uniform thickening of the distal esophageal wall, or a patulous esophagus as well as fluid in the esophagus. The presence of a hiatal hernia, although not definitive, is associated with an increased incidence of reflux.

The complications of chronic GERD are Barrett's metaplasia (a condition in which the esophageal squamous mucosa begins to take on a somewhat disordered appearance of gastric or intestinal mucosa). Barrett's metaplasia is a precursor of adenocarcinoma in the distal esophagus and GE junction. The other important complication is ulceration and stricture formation seen almost exclusively in the distal esophagus.

It is probably correct to assume that everyone, at some time or another, refluxes acid from the stomach up into the esophagus. However, the natural protective mechanisms, the lower esophageal sphincter (LES) and the secondary esophageal clearing wave which strips the acid back into the stomach, are usually sufficient to protect us from damage. Why this protective mechanism fails in some patients is not fully understood at this time. However, the incidence of GERD is increasing. Some have attributed the rise to increasing obesity in the general population and others have questioned the untoward side effect of many of the newer hypertensive and cardiac medications of lowering the LES. At this time the question awaits definitive answers.

Notes

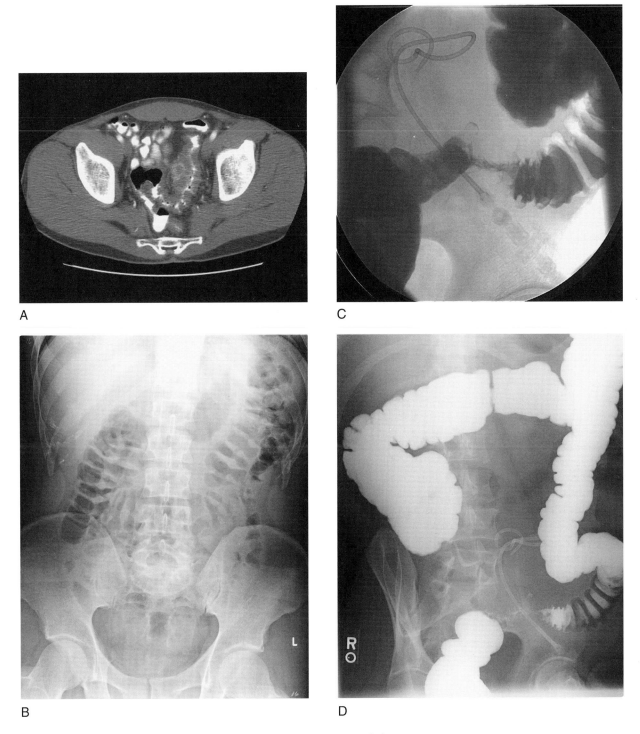

A

C

B

D

1. Where is the area of interest in the provided images of this case?

2. What is the most common cause of rectal bleeding?

3. Given chronic abnormal motility, elevated intraluminal pressures, and prolonged transit times, what conditions are likely to occur?

4. How would these conditions vary in different parts of the world?

Sigmoid Diverticulitis

1. The area of interest, both on the plain film and CT image, is the sigmoid colon.

2. The most common cause of rectal bleeding is hemorrhoids. The most common serious cause of rectal hemorrhage is bleeding from colonic diverticula.

3. With these changes, the most likely pathologic condition is diverticulosis. These changes would also be indications of stasis, which increases the possibility of neoplasm.

4. The highest incidence of diverticulosis and diverticulitis are seen in the industrialized West. They are far less common in Third World countries, as is colonic cancer.

Cross-Reference

Gastrointestinal Imaging: THE REQUISITES, ed 3, p 302.

Comments

The CT image shows thickening and irregularity of the sigmoid colon as well as a small paracolonic abscess containing some air. The plain film is nonspecific, but does show air throughout the colon with a relative paucity of air in the sigmoid region.

Between 60% and 70% of patients over the age of 60 years will have some colonic diverticula. Most of these will be asymptomatic. Some will experience episodic bleeding (in some cases serious bleeding). Some will experience recurrent vague abdominal discomfort (spastic bowel), which may represent mild inflammatory (preceding frank diverticulitis) changes around the diverticula. Others will experience peridiverticular perforations and frank diverticulitis with all the expected symptoms of diverticulitis as well as possible bowel obstruction. Some patients with diverticulitis present with colonic obstruction. A barium enema with narrowing in the sigmoid colon without mucosal destruction is shown in Figure 5C and 5D.

Notes

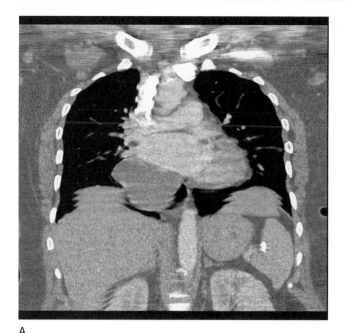

A

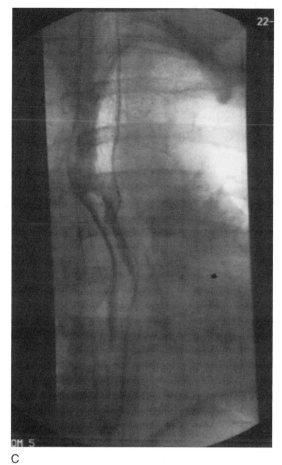

C

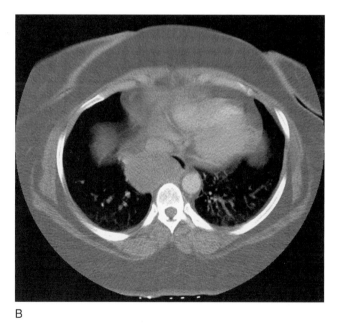

B

1. Does this finding demonstrate a mucosal, intramural, or extrinsic process?

2. What are the three most common foregut congenital cysts?

3. What is the most common enteric cyst?

4. What are the symptoms of a cyst in the lower mediastinum?

Duplication Cyst of the Esophagus

1. Extrinsic.

2. Enteric duplication cysts, bronchogenic cysts, and neurogenic cysts.

3. Esophageal duplication cysts.

4. Usually symptomatic, mostly seen as inadvertent finding except when infected.

Cross-Reference

Gastrointestinal Imaging: THE REQUISITES, ed 3, p 10.

Comments

The images disclose an extrinsic impression on the lower esophagus. The angles of the impression are obtuse, the mucosa is smooth and intact, and the lumen is somewhat compromised. There is no evidence of ulceration or mucosal destruction. All these findings suggest an extrinsic origin. In fact, the lesion is a noncommunicating duplication cyst of the esophagus. A small percentage of cysts communicate with the esophagus and may act like an epiphrenic diverticulum if the cyst is located in the lower esophagus. Esophageal duplication cysts of the gut are the most common enteric cyst (25%). Duplication cysts are one of the cystic manifestations of foregut malformations. CT demonstrates a para-esophageal cystic mass, which usually is not communicating with the lumen (Fig. 6A, 6B). A small percentage will communicate.

Bronchogenic and neurogenic cysts are the other two foregut malformation cysts, and all can affect the esophagus. These cysts tend to be unilocular and bear a close embryologic relationship to congenital cystic adenomatoid malformation of the lung. Duplication cysts are usually lined with squamoid cells with some columnar elements and are usually seen in the lower esophagus. Bronchogenic cysts are usually indistinguishable and are most commonly seen in the mediastinum in a subcarinal location. They usually contain some cilated columnar epithelium and are thought to be the result of abnormal bronchial budding during lung development. They never communicate with the esophagus. Neurogenic cysts are usually located in the posterior mediastinum and in a more posterior position than either duplication or bronchogenic cysts. They are thought to be an embryologic abnormality associated with incomplete separation from the notochordal structures. Neurogenic cysts are commonly associated with vertebral abnormalities such as hemivertebrae or butterfly vertebrae.

Notes

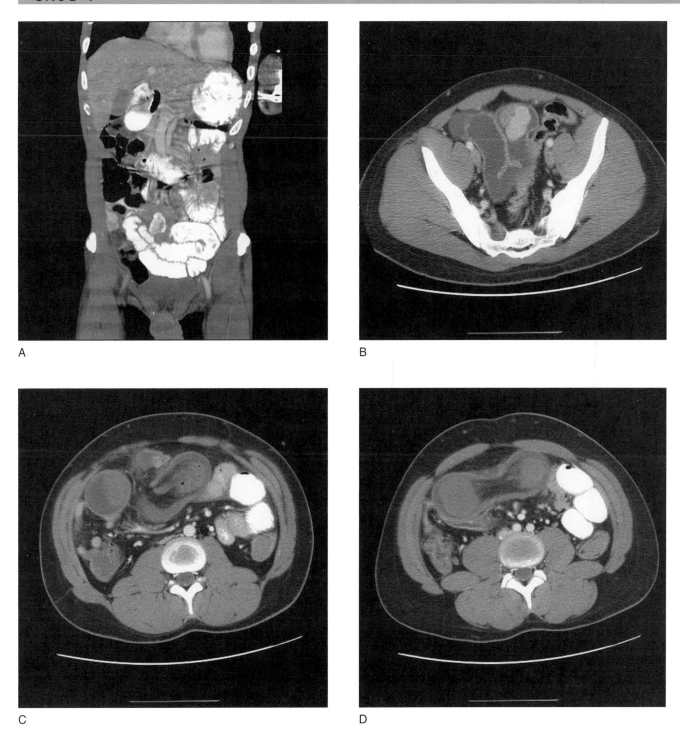

A

B

C

D

1. What is the most common tumor of the small bowel?

2. What symptoms may be associated with the presence of a benign small bowel tumor?

3. What is the most common site of lymphomas of the small bowel?

4. What polyposis syndromes most commonly affect the small bowel?

Intussusception of Small Bowel

1. The most common tumor of the small bowel is a leiomyoma (benign stromal cell tumor).

2. There may be no symptoms associated with small benign tumors of the small bowel. Larger tumors may bleed or result in intussusception.

3. The terminal ileum.

4. Familial polyposis, Peutz-Jeghers syndrome, Cronkhite-Canada syndrome, Cowden disease.

Cross-Reference

Gastrointestinal Imaging: THE REQUISITES, ed 3, p 78.

Comments

Tumors of the small bowel are not commonly encountered because they tend to occur with less frequency than esophageal, gastric, or colonic lesions; are harder to detect; and are often asymptomatic. Except for the polyposis syndromes, they are usually seen in the older population and may present with bleeding, intussusception, and bowel obstruction type symptoms. The most common benign small bowel tumor is the leiomyoma (GIST) followed by lipomas. Both lesions, as well as other benign and malignant polypoid processes, can result in a bowel intussusception. Lymphoid hyperplasia can act as the nidus for intussusception in small children.

Most cases are seen in children; only 5% to 15% of all cases of intussusception are seen in adults. Intussusception in adults is commonly seen when symptomatic and obstructed in nature. However, prior to this, most intussusceptions are probably transient, causing chronic vague abdominal symptoms that usually subside over time. Of course, when the intussusceptum (the telescoping part of the bowel) becomes locked into the intussuscipiens (the receiving part of the bowel), the symptoms are immediately evident and the situation is worsened by edema and vascular congestion, making reduction difficult (Fig. 7C, 7D). In children especially, most intussuceptions are ileocolonic and can often be reduced by slow and careful distention of the colon via a barium enema. In adults the intussusceptions tend to be ileo-ileum and require surgical intervention. Invariably, an adult intussusception will have a polyp (Fig. 7B), benign or malignant, as the leading nidus of the intussusception.

Notes

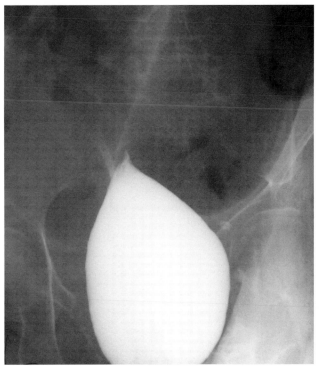

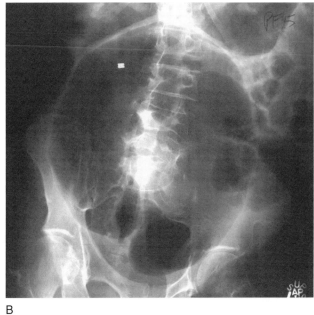

A   B

1. What condition is demonstrated in these images?

2. What is the most common form of volvulus seen in the colon?

3. What is the name of the radiologic sign seen at the site of torsion in these images?

4. What is the fastest way to make this diagnosis?

C A S E   8

Sigmoid Volvulus

1. Sigmoid volvulus.

2. Sigmoid volvulus.

3. The "beak sign."

4. Plain film of the abdomen. If the plain films are not definitive, a water-soluble enema remains the fastest, easiest, and most inexpensive way of making the diagnosis. However, the enema could degrade any CT study done in the next several hours.

Cross-Reference

Gastrointestinal Imaging: THE REQUISITES, ed 3, p 310.

Comments

Sigmoid volvulus is the most common type of volvulus seen in the GI tract, accounting for 8% to 10% of cases. The incidence is higher in areas of the world where roundworm infestation is endemic. In the West, the condition tends to occur in older patients (slightly higher rate in males) with a mortality rate of about 20%. Ultimately the mortality rate depends upon the degree of torsion and the time between the onset of symptoms and diagnosis and treatment. The amount of torsion around the sigmoid mesentery can vary from 180 to 540 degrees and usually occurs about 20 to 25 cm from the anal verge. The torsion is counterclockwise. Patients commonly present with abdominal distention and pain and inability to pass stool or gas.

Plain films of the abdomen are often enough to make the diagnosis in 70% of patients. They will show a grossly dilated sigmoid colon in the well-known "coffee bean" configuration arising out of the pelvis. The sigmoid haustra will be effaced and there may be evidence of proximal obstruction if the amount of torsion is so great as to become an obstruction above the volvulus. Most of the time the torsion will allow proximal air to pass into the volvulus, but will not permit retrograde or distal escape of air, and evidence of proximal obstruction may not be present in such cases.

If there is no free air present, nor evidence of pneumatosis or clinical evidence of peritonititis, a water soluble-enema is the best choice among contrast examinations. Contrast material will demonstrate a normal caliber distal sigmoid and rectum, but will taper to the diagnostic "beak" sign at the site of torsion.

Notes

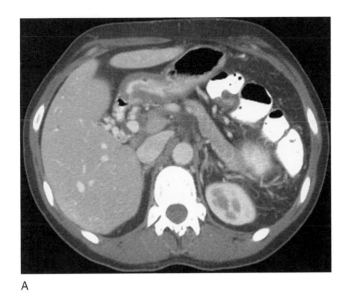

A

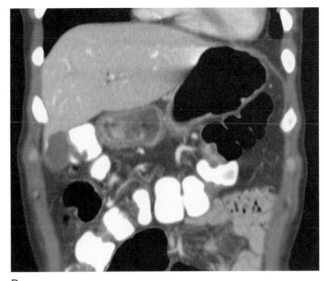

B

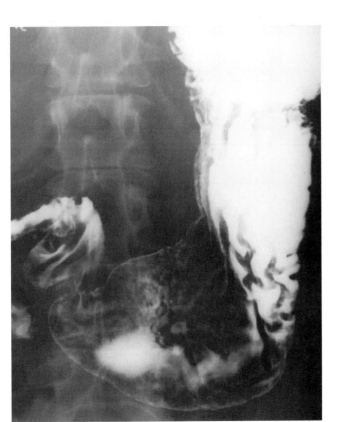

C

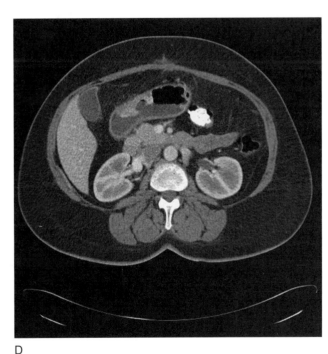

D

1. Into what three general radiologic categories can gastric ulcers be divided, based on double contrast studies of the stomach?

2. Name five radiologic characteristics of a malignant gastric ulcer.

3. What is the best imaging method to evaluate known gastric malignancy?

4. Can a benign gastric ulcer convert into malignant ulcer?

Malignant Ulcer of Stomach

1. Radiologically, gastric ulcers may be divided into malignant, benign, and indeterminate (containing characteristics of both benign and malignant).

2. Ulcer is projected within luminal confines of stomach; folds do not progress up to the edge of the ulcer crater; folds are thickened, clubbed, fused, or amputated; ulcer is asymmetrically positioned on gastric mass; ulcer is not rounded and well defined, but instead is irregularly shaped with poorly defined margins.

3. CT is the image method of choice. It not only shows the stomach lesion but also evaluates for adenopathy spread as well metastatic spread to the liver.

4. No. Although this was once considered the natural etiologic pathway for gastric malignancy, it is now known not to be the case.

Cross-Reference

Gastrointestinal Imaging: THE REQUISITES, ed 3, pp 77–78.

Comments

Today, potential gastric malignancy is almost exclusively evaluated by endoscopy and CT. However in asymptomatic screening situations, high-quality double contrast barium studies are still quite useful. Superficial spreading mucosal lesions with little or no mass can be missed on CT. Lesions such as those shown in the image from a double contrast upper GI study included with this case are best augmented with CT evaluation, which allows for much more accurate grading of the lesions. Perigastric involvement as well as lymph node spread and metastatic spread are well evaluated on MDCT of the thorax, abdomen, and pelvis (Fig. 9A, 9B).

Some of the characteristics of benignity of a gastric ulcer would include the following: (1) Hampton's line (well-defined thin lucency seen at the base of the ulcer, an ulcer collar); (2) ulcer crater is projected outside the gastric lumen; (3) ulcer is symmetrically placed on a gastric mass such as might be seen is surrounding edema of GIST tumor; (4) gastric folds flow right up to the crater edge, and although there may be thickening of the fold due to inflammation, there is no evidence of clubbing (where the termination of a fold swells into a "club-like" configuration).

Clubbing as well as fusion of fold and failure of folds are all seen on the double contrast image included in this case (Fig. 9C).

Notes

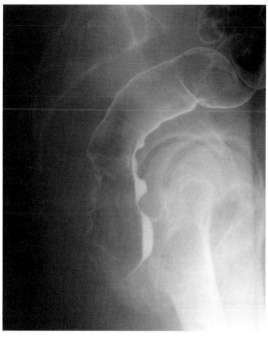

A

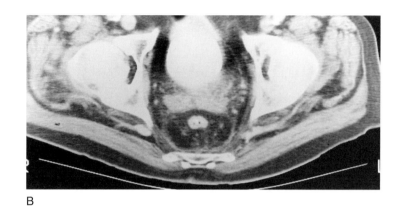

B

1. What is considered to be the normal amount of space between rectum and sacrum?

2. At what level should this space be measured?

3. In patients with inflammatory bowel disease such as ulcerative colitis, what causes widening of the presacral space?

4. Name common iatrogenic causes for presacral space widening.

C A S E   1 0

Presacral Widening

1. 1.5 to 2.0 cm.

2. Lower sacrum or midrectum.

3. Mostly normal connective tissue.

4. Radiation or pelvic surgery.

Cross-Reference

Gastrointestinal Imaging: THE REQUISITES, ed 3, pp 315–316.

Comments

The presacral space between the midrectum and sacral bone (measured below the peritoneal reflection) can be variable and sometimes is a dilemma for radiologists. This space is taken up with fascia and some fatty tissue in most people. The measurement is valid only when the rectum is fully distended, and the lack of distention in inflammatory disease involving the rectum is usually what accounts for the widening. In Crohn's disease perirectal inflammatory changes will also be present.

Widening can be due to processes that involve the rectum (most common), causes that affect the sacral bone, and processes that affect the retroperitoneum. Rectal causes can be both inflammatory and neoplastic (Fig. 10A). Retroperitoneal causes can include retroperitoneal lipomatosis (Fig. 10B) or fibrosis. Sacral diseases that can result in widening include sacral bony tumors (metastatic disease, as well as chordomas and neurofibromas) and sacral inflammation such as osteomyelitis.

Notes

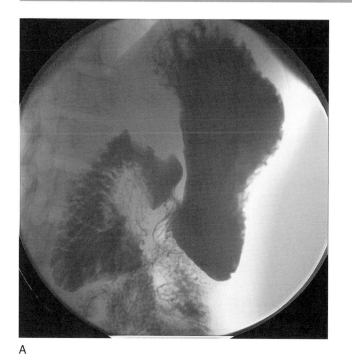

A

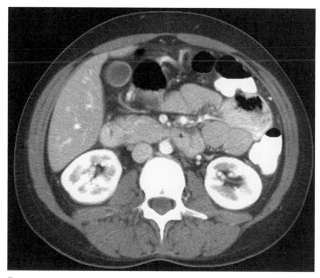

B

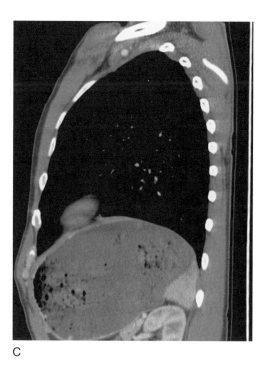

C

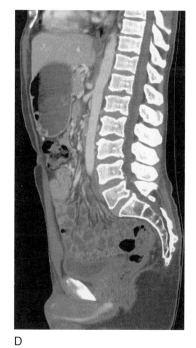

D

1. What is the abnormality demonstrated in these images?

2. What are the anatomic changes thought to be responsible?

3. What types of patients are most susceptible to this condition?

4. What simple mechanism might ameliorate the symptoms?

SMA Syndrome

1. SMA (superior mesenteric artery) syndrome.

2. Narrowing of the aortic-SMA angle, resulting in a degree of duodenal obstruction.

3. The SMA syndrome has been described in those with severe illness and sudden weight loss, burn patients, patients in body casts, children with unusually rapid growth, and young women with eating disorders.

4. Turning the patient supine will open the aortic-SMA angle in some patients.

Cross-Reference

Gastrointestinal Imaging: THE REQUISITES, ed 3, p 90.

Comments

The transverse retroperitoneal portion of the duodenum is nestled in an angle created by the aorta posteriorly and the superior mesenteric artery anteriorly. This angle can vary in size and hence this condition is sometimes controversial. There are some who refuse to accept that SMA syndrome is a real condition. Given the narrowness of the angle we are now able to measure on MDCT sagittal images in asymptomatic patients, this is quite understandable. However, from time to time we are faced with the so-called syndrome and its symptoms and findings cannot be denied. Patients will complain of abdominal pain, nausea, weight loss, and especially vomiting. Imaging of the abdomen will often show a dilated stomach and proximal duodenum (Fig. 11C). The duodenum will be narrowed at the level of the aortic-SMA angle and the distal duodenum will be normal caliber. MDCT sagittal imaging now permits us to measure the angle (Fig. 11D). In this case the angle measures 18 degrees. A normal angle is not easy to define but is probably in the 25- to 30-degree range. In severe unremitting cases surgical intervention, such as gastrojejunostomy, may be required.

Notes

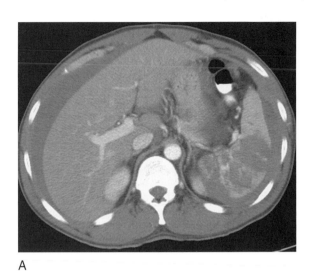

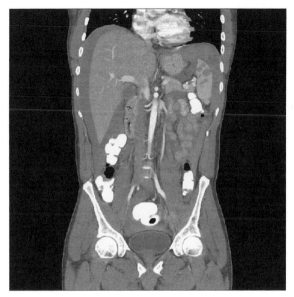

A   B

1. What important finding is demonstrated on these images?

2. What findings will increase the urgency of surgical intervention?

3. What percentage of splenic lacerations will require surgical treatment?

4. What percentage of patients with splenic injury will exhibit the classical findings of RUQ pain and hypotension?

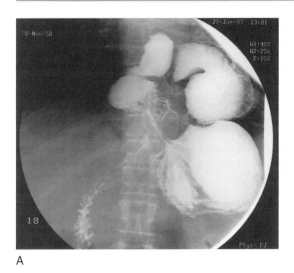

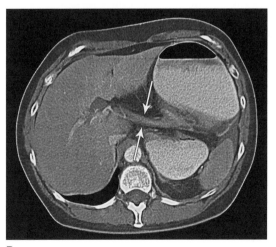

A   B

1. What is the abnormality depicted in these images?

2. What surgical emergency is this patient at risk for?

3. Name the two types of torsion abnormality that are seen in this condition.

4. What prior history might be associated with this condition?

CASE 12

Splenic Laceration

1. Splenic laceration.

2. The quantity of hemorrhage and the CT demonstration of continued bleeding.

3. This answer is rapidly changing owing to the impact of CT. Prior to CT, if diagnostic peritoneal lavage was positive, patients often underwent splenectomy. Today, with MDCT, an organ injury scale has been developed and the numbers of splenectomies has significantly decreased. Additionally, many potential splenectomies have been replaced by less invasive interventional embolization of the splenic artery.

4. Splenic injury can be deceptive and subtle. Only about 50% of patients will have abdominal pain and distention, and hypotension is seen in only 35% of presenting patients.

Cross-Reference

Gastrointestinal Imaging: THE REQUISITES, ed 3, p 211.

Comments

The spleen is the most commonly injured organ in the abdomen as a result of blunt trauma. Patients who are hemodynamically stable will routinely receive a CT examination. The degree of splenic injury is assessed and assigned a grade. The grade will help in determining whether the patient will or will not require intervention and the need for continued evaluation of the spleen. The grading method is dependent on size and depth of the tear, number of tears, amount of extravasation, and whether there is continued bleeding. A grade I injury is a small capsular tear, nonexpanding, nonbleeding, and no deeper than 1 cm, and a grade V tear is a shattered spleen with involvement of the splenic vascular pedicle.

The patient shown in this case is a young man involved in a motor vehicle accident with a grade III splenic injury. You will note several deep splenic tears (shattered spleen) with both intra- and extrasplenic bleeding. Although there is intrasplenic segmental arterial injury, the splenic hilum and splenic artery are intact. There is bleeding in the upper abdomen around both the liver and spleen. The patient was successfully treated with vascular volume stabilization and splenic artery embolization.

Notes

CASE 13

Gastric Volvulus

1. Gastric volvulus.

2. Impairment of the vascular pedicle and necrosis of the stomach.

3. Organoaxial and mesenteroaxial rotations or torsion of the stomach.

4. Prior diaphragmatic trauma.

Cross-Reference

Gastrointestinal Imaging: THE REQUISITES, ed 3, pp 54–55.

Comments

Gastric volvulus is a condition in which most or all of the stomach herniates into the chest. Although not common, it is an important condition to recognize before complications set in. The patent is quite often older in age and often asymptomatic. The condition becomes a serious surgical emergency when rotation of the stomach occurs around its long axis or its mesenteric axis and compromises the stomach so that it become sufficiently tight that gastric blood supply is compromised, leading to necrosis. Quite often these patients may have a long-standing history of hiatal hernia in which the diaphragmatic hiatus has become so lax and enlarged that the entire stomach may be found in the chest at the time of examination. The other past medical history that is sometimes associated with this condition is traumatic diaphragmatic injury.

There are two varieties of gastric volvulus. Organoaxial volvulus occurs when the stomach rotates around its long axis, an imaginary line drawn between the gastroesophageal junction and the pylorus. This is the most common type; it is usually chronic and asymptomatic and seen in older patients. Strangulation and necrosis have been reported in 5% to 25% of patients with this type. A mesenteroaxial volvulus occurs when the stomach rotates around the mesenteric axis (gastrohepatic ligament) so the distal stomach may be projected over or above the fundus. It is usually not associated with diaphragmatic disorders.

Radiologically, the diagnosis is possible on plain film when two large collections of air with air-fluid levels may be seen above the diaphragm. On CT the actual twist (torsion segment) may be visible (Fig. 13B).

Some patients may have little or no symptoms and have the condition a long time. However, when the torsion begins to obstruct or affect the vascular supply, the patient will present with symptoms ranging from nausea and vomiting to severe pain to cardiovascular collapse from gastric necrosis. Because of these potential risks, it is imperative that the referring service be made aware of an asymptomatic or minimally symptomatic gastric volvulus.

Notes

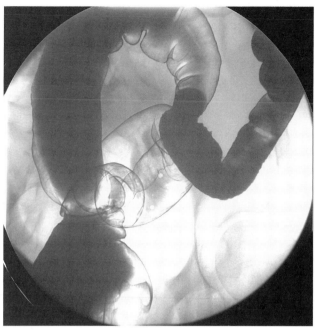

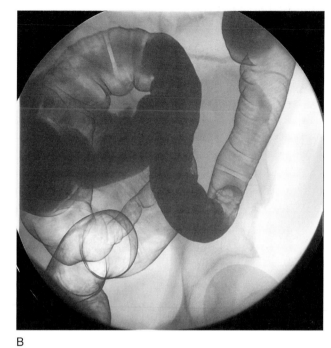

A

B

1. What pathologic feature is shown in these two spot films from an ACBE?

2. Which is more dangerous: a pedunculated adenomatous polyp or a sessile polyp?

3. What percentage of adenocarcinomas arise from polyps?

4. If one colonic polyp is discovered during an examination, what is the risk of finding a second?

Adenoma of the Colon

1. A pedunculated polyp on a long stalk at the junction of the descending and sigmoid colon.

2. A sessile polyp is more dangerous because a malignant focus within the polyp will be capable of reaching the colonic mucosal surface much faster than in a polyp with a stalk.

3. 99%.

4. 25%.

Cross-Reference

Gastrointestinal Imaging: THE REQUISITES, ed 3, p 272.

Comments

Colon adenomas are found in the colons of 15% to 30% of patients over 60 years of age, with the prevalence very dependent on age, heredity, and risk factors. Polyps come in at three histologically identifiable forms. The first, and most common (80%), is the tubular adenoma. These polyps are usually small and carry very little risk for malignant degeneration. They can be on long stalks (such as this case). However, the fact that the stalk permits the polyp to move with the patient, can occasionally make detection on both ACBE and CT quite difficult. The other two types are tubovillous adenomas and villous adenomas. Villous adenomas have the greatest risk for developing into a malignancy. Some researchers and clinicians consider a colonic villous adenoma a low-grade malignancy regardless of what the histologic picture shows. Polyps under 0.5 mm (diminutive polyps) have little or no malignant potential. Polyps 1 to 2 cm in size carry about a 10% risk. Polyps greater than 2 cm are generally thought to have a 30% to 40% risk of malignancy. The anatomic distribution of colonic adenomas seems to be an equal distribution throughout the colon. However, the larger the polyp, the more likely it will be in the distal colon. Moreover, in patients over age 60, the number of polyps detected in the right colon is on the rise.

Notes

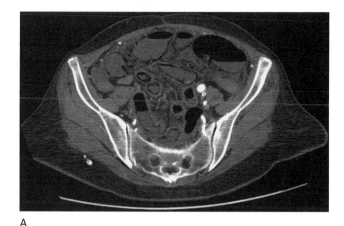

A

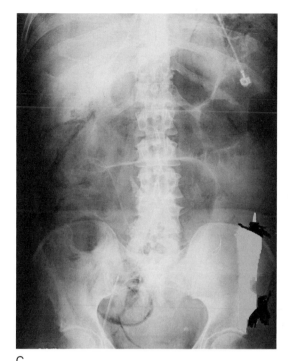

C

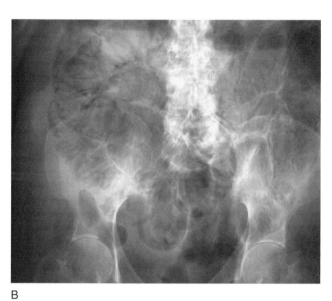

B

1. What is unusual about the bowel air in these plain film images?

2. What are some of the causes of this condition?

3. Is this condition always serious?

4. In an older patient with abdominal pain, what condition must be considered first?

Pneumatosis Intestinalis

1. The air is streaky and submucosal in location.

2. Bowel necrosis, aftereffect of bowel surgery or instrumentation, ulceration.

3. It should always be considered serious, but can be seen in asymptomatic patients who have had surgery to bowel or endoscopic instrumentation.

4. Bowel ischemia and necrosis.

Cross-Reference

Gastrointestinal Imaging: THE REQUISITES, ed 3, p 335.

Comments

Pneumatosis intestinalis of the bowel describes a condition in which air collects in the layers of the wall of the bowel. The most plausible cause for this condition is a breakdown of the mucosal integrity, allowing bowel air to pass through the mucosa into the submucosa. To gain access to the bowel wall, there must be some disruption of the mucosal integrity, such as mucosal tears or ischemic or necrotic disease of the bowel.

Ischemia is a common and most serious cause. Inflammatory conditions, such as necrotizing enterocolitis, pseudomembranous colitis, Crohn's disease, and even infectious agents also are known to produce pneumatosis. It may affect individuals who take steroids. Also, obstruction, trauma, prior endoscopy, malignancies, chemotherapy, and bowel surgery are associated with the development of pneumatosis. CT is a wonderful method for demonstrating even minor amounts of pneumatosis (Fig. 15A).

The radiologic appearance may be one of multiple linear submucosal air lucencies in nature. Portal venous gas in a patient with pneumatosis often indicates the presence of bowel necrosis, which is probably the most significant associated finding. A benign form of pneumatosis, referred to as pneumatosis intestinalis cystica, is a condition in which subserosal blebs are seen in the distal bowel, usually having no clinical significance. The patients are asymptomatic and the condition has been associated with air tracking along bronchovascular pathways into the retroperitoneum, out the mesentery, and finally to the subserosal layer of the distal bowel (Macklin's pathway).

Notes

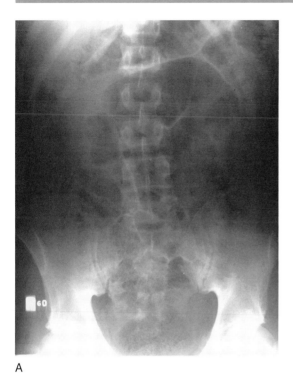

A

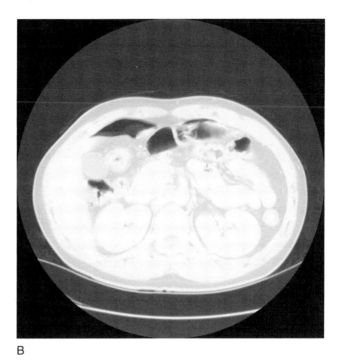

B

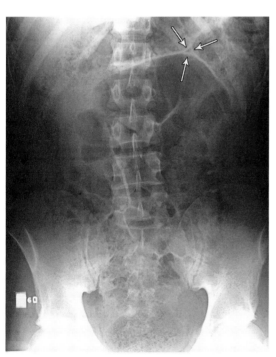

C

1. What is the minimal amount of free intraperitoneal air visible on an upright chest film?

2. Explain Rigler's sign. What is Rigler's triangle?

3. What imaging procedure is best for demonstrating free intraperitoneal air?

4. What factors affect the absorption of intraperitoneal air in the abdomen after surgery?

Pneumoperitoneum

1. 1 to 2 mL of air.

2. Air is present on both the mucosal and serosal sides of the bowel wall, creating a linear stripe. Rigler's triangle is a sign of pneumoperitoneum in which three loops of bowel meet with a lucent (air-filled) triangular center (Fig. 16C).

3. Computed tomography is considerably more sensitive to the detection of pneumoperitoneum as well as pneumothorax and pneumoretroperitoneum.

4. The amount of air introduced during surgery, the amount of body fat, the presence of inflammation, and ileus.

Cross-Reference

Gastrointestinal Imaging: THE REQUISITES, ed 3, p 344.

Comments

Intraperitoneal air is frequently encountered in the abdominal cavity. The most common cause of the free air is surgery or surgical laproscopy. Air that is introduced into the abdomen during surgery usually takes 3 to 10 days to reabsorb. Under certain circumstances, this process may take several weeks. The more air introduced, the longer it takes to reabsorb. Thin patients take longer to reabsorb air. This finding may relate to the fact that obese patients usually have more omental fat, which decreases the amount of air that can be introduced. If the patient has postoperative ileus or peritonitis, the ability of the peritoneum to absorb the air is also reduced.

For many years, the upright chest film and the left lateral decubitus view of the abdomen were considered the best for demonstrating even minute amounts (1 to 2 mL) of air. However, CT has been shown to demonstrate free air even when these views cannot. MDCT is now considered, by far, the best modality for demonstrating even the tiniest amounts of free air.

Several signs have been described regarding the appearance of free intraperitoneal air on a conventional supine abdominal image. (Often the patient is too sick for upright or decubitus views to be obtained, and the only view that can be obtained is a supine film.) In this situation one or more of these signs may be seen. Rigler's sign refers to the ability to see both sides of the bowel wall because there is air on both sides. What we routinely see on abdominal images when we see intestinal air is actually a tissue-air interface; specifically a mucosal-air interface. The serosal side of the bowel cannot be seen without the presence of free air in the peritoneum. Thus, when we are seeing both a mucosal-air interface

and a serosal-air interface, we are seeing Rigler's sign. When three loops of bowel touch each other we may see a lucent triangle in the center representing three serosal-air interfaces; this is known as Rigler's triangle. This sign is difficult to see unless there is a sufficient amount of free air. Ability to see the patient's falciform ligament is another sign indicating free air. Also, free air beneath the liver margin in Morrison's pouch results in a tissue-air interface with the liver margin as well as lucency that typically is not present on a supine film. Occasionally we may see the lateral pelvic ligament, which becomes visible with the presence of sufficient amounts of free air. CT is considerably more sensitive in the detection of free intraperitoneal air (Fig. 16B).

Notes

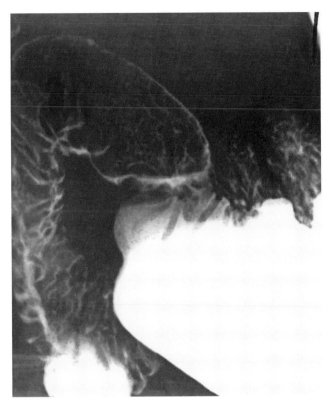

1. What causes benign lymphoid hyperplasia of the duodenum?

2. Approximately what percentage of people have heterotopic gastric mucosa in the duodenal bulbs?

3. What may occur as a response to increased acidity in the duodenal bulb?

4. Where do most benign tumors of the duodenum occur?

Heterotopic Gastric Mucosa of the Duodenum

1. Unknown. Although sometimes it may be seen in conditions such as hypogammaglobulinemia.

2. Some authors claim as many as 20%.

3. Brunner's gland hyperplasia.

4. Proximal half of the duodenum.

Cross-Reference

Gastrointestinal Imaging: THE REQUISITES, ed 2, p 96.

Comments

It is not uncommon to encounter nodular filling defects within the duodenal bulb. These may be solitary or multiple and are of variable size. Certain distinguishing features may help differentiate the conditions that are known to produce this radiologic appearance.

Heterotopic gastric mucosa in the duodenal bulb occurs more frequently than most radiologists recognize, occurring in up to 20% of patients in some pathologic series but seen in less than 1% of patients in radiologic series. The radiologic appearance is that of slightly elevated lesions of varying sizes measuring only a few millimeters in diameter and often clustered in a mosaic pattern in the base of the duodenal bulb. A distinguishing feature is their sometimes angulated or plaque-like margins. These lesions are believed to have no clinical significance. Benign lymphoid hyperplasia of the bulb and proximal duodenum is characterized by multiple tiny (1- to 2-mm), smooth filling defects, which are usually diffuse throughout the region. Often there is no known reason for their appearance, but they occur more frequently in patients with decreased immune competence, such as those with hypogammaglobulinemia or agammaglobulinemia. Brunner's gland hyperplasia has a different radiologic appearance than the two aforementioned entities.

The filling defects in this condition are larger, often ranging up to 1 cm. These lesions are smooth and diffuse, often producing a cobblestone appearance. They may be associated with hyperacidity, although this belief is not universally accepted, given the frequency of hyperacidity disease and infrequency of Brunner's glands hypertrophy. However, it may be that acidity is a contributing factor.

The possibility of pancreatic rests, either single or multiple, giving rise to a polypoid filling defect in the duodenal bulb, should also be considered. A tiny barium collection, which may at times be seen in the center of these filling defects, is the orifice of a duct, and such a finding is an extremely important diagnostic finding.

Benign tumors of the duodenum, such as leiomyomas (GIST), adenomas, and neurofibromas, occur more frequently in the proximal duodenum, particularly the duodenal bulb. Also, polyposis syndromes, such as Peutz-Jeghers, Cronkhite-Canada, and familial polyposis syndromes, are known to cause multiple polyps in the duodenum.

Notes

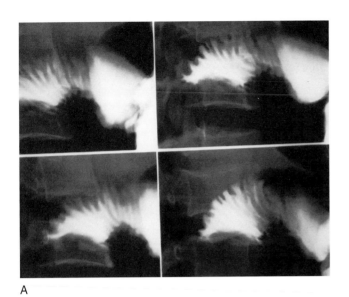

A

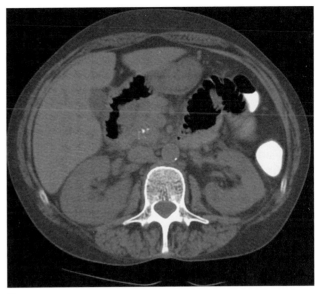

B

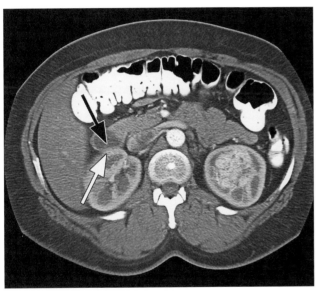

C

1. What are the findings in the barium image and CT image of the upper abdomen?

2. What is the most common malignant lesion of the small bowel?

3. How does the right kidney affect the duodenum?

4. What is the most common cause for duodenal inflammation?

C A S E   1 8

Duodenal Narrowing Secondary to Pancreatitis

1. Narrowing and spasm of the second portion of the duodenum. Note lack of proximal dilatation. The CT images show thickened duodenal folds through this area.

2. Lymphoma.

3. The right kidney abuts the duodenum at the junction of the descending and transverse portions of the retroperitonel duodenum.

4. Hyperacidity/peptic ulcer disease.

Cross-Reference
Gastrointestinal Imaging: THE REQUISITES, ed 3, p 99.

Comments
Thickened folds and spasm of the duodenal bulb and sweep can be seen in a number of conditions both primary in the duodenum or in the adjacent structures in the periduodenal area. In the duodenum the commonest is the result of peptic ulcer disease. Although spasm is not always a component, thickened fold can be seen in such conditions as Zollinger-Ellison syndrome, eosinophilic enteritis, Crohn's disease, Whipple's disease, and amyloid, as well as intramural bleeding and hypoproteinemia. Also to be considered, in the malignant category, is lymphoma (Fig. 18A, 18B).

Pancreatitis affecting the pancreatic head will almost always affect the folds of the second portion of the duodenum. The folds will appear thick and irregular, especially on the pancreatic side. There may also be tethering of folds (Selleck's folds), also seen on the same side.

The most common malignancy is lymphoma (mostly non-Hodgkin's). It is most common in the distal small bowel, but lesions of the duodenum are encountered on rare occasions.

Besides the pancreas, the right kidney bears a close and, in many patients, a contiguous relationship to the duodenum. Figure 18C shows the right kidney (*black arrow*) and adjacent duodenum (*white arrow*) touching the kidney—note the lesion present in the left kidney. It is not unusual to see a large right-sided upper pole renal malignancy affect the adjacent duodenum.

Notes

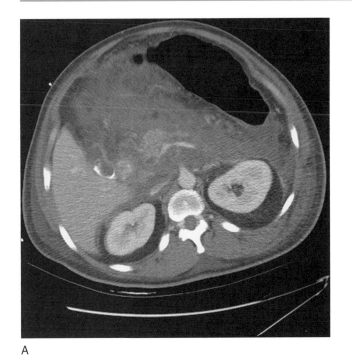

A

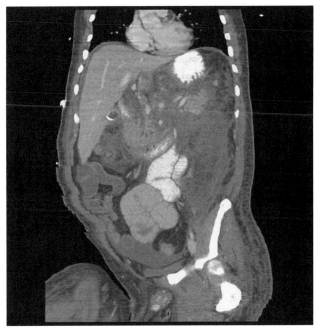

B

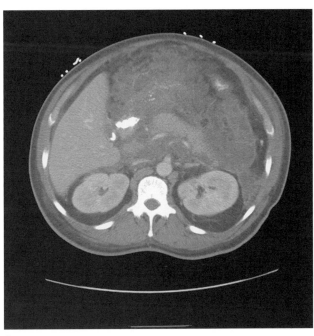

C

1. What is the most common cause of pancreatitis in North America?

2. What is the pathologic etiology of alcoholic induced pancreatitis?

3. What are the CT findings in acute pancreatitis?

4. Describe the appearance of the left lung base in patients presenting with acute pancreatitis.

Acute Pancreatitis

1. Alcohol abuse accounts for about 40% to 50% of cases in the Western world.

2. It is not definitely known. There are several theories.

3. Usually peripancreatic edema and fluid collections. With hemorrhagic disease (as shown in this case), there will be denser collections of fluid representing blood. Small bubbles may be seen in necrotic pancreatitis.

4. Almost all patients with acute pancreatitis will have left basilar changes ranging from pleural effusion to linear atelectasis.

Cross-Reference

Gastrointestinal Imaging: THE REQUISITES, ed 3, pp 171–172.

Comments

Acute pancreatitis is a serious condition, the frequency of which varies from country to country. The incidence has slowly declined in the United States over the last 10 years. The disease is associated with a 10% to 15% mortality rate, is more common in the black population, and affects males more than females. Alcoholic pancreatitis is seen in younger adults, and biliary related etiologies are more commonly seen in an older population. Other causes of pancreatitis include trauma, drug-related, iatrogenic (ERCP), and idiopathic. These patients present with abdominal tenderness and guarding as well as fever and tachycardia. In hemorrhagic pancreatitis both the Cullen sign (a bluish discoloration around the umbilicus) and the Grey Turner sign (discoloration along the flanks) may be seen as blood collects in the peritoneum and dissects along tissue planes. Associated with virtually every case of pancreatitis will be some change at the left lung base. They may be prominent or minimal, depending on the severity of the case. The inflammatory process in the right upper quadrant results in diminished diaphragmatic excursion on the left, hypoventilation of the left lung base with resultant degrees of atelectasis, effusions, and air-space disease. Passed gallstones lodged in the sphincter of Oddi is a common cause of pancreatitis. The size of the stone and duration of occlusion will determine the severity of the pancreatitis. Approximately 5% of post-ERCP patients will develop some degree of pancreatitis. The case shown here demonstrates the dramatic inflammatory changes and blood around the pancreas as well as in the peritoneal cavity and along the left flank (Fig. 19C).

Notes

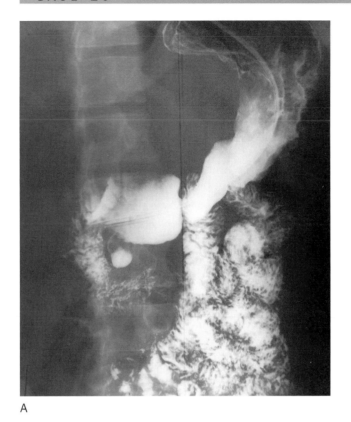

A

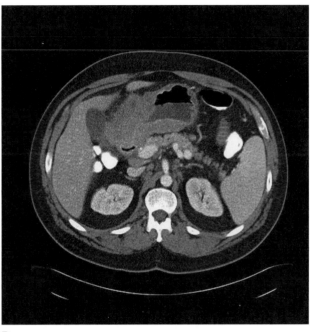

B

C

1. Which crosses the pylorus more frequently, adenocarcinoma or lymphoma?

2. What is the frequency of lymphoma limited just to the stomach?

3. Intraperitoneal metastases tend to invade the stomach on which curvature?

4. What percentage of gastric lymphomas are of the non-Hodgkin's type?

Gastric Lymphoma

1. Both carcinoma and lymphoma cross the pylorus. However, adenocarcinoma crosses more commonly because of its much greater incidence. Nevertheless, the incidence of breaching the pylorus is greater in lymphomas.

2. In approximately one half of patients, lymphoma of the stomach involves only the stomach and the adjacent lymph nodes.

3. Greater curvature, usually because of access to the stomach via the omentum.

4. This is the most common type, usually involved in about 90% of cases.

Cross-Reference
Gastrointestinal Imaging: THE REQUISITES, ed 3, p 60.

Comments
The stomach is the area of the gastrointestinal tract most commonly affected by lymphoma. It may be part of generalized lymphoma involving other portions of the body and lymph system, or it may be primary, involving only the stomach and associated lymph nodes. Approximately half of all cases are primary lymphoma and half are associated with generalized disease. Lymphoma accounts for only 5% or less of primary gastric malignant neoplasms. Most lymphomas of the stomach are of the non-Hodgkin's variety, with Hodgkin's disease being the least common. Hodgkin's lymphoma typically accounts for less than 10% of cases. The disease predominantly affects men and is typically seen in an older age group (50 years and up).

Lymphoma has a variety of presentations in the stomach. It may appear as thickened gastric folds (Fig. 20B, 20C) and be indistinguishable from gastritis and other causes of rugal fold thickening. It may also present as a solitary mass or as multiple masses and polyps. These masses are known to ulcerate. Rarely, it may infiltrate the entire stomach and produce more of a linitis plastica appearance (Fig. 20A), but this is more typically seen with Hodgkin's lymphoma because of the cellular desmoplastic reaction associated with it. Lymphoma will readily cross the pylorus into the duodenum, somewhat more readily than does carcinoma. However, both are known to cross the pylorus, carcinoma in greater numbers because of its greater incidence. It is not a specific distinguishing feature.

Surgical resection of the involved stomach is still the best treatment and may be supplemented by chemotherapy, depending on the situation. Patients with advanced primary disease or systemic lymphoma are best treated by chemotherapy first.

Notes

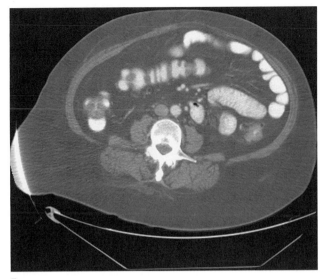

B

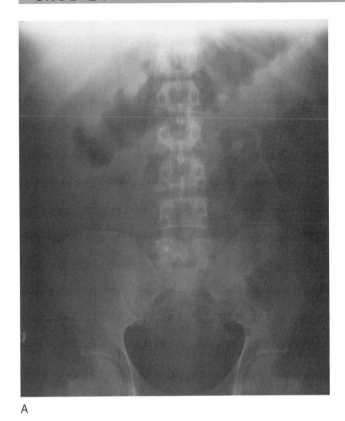

A

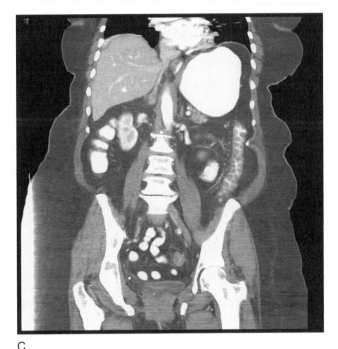

C

1. What descriptive terms would you use to describe the abnormalities on the plain film of the abdomen?

2. What modality is best for evaluating intestinal ischemia?

3. Where is the "watershed" region in the colon?

4. Small emboli to the colon may resemble what disease?

Ischemic Colitis of Transverse Colon

1. Thickened colonic folds; thumbprinting.

2. CT.

3. Splenic flexure.

4. Carcinoma of the colon.

Cross-Reference
Gastrointestinal Imaging: THE REQUISITES, ed 3, p 298.

Comments
Ischemic bowel disease is a common clinical problem, especially in the elderly. Most often it is produced by low flow to the intestines, which occurs in patients who are in hypotensive states, those who are experiencing cardiac failure, and patients who have just had surgery, as well as in those with other conditions. Arterial obstruction is less common but can affect elderly patients with athero-sclerotic disease that obstructs mesenteric vessels or those with embolic disease who have cardiac abnormal-ities. Also, a small percentage of patients have ischemia caused by venous obstruction.

Arteriography is being used less frequently with the advent of high-quality MDCT in patients with ischemia. Angiography will often not demonstrate obstructing ves-sels. CT is probably the best modality for defining the involved segments and identifying underlying pathologic conditions or complications.

Ischemic disease of the colon is often segmental in nature and rarely involves the entire colon. The different regions of the colon have separate blood supplies, although they are interconnected to some extent. The watershed regions are defined as the areas of transition between the superior and inferior mesenteric blood sup-plies. This term frequently applies to the splenic flexure, although sometimes it can include parts of the rectosig-moid junction as well. The splenic flexure is thought by some to be the most susceptible area for ischemia in patients with low flow states because it is the most distal point of arterial flow to the colon. On the other hand, some think that being supplied by two arterial systems confers some protection. Interestingly, most dis-ease seems to occur in the descending and sigmoid regions. The right colon also is commonly involved because it is prone to ischemia resulting from pathologic distention. The right colon is the most distended segment of colon under most conditions.

Radiologically, ischemia first can be identified as thick-ening and edema of the bowel wall. Nodularity of the bowel wall could be the result of either multiple areas of focal edema or hemorrhage (thumbprinting, Fig. 21C). The mucosa may become shaggy and begin to resemble inflammatory bowel disease. As ischemia heals, the colon may become fibrotic, with loss of haustral pattern and even pseudodiverticula formation. This fibrosis can be multifocal in nature. However, in at least 50% of cases healing will be complete without stricture.

Notes

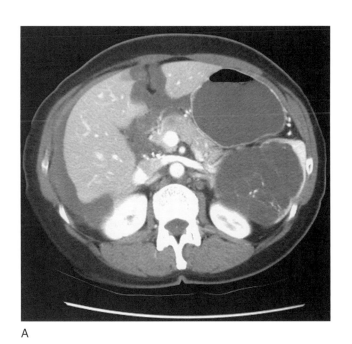

A

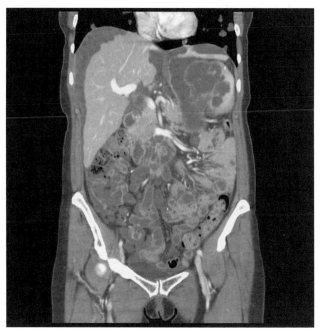

B

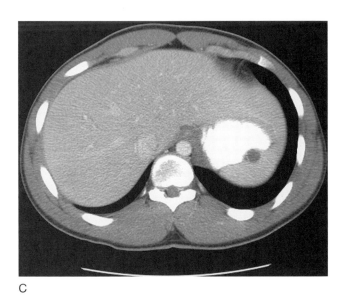

C

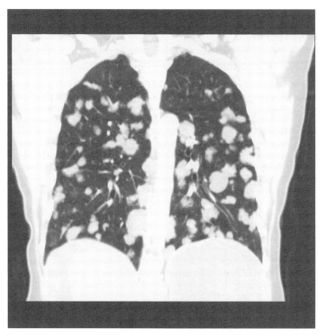

D

1. Using precise and concise radiologic terminology, how would you describe the appearance of the spleen in these images?

2. What are the two most common causes for benign splenic cysts?

3. What percentage of metastatic disease involves the spleen?

4. What is the most common benign neoplasm of the spleen?

C A S E   2 2

Metastatic Disease to the Spleen

1. Most of the substance of the spleen has been replaced by a large expansile septated, inhomogeneous cystic lesion. A small rim of functioning spleen remains.

2. Acquired and epidermoid cysts.

3. Less than 4% of metastatic disease.

4. Hemangiomas.

Cross-Reference

Gastrointestinal Imaging: THE REQUISITES, ed 3, p 215.

Comments

The most common cystic lesions that affect the spleen are the traumatically acquired lesions and epidermoid cysts. Acquired cysts are thought to be mostly traumatic in origin (the small splenic laceration that heals, leaving a hematoma, seroma, and finally a cystic fluid collection that may remain indefinitely). These cysts are without a well-defined lining and calcify over the years. They account for about 80% of benign cystic lesions of the spleen and are best left alone. Epidermoid cysts have a well-defined epithelial lining and are probably congenital in origin. These cysts are also often an incidental finding on CT examinations.

Occasionally a pancreatic tail pseudocyst can be confused with a splenic cyst. However, with MDCT and multiplanar evaluation of the abdomen, these can usually be sorted out. Primary neoplasms of the spleen are rare, with hemangioma being the most common (Fig. 22C). Metastatic disease involving the spleen is also very uncommon. However, as seen in the images, it should not be neglected in the differential diagnosis for splenic defects in patients with known primary neoplasms. In this case the primary cancer is ovarian carcinoma, and there has been widespread dissemination of tumor throughout the peritoneal cavity with ascites and invasion of the spleen as well as involvement of the thoracic cavity (Fig. 22D).

Notes

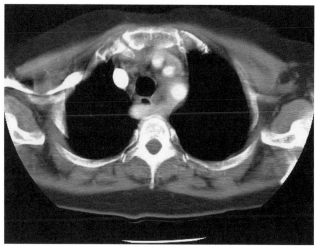

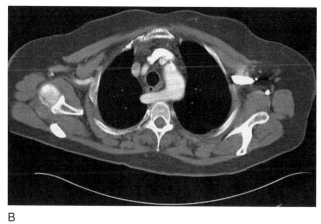

A   B

1. What might this patient's presenting complaint be?

2. What is the origin of the right subclavian artery in most people?

3. What other vascular structures may cause esophageal symptoms?

4. What is the general name given to vascular conditions that result in dysphagia?

Aberrant Right Subclavian Artery

1. Dysphagia.

2. The right common carotid artery.

3. Enlarged left atrium, marked aortic tortuosity, pulmonary sling, double aortic arch, and thoracic aortic aneurysm.

4. Dysphagia lusoria.

Cross-Reference

Gastrointestinal Imaging: THE REQUISITES, ed 3, p 14.

Comments

The normal extrinsic impressions one expects to see on the esophagus are (1) the aortic arch, (2) the left main bronchus, and (3) the left atrium of the heart. Congenital malplaced right subclavian artery originating from the distal aspect of the aortic arch (instead of its usual origin off the right common carotid artery) is seen in slightly less than 1% of the population. In crossing back from left to right across the mediastinum to reach the right limb, the aberrant right subclavian artery passes behind the esophagus. In a small number of cases, it passes anterior to the esophagus, although this is uncommon.

The posterior-crossing artery shown here impressed the posterior wall of the upper esophagus and may produce dysphagia. A barium esophagogram is the simplest and least expensive way of making the diagnosis. However, if necessary, MDCT can demonstrate the anomaly, as in the images presented in this case. Here one can see the aberrant subclavian artery cross to the right of the mediastinum behind the esophagus, which conveniently contains a small amount of air. The term dysphagia lusoria was historically meant to apply to the impression of a greatly enlarged left atrium of rheumatic heart disease. However, today it is generally used to describe dysphagia caused by any impression by any vascular structure.

Notes

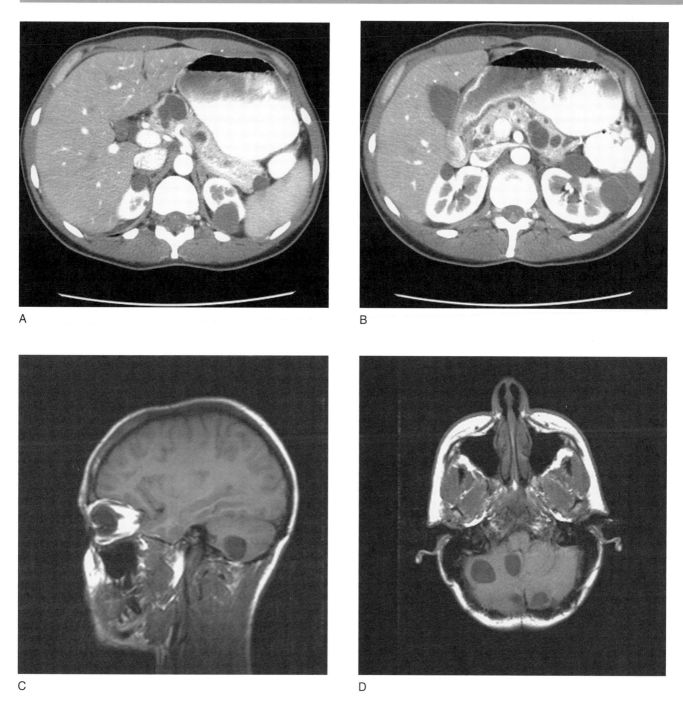

A

B

C

D

1. What percentage of patients with pancreatitis will develop pseudocysts?

2. Multiple congenital cysts of the pancreas are associated with what disease?

3. Cystic fibrosis always produces pancreatic cysts. True or false?

4. Pancreatic trauma could likely produce the images shown with this case. True or false?

von Hippel–Lindau Disease

1. Approximately 10% of cases of pancreatitis will develop pseudocysts; chronic disease produces slightly more and acute disease slightly less.

2. Familial polyposis primarily involving the kidneys.

3. False. Although these cysts may occur early in life, the usual finding is marked atrophy of the gland.

4. False.

Cross-Reference
Gastrointestinal Imaging: THE REQUISITES, ed 3, p 168.

Comments
The images shown in this case show multiple pancreatic cysts of varying size. The CT images are from a patient with von Hippel–Lindau (VHL) disease. VHL disease is an autosomal dominant inherited disease of capillary angiomatous hamartomas with CNS involvement of the brain and retina. In the brain the lesion is usually a hemangioblastoma of the posterior fossa (Fig. 24C, D).

Visceral abdominal tumors also seen in this condition include renal cell carcinoma, pheochromocytoma as well as increased incidence of cystic malignancy of the pancreas.

Multiple pancreatic cysts are seen in almost three quarters of patients with VHL disease and are highly suggestive of the diagnosis. Solid islet cell tumors may be seen in VHL disease. Most of the cases are discovered in the third and fourth decades of life. If malignancy is present at the time of diagnosis, the prognosis is usually poor. Thus, any patient undergoing a CT of the abdomen who demonstrates multiple pancreatic cysts should arouse suspicion, and the abdomen should be carefully searched for such neoplasms as pheochromocytomas and renal cell cancers.

Notes

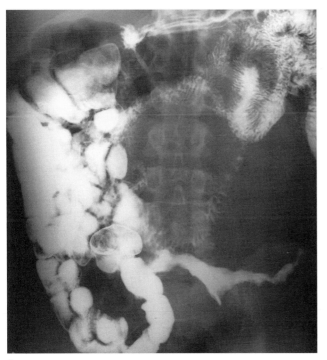

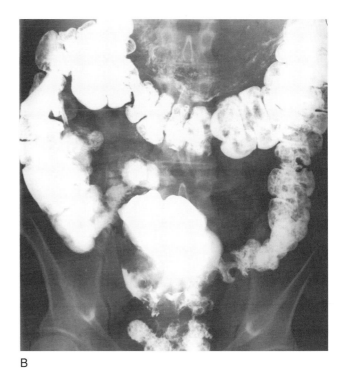

A   B

1. What are the radiologic findings in the two images shown?

2. What lesion is known to cause large masses involving the gut without bowel obstruction?

3. In question 2, what is that the reason for lack of obstruction?

4. What small bowel lesion results in elevated levels of 5-hydroxyindoleacetic acid (5-HIAA) in the urine?

Aneurysmal Dilatation of the Small Bowel Lymphoma

1. Figure 25A shows a long, highly abnormal segment of small bowel with mucosal destruction and without evidence of bowel obstruction. Figure 25B demonstrates a large irregular cavitary lesion of the small bowel without obstruction.

2. Lymphoma, especially the non–Hodgkin's type.

3. Aneursymal dilatation.

4. Carcinoid.

Cross-Reference

Gastrointestinal Imaging: THE REQUISITES, ed 3, p 133.

Commentary

Non-Hodgkin's lymphoma is the most common malignancy of the small bowel. It mostly occurs in the distal small bowel and can often grow to large masses, which, quite often, do not obstruct the bowel. This phenomenon is due to a particular characteristic of lymphoma called "aneursymal dilatation" in which the gut lumen is channeled through the lesion, leaving a false channel surrounded by tumor (Fig. 25A) but without obstruction. This condition may be rarely seen in other small cell lesions of the gut, such as melanoma, but 99% of the time is indicative of lymphoma. It does not seem to occur in Hodgkin's disease and the mechanism is not understood. As a result, patients may present with large abdominal masses, possibly with constitutional symptoms, but no complaints related to bowel obstruction. CT findings would include large masses involving the bowel most often with large foamy lymphomatous nodes in the peritoneum, retroperitoneum, and at the base throughout the mesentery.

Notes

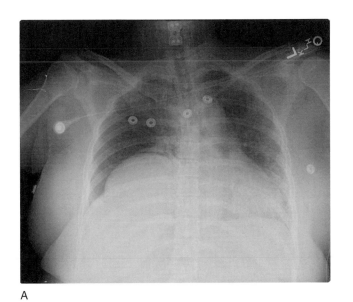

A

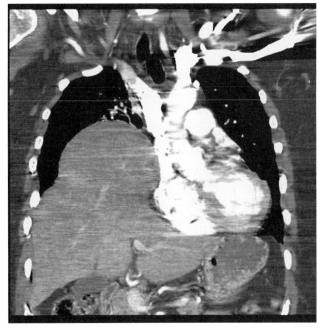

B

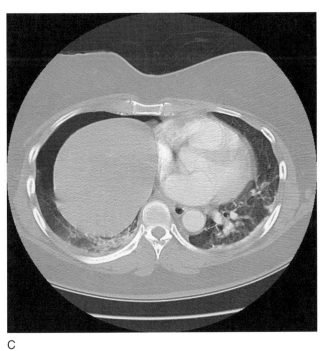

C

1. This person has been in an MVA. Describe the findings on the plain film.

2. On which side is diagrammatic rupture and visceral herniation most common?

3. What structure is seen in the right chest on Figure 26C?

4. What other conditions should be considered in this case?

Traumatic Diaphragmatic Injury

1. Prominent focal right-sided elevation of the diaphragm and shift of the heart and mediastinum to the left.

2. The left. They are closer to equal in occurrence, but right-sided injuries are more often associated with vascular injuries and thus those patients are less likely to survive and reach the ER.

3. CT shows the focal elevation of the diaphragm seen on plain film to be the dome of the liver in the chest.

4. Diaphragmatic injuries rarely occur as an isolated finding. Such things as splenic and liver lacerations are seen in 25% of patients, and pelvic and spinal fractures may be seen in as many as 40% of patients. A smaller number of patients, approximately 5%, may have aortic trauma.

Cross-Reference
Gastrointestinal Imaging: THE REQUISITES, ed 3, p 193.

Comments
Most traumatic diaphragmatic ruptures are associated with high-velocity, high-impact motor vehicle accidents (85%), and the remainder are usually associated with falling from ladders and roofs, or penetrating trauma. Diagnosis of diaphragmatic trauma is often delayed or missed, even with the current advances in imaging (Fig. 26C). This is often the case with penetrating injuries. The more severe the diaphragmatic trauma, the easier the diagnosis. However, the more severe the trauma, the less likely is survival. This is especially true of right-sided trauma because of the increased incidence of aortic tears associated with it.

The size of the diaphragmatic tear can vary from 1 cm to almost the entire diaphragm (about 15 cm), such as in this case.

Notes

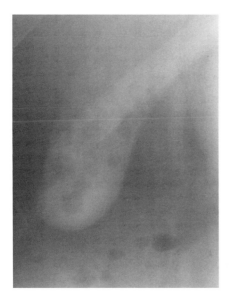

1. What can produce multiple mural and intramural lesions of the gallbladder?

2. What is the most common type of gallbladder polyp?

3. What types of tumors may produce mural nodules?

4. What benign condition can produce nodularity of the wall of the gallbladder?

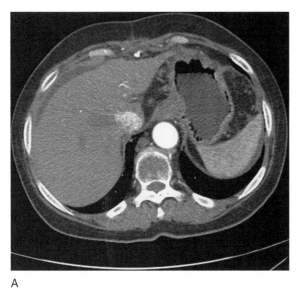

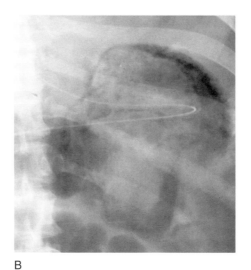

A   B

1. What infectious processes can produce this abnormality?

2. Ingestion of what type of substance may cause this problem?

3. What aspect of the patient history is pertinent when this finding is discovered?

4. What other conditions can be associated with this finding?

Gallbladder Polyps

1. Polyps, adherent stones, metastases, adenomyomatosis, and blood clots.

2. Cholesterol.

3. Metastases.

4. Adenomyomatosis.

Cross-Reference
Gastrointestinal Imaging: THE REQUISITES, ed 3, p 246.

Comments
Although calculi are by far the most common cause of filling defects within the gallbladder, several noncalculous lesions can produce filling defects within the gallbladder lumen. One of the more common noncalculous causes is a gallbladder polyp. Polyps in the gallbladder produce echogenic filling defects within the lumen but are fixed, often along the nondependent surface of the gallbladder. They do not move with changes in position. Polyps of the gallbladder, particularly when they are multiple, are most often cholesterol polyps. The patient with multiple cholesterol polyps is considered to have a type of cholesterolosis. If the polyp is solitary, it could be cholesterol, an adenoma, or a papilloma.

Rarely, other conditions produce multiple mural nodules or protrusions that simulate gallbladder polyps. Adenomyomatosis with prominence of the Rokitansky-Aschoff sinuses sometimes results in some mural nodularity. Adherent stones may also produce polyp-like lesions that can be difficult to differentiate from true polyps. Metastases are quite uncommon in the gallbladder, but when they occur, they can produce mural polyps. Melanoma, breast cancer, and lymphoma infiltrating the gallbladder can cause gallbladder metastases. Primary gallbladder carcinoma can result in the formation of a solitary polypoid lesion but rarely results in multiple mural polyps. Potentially, blood clots, hemorrhage, and even varices could produce mural polyps or nodularity, but this is quite uncommon.

Notes

Emphysematous Gastritis

1. Hemolytic streptococci, *Clostridium* species, and coliform bacteria.

2. Corrosives.

3. Recent endoscopy or surgical procedure.

4. Peptic ulcer disease, gastric outlet obstruction, and pulmonary disease.

Cross-Reference
Gastrointestinal Imaging: THE REQUISITES, ed 3, p 88.

Comments
The finding of air in the wall of the stomach is quite frequently an ominous sign. Although air in the stomach wall can be a sequela of recent endoscopy or gastric surgery, it is a rare complication. Despite the thousands of endoscopic procedures performed, a radiologist rarely encounters air in the gastric wall as a result of them.

Most commonly the occurrence of air in the wall represents a severe infection of the stomach, a type of phlegmonous gastritis. Although many organisms have been isolated in these infections, the most common are hemolytic streptococci, *Clostridium welchii*, and coliform bacteria. Infection may be slightly more common in severe diabetes, relating to the overall systemic disease process as well as local diabetes-induced vasculitides. Infection has been identified in otherwise healthy patients, as well as in those with a variety of chronic, debilitating conditions (e.g., transplant recipients, postoperative patients, those with AIDS). The process by which the infection develops is uncertain, but it is believed that ulcers or other breaks in the mucosa allow bacteria access to the submucosal tissue, with resultant spread of infection. Discovery of phlegmonous gastritis probably indicates impending necrosis of the gastric wall. Prompt therapy, including gastrectomy and antibiotics, is necessary because the mortality rate is quite high.

Emphysematous gastritis also can be encountered in patients with gastric outlet obstruction, in whom elevated intraluminal pressures may force air into the gastric wall. Rarely, the condition is seen in patients with pulmonary disease who also develop pneumatosis in other parts of the gastrointestinal tract. Patients who ingest corrosive agents in an attempt to commit suicide also can develop this complication, which heralds necrosis of the gastric wall. As is true of other radiologic findings, the clinical history is the most important factor in establishing the correct diagnosis.

Notes

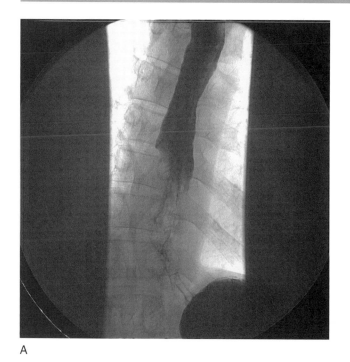

A

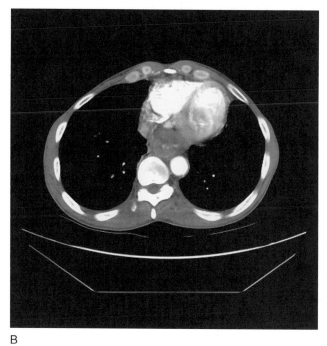

B

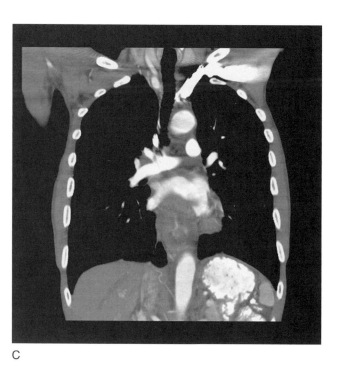

C

1. Describe the findings on the shown images.

2. What is most common type of malignancy seen in the esophagus?

3. What inflammatory processes could give this pattern?

4. What predisposing processes can be associated with this lesion?

Adenocarcinoma of the GE Junction

1. Thickening and irregularity of the distal esophagus. The barium study is more suggestive of mass and ulceration and luminal narrowing.

2. Adenocarcinoma.

3. Chronic and acute reflux esophagistis.

4. Barrett's metaplasia.

Cross-Reference

Gastrointestinal Imaging: THE REQUISITES, ed 3, p 23.

Comments

Adenocarcinoma of the esophagus has become the most common form of cancer of the esophagus in the Western world over the last 30 years. Its incidence has increased almost 500% over that period. Once squamous cell carcinoma was by far the most common (80–90%), but in the last three decades the dramatic increasing incidence of adenocarcinoma has reversed the numbers. At this time the relative incidence of adenocarcinoma to squamous cell carcinoma is approximately 55% to 45%.

This change is due directly to the increased incidence of Barrett's metaplasia now seen in the distal esophagus. Patients with Barrett's metaplasia have a 40% or greater risk of malignancy, and almost all adenocarcinomas of the distal esophagus and gastroesophageal junction are a result of pre-existing Barrett's metaplasia. These patients are usually younger than those with the typical squamous cell lesion of the esophagus. They will often have a long history of heartburn symptoms and will present with dysphagia to solid foods. The correlating factors of smoking and alcohol seen with squamous cell carcinoma may not apply to this lesion. Although almost all adenocarcinomas arise from underlying dysplastic disease (Barrett's), there may be a tiny percentage that arise from the sparse adenomatous glands of the esophagus directly. In general, the more distal the lesion, the more lightly the predisposing factor is Barrett's metaplasia.

The 5-year survival rate in general for this lesion is 10% to 12%. But this, too, is to a great extent related to the spread of the disease. It can be very local, or may spread via the adjacent lymph node chain (upper celiac in the gastrohepatic ligament, Fig. 29C), or can present with distal metastatic disease to the lung and elsewhere.

Radiologic findings include mass, narrowing, and irregularity at the GE junction. This may be associated with some chronic inflammatory changes on barium studies. CT images will reveal a thickened esophageal wall (greater than 5 mm) as well as the possibility of nodes in the mediastinum and paragastric areas.

Notes

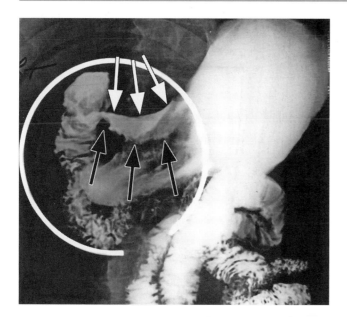

1. In what condition is the Carmen meniscus sign (CMS) found?

2. What is the Kirkland complex?

3. Where must the lesion be located for the CMS to be seen?

4. The CMS is best seen in the double contrast UGI. True or false?

Carmen Meniscus Sign

1. Ulcerated gastric malignancies.

2. The concave lucent margin around the ulceration.

3. The lesion must occur on the lesser curvature of body or antrum.

4. False. It is best seen on single contrast studies or biphasic studies.

Cross-Reference

Gastrointestinal Imaging: THE REQUISITES, ed 3, p 84.

Commentary

The Carmen meniscus sign was first described by Dr. Carmen in the late 1930s before double contrast studies were in routine use. It is a sign that is considered to be pathognomic for an ulcerated gastric malignancy. The sign is confusing and not well understood. This is because certain conditions must be present for the sign to occur. First, the lesion must be a flat infiltrating ulcerative lesion with heaped up margins. Second, the lesion must be in the "saddle" region of the stomach, the lesser curve of the body or antrum. The examination should be a single contrast or at least a biphasic study (when both single contrast and double contrast evaluation are used). The sign may be seen on a double contrast study but is often not recognized. Finally, compression must be applied to the stomach so that the ulcerated margins of the ulcer are forced together to entrap barium in a curved semilunar configuration with the convexity directed toward the lumen of the stomach. The lucency that results from the heaped up walls of the ulcer touching each other is called the Kirkland complex.

Notes

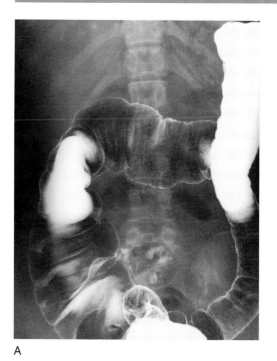

A

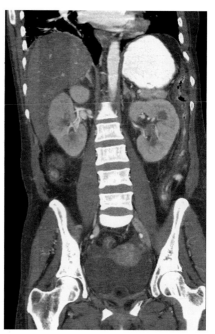

B

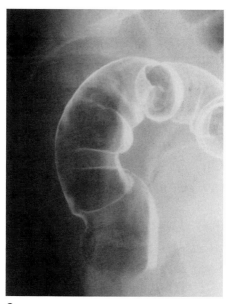

C

1. Describe the pertinent findings in the three images.

2. What parts of the colon are most involved with acute ulcerative colitis?

3. Which inflammatory bowel disease (IBD) is most likely to cause fistula formation?

4. Which IBD has the greatest risk for malignancy?

Acute Ulcerative Colitis

1. The lateral rectal image shows fold thickening and widening of the presacral space. The double contrast image of the colon shows granularity and loss of haustra involving the distal colon. The right colon appears normal. The coronal CT image shows inflammatory changes in the descending colon.

2. The rectum and distal colon.

3. Crohn's disease.

4. Chronic ulcerative colitis.

Cross-Reference

Gastrointestinal Imaging: THE REQUISITES, ed 3, p 292.

Comments

Ulcerative colitis (UC) is a superficial inflammatory disease usually affecting the distal colon. It begins as a granularity, hyperemia, and edema of the mucosa and progresses to multiple widespread evenly distributed tiny ulcerations. The patient presents with abdominal pain, diarrhea, and blood per rectum. The disease may spontaneously disappear (in which case one ought to reconsider the diagnostic possibilities) or go on to simmering chronic disease with occasional flare-ups. The entire colon may be involved in about a third of patients presenting with severe disease. Differentiating between ulcerative colitis and Crohn's disease can sometimes be very difficult clinically and histologically. Radiologic examinations can sometimes be more specific. In ulcerative colitis the disease starts distally and progresses proximally. The terminal ileum is never involved with UC, although it may appear patulous (backwash ileitis). The skip lesions and asymmetry seen in Crohn's disease are not present in UC. The fistula formation commonly seen in Crohn's disease is not seen with UC. Involvement of other parts of the gut, such as may be seen with Crohn's disease, is never seen in UC. Extracolonic manifestations can be seen in both diseases. The risk for malignancy is much higher in UC than in Crohn's disease.

Notes

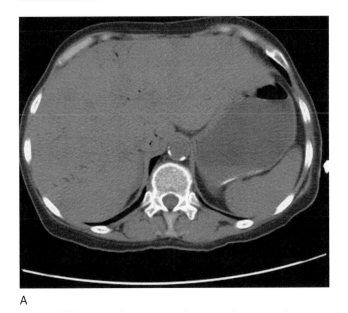

A

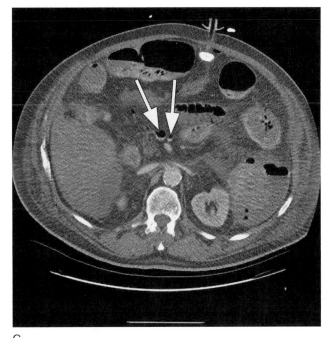

C

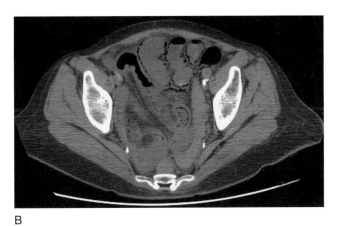

B

1. What common finding links these three images?

2. Name some benign causes for air in the portal venous system.

3. How does one distinguish air in the portal venous system of the liver from air in the biliary system?

4. In situations when air is seen in branching patterns *both* in the periphery and centrally in the liver, is the air in the portal venous system or the biliary system?

Air in the Portal Venous System

1. Air in the portal venous system of the liver (Fig. 32B) and in the structures that feed the portal system, in the bowel wall (Fig. 32A) (pneumatosis), and in the superior mesenteric vessels (Fig. 32C).

2. Bowel surgery (the most common), instrumentation, ulceration of the bowel, obstruction and distention of the bowel.

3. Air in the portal venous system flows with the portal blood in a centrifugal direction. Thus, the air will be seen mostly in the periphery of the liver. Air in the biliary system flows with the bile in a centripetal direction and thus we see the air in the region of the porta hepatitis.

4. When air is seen both centrally and peripherally in the liver, it is a large amount of portal venous air and an ominous finding. In such situations one may see air in the splenic vein and even the spleen.

Cross-Reference

Gastrointestinal Imaging: THE REQUISITES, ed 3, p 210.

Comments

Air in the portal venous system can be a serious finding, especially in the elderly. However, as mentioned earlier, there are benign causes for this finding. Nevertheless, the identification of potential air in the portal venous system always requires immediate communication with the clinical service to consider the catastrophic issue of bowel necrosis. A careful evaluation of the bowel for pneumatosis is also required. Occasionally air can be seen in the mesenteric vessels, as in this case (Fig. 32C).

Air in the biliary system is almost never a life-threatening event. The only exception might be air in the biliary system due to gas-forming pyogenic infection. This is exceedingly rare and the patient would be extremely ill. Most air in the bilary system is the result of surgery (choledochoenterostomies), erosion of gallstones through the wall of a chronically inflamed gallbladder into adjacent hollow viscus, or ERCP and papillotomies.

Notes

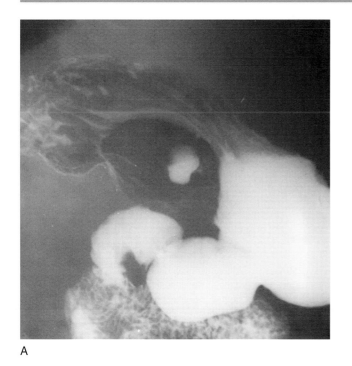

A

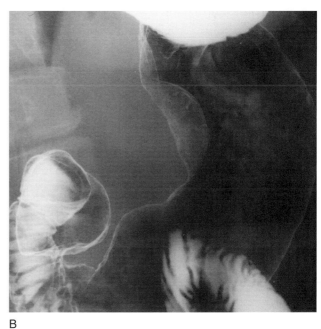

B

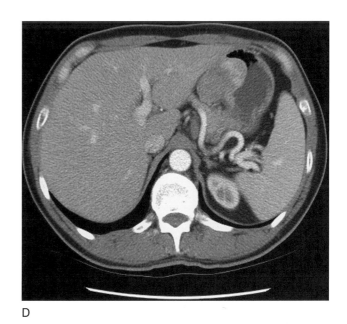

C

D

1. What neoplasms of the stomach grow exophytically?

2. What is the most common benign submucosal tumor of the stomach?

3. How is a leiomyoma distinguished from a leiomyosarcoma?

4. What congenital abnormality may mimic a leiomyoma?

C A S E   3 3

Large Gastrointestinal Stromal Tumor of the Stomach

1. Generally, tumors of stromal cell origin, such as leiomyosarcomas, leiomyomas, and leiomyoblastoma; and rarely, neurofibromas or even lymphomas.

2. Benign GIST of stomach (leiomyoma).

3. Mitotic activity identified on pathologic examination (or the presence of metastases).

4. Rarely, an ectopic pancreatic rest or duplication cyst.

Cross-Reference
Gastrointestinal Imaging: THE REQUISITES, ed 3, p 76.

Comments
Smooth muscle or gastrointestinal stromal tumors are among the more commonly encountered tumors of the stomach. They account for almost half of all benign stomach tumors. Only a small percentage (<10%) are malignant in nature. Benign GISTs occur equally among men and women, whereas malignant GISTs are more common in men. There tends to be a slight increase in the number of tumors with increasing age.

It is difficult to radiologically distinguish between benign and malignant GISTs and other submucosal tumors. The benign GIST can be found anywhere in the stomach, whereas its sarcomatous counterpart is usually more proximal. The pattern of growth is variable. The majority of both types of lesions grow endogastrically, or into the lumen. However, a small but significant percentage grow exophytically, or into the perigastric abdominal cavity, creating only a mild extrinsic mass impression on the stomach. This growth is fairly unique but should be considered whenever a large intra-abdominal mass with growth into the abdominal cavity is encountered in the vicinity of the stomach. The tumors that grow into the lumen may ulcerate and can be large or even, rarely, multiple. Because these tumors are vascular in nature, ulceration over the stretched and thinned mucosa can occur, and patients may present with a GI bleed. Distinguishing benign from malignant smooth muscle tumors is difficult even for the pathologist. The classic criterion has been the number of mitotic figures visible per high power field (>10 for malignant GIST). However, the nature of the histologic activity of the tumor is variable in different parts, and sampling can have a significant impact on the mitotic activity and pleomorphism viewed by the pathologist. Some believe that size of the tumor is just as important. Tumors less than 5 cm in diameter are more likely to be malignant. Finally, the absolute criterion is evidence of metastatic disease.

If the lesion is indeterminate based on pathologic findings, CT often becomes an absolute necessity to determine the exact nature of the tumor (Fig. 33C, D).

Notes

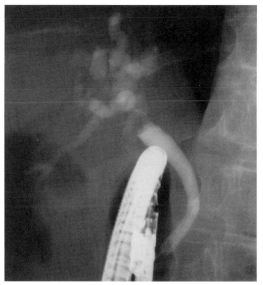

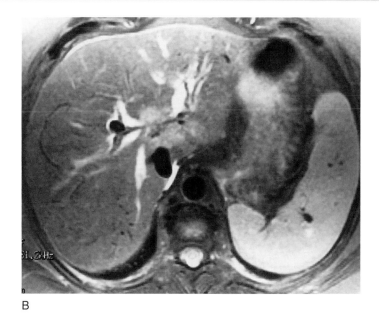

A   B

1. What is the most likely diagnosis?

2. What is this condition called?

3. What conditions predispose a patient to cholangiocarcinoma?

4. In what forms can this tumor appear?

Bile Duct Malignant Stricture (Klatskin Tumor)

1. Cholangiocarcinoma.

2. Klatskin tumor.

3. Sclerosing cholangitis, choledochal cyst, congenital hepatic fibrosis, and recurrent parasitic infection.

4. Strictures, polyps, and liver masses.

Cross-Reference

Gastrointestinal Radiology: THE REQUISITES, ed 3, p 232.

Comments

Cholangiocarcinomas are adenomatous tumors that arise from the lining of the bile ducts. Because they can arise from any portion of the biliary system (even the tiniest branches in the liver), the appearance of cholangiocarcinomas can be quite variable. They most often form nontumorous strictures, which are malignant cells spreading down the walls of the bile duct in a scirrhous pattern. They may also form polypoid masses that project into the lumen of the ducts. In the liver parenchyma itself, cholangiocarcinomas are often identified as liver masses and are indistinguishable from other liver tumors. Those patients in whom these growths arise in the extrahepatic bile ducts have the best prognosis. Cholangiocarcinomas may produce jaundice or other symptoms before they spread to adjacent structures. Cholangiocarcinoma is often fatal because it invades adjacent critical structures in the region, such as the bile ducts and portal vein. Distant metastases are not common.

CT inspection of the bile ducts will reveal proximal ductal dilation (Fig. 34A), an area of narrowing (Fig. 34B), or a polypoid lesion in the duct lumen. Proximal ductal dilation is often evident. On CT examination the tumors themselves are typically evident only when they are in the liver parenchyma and mass effect is visible. Approximately one third of cholangiocarcinomas present as liver masses because they grow exophytically into the liver parenchyma.

The type of cholangiocarcinoma that arises at the confluence of the right and left bile ducts is termed a *Klatskin tumor*. This tumor is typically scirrhous cholangiocarcinoma that grows along the ducts, producing thickening of the wall of the ducts and progressive narrowing of the lumen. As the tumor grows, focal lobar atrophy may become evident. CT may demonstrate a mass in the region. The condition is almost invariably fatal within 6 to 8 months because critical structures in the region, such as the portal vein, are often invaded. Enlarged lymph nodes in the porta hepatis and Mirizzi syndrome caused by an impacted stone in the cystic duct may mimic this condition.

Notes

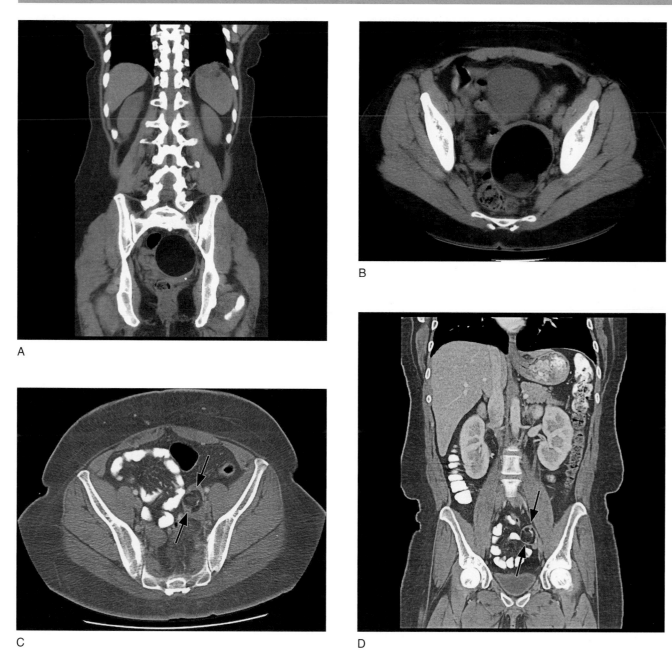

A

B

C

D

1. What abnormality is shown in the axial and coronal images of this 24-year-old woman complaining of abdominal pain?

2. What percentage of dermoid cysts are bilateral?

3. What are the internal components of most benign dermoid cysts?

4. Under what circumstances might you be concerned about malignancy?

C A S E 3 5

Pelvic Ovarian Teratoma

1. The CT images show a large, well-defined fat-filled lesion arising from the left pelvis. There is debris in the dependent portion of the lesion.

2. Somewhere between 10% and 15% are bilateral.

3. Sebaceous fatty material, hair and even rudimentary teeth can be seen within the lesion.

4. A lesion exceeding 10 cm in size, irregularity, loculation, and increased soft tissue content should raise suspicion.

Cross-Reference

Gastrointestinal Imaging: THE REQUISITES, ed 3, p 306.

Comments

Benign dermoid cysts (also called mature cystic teratomas) are the most common pelvic masses in young women. They usually are asymptomatic and bilateral in 10% to 15%, but can cause discomfort in some patients. The reasons are not clear. It may relate to a contiguous position of the lesion or possibly to degrees of torsion. On the other hand, it may also be a sign of possible malignancy. Fatty density is seen in almost 100% of ovarian dermoids along with hair and rudimentary teeth.

CT of the pelvis will show these findings, usually as an incidental finding in most patients. Extragonadal germ cell tumors, which include dermoid cysts, are not uncommon and are among the important differential diagnoses in upper anterior mediastinal masses. Malignant degeneration is rare, but increases with the age of the patient. The size of the lesion and the amount of soft tissue and fatty material held by the lesion are variable (Fig. 35C, D). Torsion is the most common complication associated with these lesions.

Notes

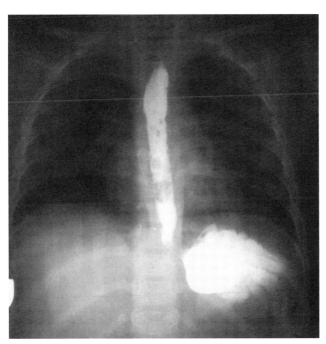

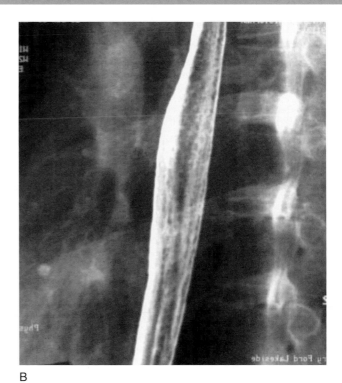

A   B

1. What is the most common cause of small nodules in the esophagus?

2. What condition produces plaque-like lesions in immunocompromised patients?

3. What condition affecting the elderly may produce this appearance?

4. What skin condition may be associated with multiple tiny esophageal lesions?

Candidiasis of the Esophagus

1. Artifact caused by the effervescent agent used in double contrast esophagography.

2. *Candida* esophagitis.

3. Glycogen acanthosis.

4. Acanthosis nigricans with esophageal papillomatosis.

Cross-Reference
Gastrointestinal Imaging: THE REQUISITES, ed 3, p 7.

Comments
Numerous small plaques or nodules of the esophageal mucosa are not an uncommon finding. A variety of conditions may produce these abnormalities. Often the correct diagnosis can be made based on the clinical information provided by the patient. These nodules are either diffuse or focal, and this determination has some bearing on the diagnostic possibilities.

The numerous filling defects commonly seen in the esophagus are usually a technical issue. Having the patient drink barium along with the CO_2 granules will almost invariably yield this artifact. It is advisable to give the granules first, followed by a small amount of water immediately after. Several infectious and inflammatory conditions may produce this true mucosal filling defect in the esophagus. The most important is *Candida* infection. These small well-defined plaques, which are identified by the radiologist, correspond to the whitish ovoid or rounded plaques that are seen in the back of the pharynx of patients with thrush. Early on, they seem to line up on the longitudinal fold of the esophagus. This is usually referred to as the colonization stage. Later, as rhizoid extension into the mucosa and submucosa occurs, some ulceration may be detected (ulceration stage) and the patient will experience odynophagia. With progression of the ulceration stage, widespread diffuse ulceration and bleeding occur throughout the esophagus (the "shaggy" esophagus).

Typically in the colonization phase the superficial plaques are only a few millimeters in diameter, but they may increase quickly to as large as 1 cm or more in diameter. In addition to immunocompromised patients, patients with scleroderma, achalasia, and other conditions associated with stasis of the esophageal contents may have *Candida* organisms visible on radiologic studies. Reflux esophagitis may produce plaque-like elevations in the distal esophagus, and these growths correspond to areas of edema and inflammation without ulceration. Very rarely, herpetic esophagitis also may produce multiple small nodular lesions. However, herpetic involvement is usually tiny punctuate ulcers rather than plaques.

A common benign condition of the esophagus is glycogen acanthosis. This condition, which consists of swelling of the epithelium caused by increased cytoplasmic glycogen, predominantly affects the elderly. It is believed to be a degenerative phenomenon and of little or no clinical significance. Some malignant and premalignant conditions also may produce multiple plaques.

Rarely, early esophageal cancer can present as a focal area of irregular, variously sized raised plaques, without a discrete mass. Superficial spreading carcinoma of the esophagus may have more diffuse nodules. Leukoplakia is a premalignant condition of the mouth that sometimes is found in the esophagus. Esophageal papillomatosis can be seen with acanthosis nigricans of the skin.

Notes

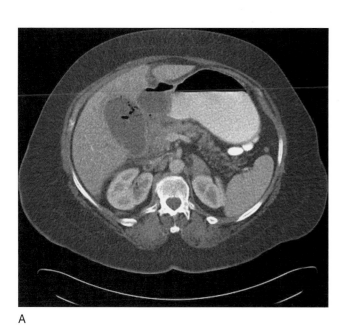

A

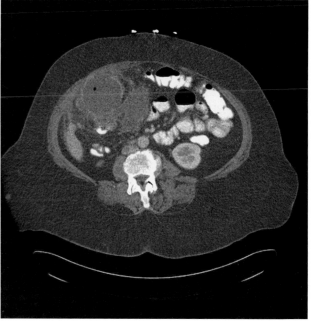

B

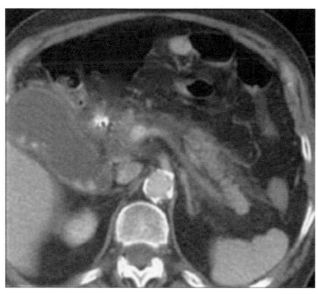

C

1. What are the CT findings in this patient presenting with severe RUQ pain and fever?

2. What might an ultrasound of the RUQ disclose?

3. What percentage of acute cholecystitis is associated with gallstones?

4. What percentage of acute cholecystitis will result in gallbladder perforation?

Acalculous Cholecystitis and Perforation

1. Distended gallbladder with thickened wall and pericholecystic fluid, as well as tiny air bubbles in the gallbladder. No gallstones are seen.

2. Distended gallbladder, thickened wall, and fluid in gallbladder fossa.

3. 90%. Acalculous cholecystitis is seen in 10% of cases.

4. Probably no more than 1% to 2%.

Cross-Reference

Gastrointestinal Imaging: THE REQUISITES, ed 3, p 252.

Comments

Acute cholecystitis is one of the most common of abdominal problems seen in ER patients. About 90% of cases are associated with gallstones in younger patients, more frequently females (Fig. 37C). It is thought to occur as a result of occlusion of the cystic duct with a gallstone, resulting in biliary colic and inflammatory changes in the gallbladder and the famous Murphy sign. Most cases of acute cholecystitis will spontaneously resolve in 7 to 10 days, and almost all patients will have had prior episodes. A small number of patients will go on to more severe disease such as gallbladder emphysema, peroration, and peritonitis. These conditions present life-threatening situations. Although the condition of acalculous cholecystitis is uncommon, it does tend to occur in older, and particularly in male, patients.

Notes

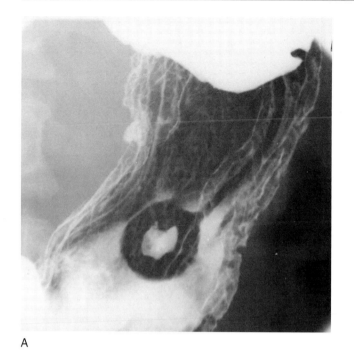

A

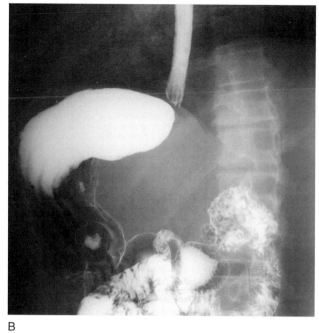

B

C

1. What is this unique pattern of gastric disease called (Fig. 38A, 38B)?

2. What are some of the causes that might result in this pattern?

3. What does the term "linitis plastica" mean?

4. Is this pattern more indicative of primary or secondary disease?

Bull's Eye Metastatic Lesions to Stomach

1. Bull's eye lesions.

2. Usually metastatic lesions to the stomach.

3. The Latin term, meaning "leather bottle," indicates widespread diffuse infiltrative disease of the stomach.

4. Secondary disease.

Cross-Reference

Gastrointestinal Imaging: THE REQUISITES, ed 3, p 74.

Commentary

Metastatic lesions to the stomach can take several forms. The form shown in this case is the classic "bull's eye" lesion; so named for the appearance of a rounded filling defect with a barium collection at its center. The mound is the metastatic mass arising from the intramural layer of the stomach and the displacement of barium. The bull's eye is the ulceration and resultant barium collection.

In this case the primary lesion is small cell carcinoma of the lung (Fig. 38C). However, hematogenous metastatic spread from other lesions can also cause a similar appearance. These lesions would include breast cancer and melanoma. In addition, a smaller number of bull's eye lesions of the stomach can occur as a result of primary gastric tumors. These tumors would include some presentations of lymphoma and Kaposi sarcoma. In recent decades the most common cause of bull's eye lesions in the stomach has been Kaposi sarcoma seen in AIDS patients.

Another benign cause of a solitary bull's eye lesion of the stomach is a GIST mass in which the mucosa over the center of the intramural lesion ulcerates. Occasionally bull's eye lesions can be seen in the small bowel, but this location is uncommon.

Notes

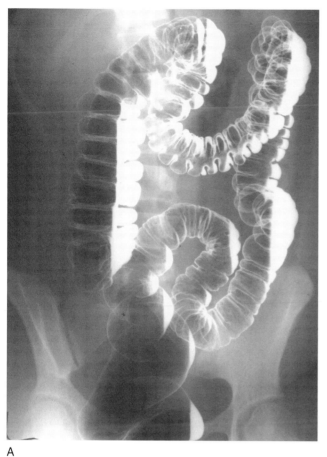

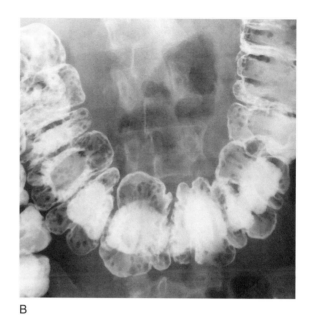

A   B

1. What is the inheritance pattern of most colonic polyposis adenomatous syndromes?

2. What bony abnormalities are seen in patients with adenomatous polyposis syndrome?

3. What syndrome includes central nervous system tumors?

4. What thyroid abnormality may develop in patients with this condition?

Familial Adenomatous Polyposis of the Colon

1. Autosomal dominant.

2. Osteomas and cortical hyperostosis.

3. Turcot's syndrome.

4. Thyroid carcinoma.

Cross-Reference

Gastrointestinal Imaging: THE REQUISITES, ed 3, p 284.

Comments

Innumerable adenomatous polyps of the colon, particularly in a young adult, usually indicate the presence of a polyposis syndrome. For years, these adenomatous polypoid conditions were classified as familial polyposis coli or (when fewer polyps) Gardner's syndrome. Patients with the latter condition were believed to develop the extracolonic manifestations. These conditions are inherited as autosomal dominant traits and cause the formation of numerous adenomatous colonic polyps. Many now believe that these two conditions represent variable penetrance of the same genetic defect and classify these entities as familial adenomatous polyposis syndrome (FAPS).

In patients with FAPS, polyps are seen primarily in the colon but can occur infrequently outside the colon, usually in the stomach or small bowel. There is also an associated increase of nonadenomatous polyps present in both colon and stomach. These growths usually are hyperplastic polyps or so-called fundic gland polyps. Adenomas also occur with slightly increased frequency in the stomach and duodenum, and there is an increased incidence of periampullary carcinoma (the second most frequent malignancy after colonic carcinoma) among these patients. In some studies the incidence of small bowel adenomas has been notably increased.

Extraintestinal manifestations include bony abnormalities. Osteomas, although classically associated with Gardner's syndrome, occur in up to 50% of patients. There also is an increased incidence of cortical hyperostosis and dental abnormalities associated with FAPS. Epidermal cysts have been described, as have pigmented lesions of the retina. The incidence of thyroid carcinoma also is believed to be increased, particularly in women. Large intra-abdominal fibrous tumors, mesenteric fibromatosis, and desmoid tumors occur sporadically. Some believe that there is a slight increase in the incidence of pancreatic carcinoma and benign liver tumors. Tumors of the central nervous system (glioblastomas and medulloblastomas) are generally associated with Turcot's syndrome, but many claim that Turcot's is just another, more deadly, variation of FAPS.

Notes

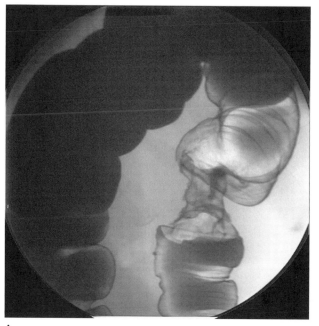

A

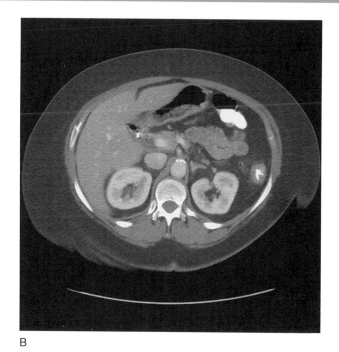

B

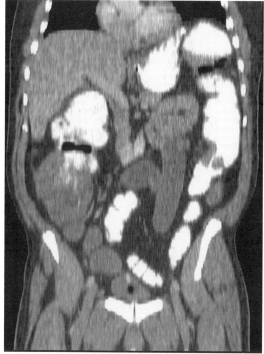

C

1. What are the pertinent findings on these images?

2. What is the generally accepted etiologic pathway for colorectal carcinoma?

3. What exceptions are there to this pathway?

4. List some of the accepted risk factors associated with colorectal cancer.

C A S E   4 0

Apple Core Lesion of Descending Colon

1. The double contrast view of the splenic flexure shows focal mucosal destruction and luminal narrowing (apple core).

2. Most colorectal cancers follow the adenoma to cancer pathway.

3. Exceptions would include spontaneous lesions arising in dysplastic bowel mucosa, such as in ulcerative colitis.

4. Risk factors would include familial history, chronic ulcerative colitis, presence of adenomatous polyps, diet, and region of the world one resides in.

Cross-Reference

Gastrointestinal Imaging: THE REQUISITES, ed 3, p 272.

Comments

Although the incidence of colorectal carcinoma (CRC) has leveled off in the United States in recent years, it is still the fourth most common cancer after prostate, breast, and lung. Its mortality rate is exceeded only by lung cancer at this time. Survival depends on early detection, which in CRC means finding and removing polyps. In polyps between 5 mm and 10 mm there is about a 1% chance of malignancy. In polyps between 1 and 2 cm there is about a 10% risk. As the size of sessile polyps increases, the cancer risks increase; polyps over 2 cm have about a 40% risk. Diminutive polyps (less than 5 mm) have little or no risk of malignancy and the search for diminutive polyps is probably a waste of time, expense, and effort. However, the screening for 1 cm or larger polyps is warranted. This can be done with colonoscopy; which has the added benefit of polyp removal at the time of discovery. However, the complication rate (perforation) is at least 10 times that of the air contrast barium enema (ACBE) and the cost is considerably higher than ACBE. If done by skilled radiologists, the detection rate of polyps 1 cm and larger, as well as CRC, approaches that of colonoscopy. MDCT is now especially useful in detection by evaluation for nodal or distant spread (Fig. 40C). As the number of sites using CT colonoscopy increases, this holds promise as being an excellent screening method in the general population with minimal examination time, no sedation, and rapid results.

Notes

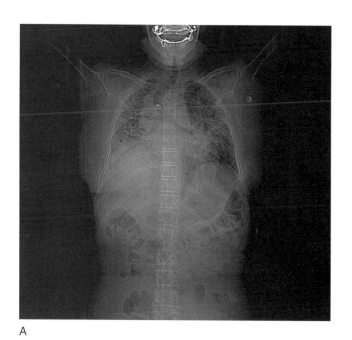

A

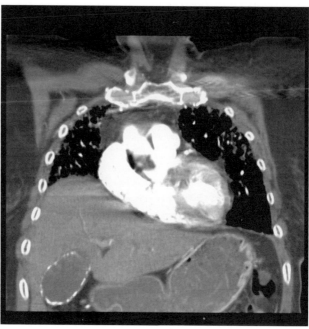

B

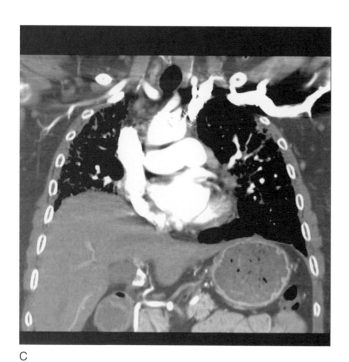

C

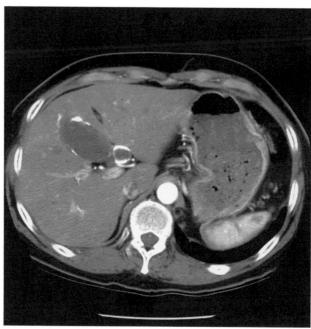

D

1. What is the large calcification seen in the right upper quadrant of the abdomen?

2. What can this finding be mistaken for?

3. What is the usual etiologic basis for this condition?

4. Name the major complication associated with this finding.

Porcelain Gallbladder

1. Porcelain gallbladder; calcification of the gallbladder wall.

2. A large calcified gallstone.

3. Porcelain gallbladder is thought to be the result of chronic cystic duct obstruction.

4. Carcinoma of the gallbladder.

Cross-Reference

Gastrointestinal Imaging: THE REQUISITES, ed 3, p 254.

Comments

It is thought that chronic cystic duct obstruction and sub-acute inflammation are the basis of gallbladder wall calcification. Quite often the calcified gallbladder is small and contracted (unlike the example in this case), and it is easy to confuse the finding with calcified gallstones. However, the porcelain gallbladder carries its own inherent risk, which much outweighs gallstones. The risk of developing carcinoma of the gallbladder in an untreated porcelain gallbladder is high, somewhere between 10% and 30%. Plain film and ultrasound may confuse calcified gallstones and a porcelain gallbladder. However, MDCT is much more adept at distinguishing the differences and may show the cystic duct obstruction as well (Fig. 41C, D in which a calcified obstructing stone is seen in the cystic duct).

Notes

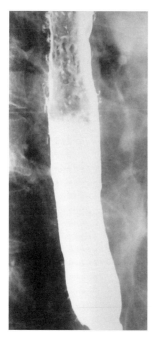

1. What structures are visible or filled by the barium?
2. Name some pathologic entities often seen in patients with this condition.
3. What common pathogen has been associated with this condition?
4. Is this pathogen ever found in a normal esophagus?

Esophageal Intramural Pseudodiverticulosis

1. Dilated excretory ducts of the esophageal mucus glands.

2. Strictures (usually benign), carcinoma, inflammation, and reflux.

3. *Candida* organisms.

4. No.

Cross-Reference

Gastrointestinal Imaging: THE REQUISITES, ed 3, p 30.

Comments

Intramural pseudodiverticulosis of the esophagus is a rare condition. Anatomically it represents barium filling the sparse adenomatous excretory ducts of the mucus glands of the esophagus. These mucus glands are normal anatomic structures of the esophagus but typically are not visible on radiologic studies. However, sometimes (thought to relate to chronic inflammation) these ducts become dilated, allowing barium to track into the ducts and glands.

Some type of inflammation must be present for these pathologic changes to occur, and the large majority of these patients have evidence of esophageal inflammation. A large proportion of patients with intramural pseudodiverticulosis also have strictures. The strictures are typically benign, but intramural pseudodiverticulosis has been reported in association with malignant strictures. *Candida* organisms have been found in patients with this condition, but the exact causal relationship is uncertain. More than likely, this finding represents a secondary infection of the glands and not a predisposing condition. Rarely this condition is found in patients with an otherwise normal esophagus. However, the very presence of intramural pseudodiverticulosis is abnormal.

Radiologically the intramural pseudodiverticulosis appears as small outpouchings, often with a flask shape. These outpouchings are most commonly mistaken for ulcers by those who are unfamiliar with the condition. Intramural pseudodiverticulosis may be either segmental or diffuse. Even intramural tracking and deep penetration may be evident. On CT, the condition produces changes of esophageal wall thickening and irregularity of the lumen, mimicking esophageal carcinoma. Because it is primarily a radiologic oddity, the condition's clinical course depends on treatment of the underlying condition. Often, treatment of the stricture or inflammation results in a decrease or even disappearance of the pseudodiverticulosis. Recently slightly increased risks of adenocarcinoma of the esophagus have been associated with this condition.

Notes

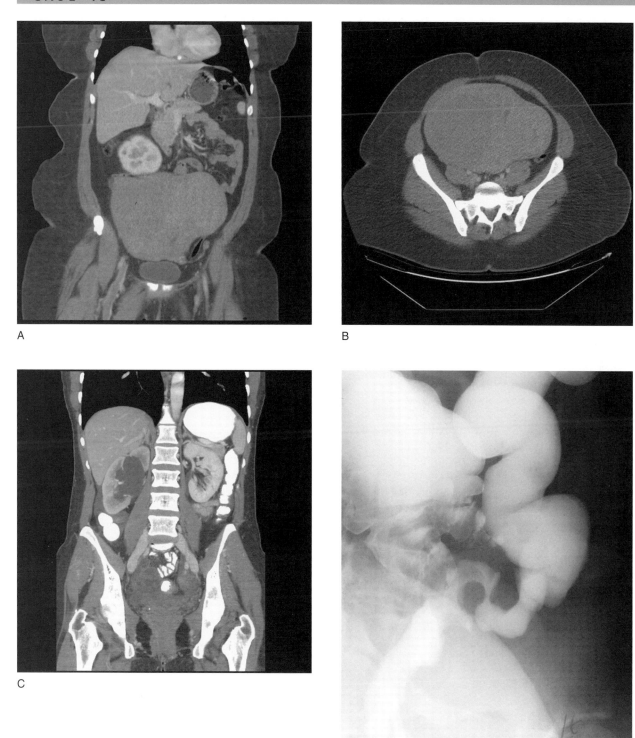

A

B

C

D

1. What might this woman's presenting complaints be?

2. What is the most likely origin of the mass?

3. Apart from her bowel, what other organ system might be compromised by the pelvic mass?

4. How do malignant and benign pelvic masses affect the bowel differently?

C A S E 4 3

Large Pelvic Mass Impressing Sigmoid Colon

1. Pelvic pain or discomfort, difficulty with bowel moments, flank pain.

2. Probably uterus, being purely solid in density. Ovarian might be cystic or a mixture of cystic and solid density. On very rare occasions an ovarian lesion may be solid. Mesenteric lesions can be cystic or solid.

3. Urinary tract. Compression on ureters resulting in obstruction and hydronephrosis. Compression on the bladder with resultant urinary frequency.

4. Benign lesions tend to cause compression of bowel while malignant lesions can result in contiguous invasion of the serosal surface of the bowel.

Cross-Reference
Gastrointestinal Imaging: THE REQUISITES, ed 3, p 291.

Comments
Large masses in the pelvis are quite common in women and are usually related to uterine fibroids. They can vary in size and appearance. Some can be solid, some have necrotic foci within them, and many have calcifications. If the mass is sufficiently large, it can compress the sigmoid or descending colon, causing symptoms by its sheer bulk such as in the images shown with this case. If the mass is malignant, it can invade the bowel from its serosal surface (Fig. 43D), causing narrowing, irregularity, and tethering of the bowel. Distention of such a segment of bowel is usually exceptionally painful, so keep this in mind when doing barium enemas as part of the workup on patients with possible malignant disease in the pelvis. The other issue (which is best addressed with CT) is the possibility of compression of one or both ureters and hydronephrosis (Fig. 43C).

Notes

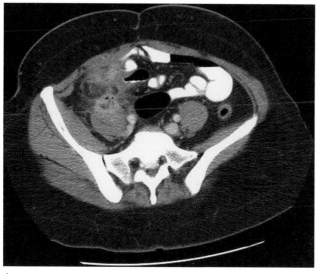

A

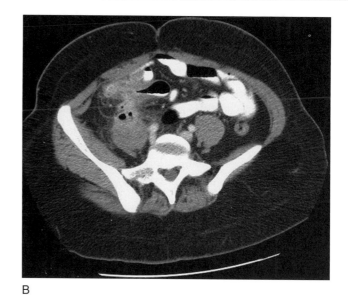

B

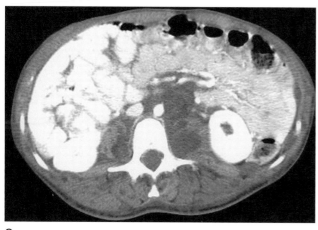

C

1. The patient is a young woman with both abdominal pain and a "psoas sign" on physical examination. From the provided images, how can you explain this pattern?

2. What is the "psoas sign"?

3. What is the disease most closely associated with a psoas abscess?

4. Can acute appendicitis cause a psoas sign?

Psoas Abscess

1. The CT images reveal inflammatory changes involving the bowel of the RLQ with extension into the retroperitoneum and psoas muscle.

2. A sign on physical examination in which leg lifting, or flexion of the right hip, on the affected side elicits pain.

3. Pott's disease. TB involvement of the spine with a "cold" abscess involving the psoas muscle.

4. Yes. Although the appendix is intraperitoneal and the psoas muscle retroperitoneal, significant inflammation in the RLQ can cause irritation of the psoas.

Cross-Reference
Gastrointestinal Imaging: THE REQUISITES, ed 3, p 340.

Comments

In the modern setting inflammation in the RLQ involving the bowel with extension through to the retroperitoneal psoas muscle has a limited differential diagnosis. Tuberculosis involving the terminal ileum and cecum is relatively uncommon, except perhaps in AIDS patients, and extension through the retroperitoneum would be unusual. Appendicitis might irritate the psoas but violation of the retroperitoneum would again be uncommon. Thus, the most likely diagnosis in a young patient with an inflammatory phlegmon in the right lower quadrant (RLQ) would be Crohn's disease with fistulous communication with the retroperitoneum as in the images shown in this case. However, even with Crohn's disease, a breach of the retroperitoneum is not common. A differential consideration should include actinomycosis, which, although uncommon, is known to routinely breach fascial and peritoneum barriers. Most of the fistulous communications seen in Crohn's disease are bowel to bowel, bowel to bladder, bowel to skin, and on rare occasions, bowel to ureter. Other conditions in which psoas infiltration may occur are metastatic disease, spinal diseases, and neuromuscular conditions such as neurofibromatosis (Fig. 44C).

Notes

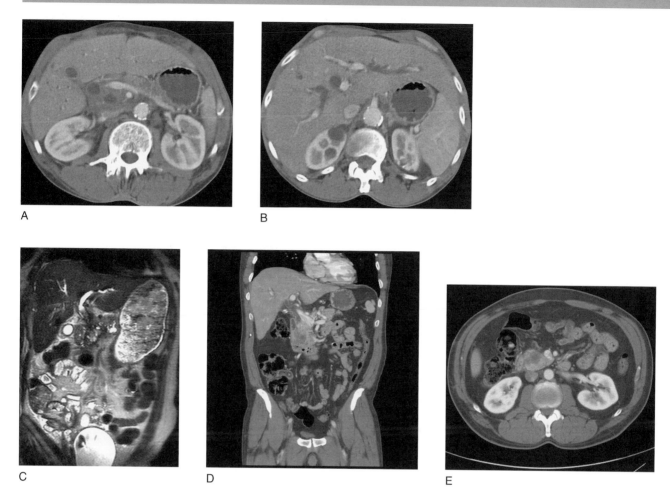

A   B

C   D   E

1. What might a physical examination and history of this patient reveal?

2. What percentage of pancreatic carcinomas occur in the pancreatic head or uncinate process?

3. Do most pancreatic adenocarcinomas arise in acinar or ductal epithelium?

4. How has improved imaging technology affected the mortality rate for pancreatic carcinoma?

Carcinoma of the Pancreatic Head

1. Jaundice, weight loss, persistent epigastric pain, loss of appetite and energy.

2. 80%.

3. Most pancreatic adenocarcinomas arise from the ductal epithelium.

4. Increasing detail and sensitivity in imaging technology has resulted in earlier diagnosis for patients with lesions located in the pancreatic body and tail, when these lesions are discovered (and they are usually discovered as an incidental finding). However, overall there has been no perceptible improvement in overall survival.

Cross-Reference

Gastrointestinal Imaging: THE REQUISITES, ed 3, p 159.

Comments

The CT images show a mixed density pancreatic head mass obstructing both the pancreatic and the common bile duct as well as encasing the superior mesenteric artery and vein and narrowing the portal vein. These findings indicate an inoperable lesion. MRI images confirm these findings (Fig. 45C), as do coronal CT images (Fig. 45D). The findings of jaundice and painless gallbladder enlargement (Courvoisier's gallbladder) are associated with this disease, as is Trousseau's syndrome (venous thrombotic disease) and occasionally new onset of diabetes mellitus. At the time of diagnosis patients with symptoms have a median survival rate of about 20 months.

On occasion, and usually as an unexpected incidental finding, one can come across a very small pancreatic head lesion, often in the uncinate process, that is asymptomatic (Fig 45E). These fortunate individuals may be candidates for resections and a Whipple procedure with an increased life expectancy.

Notes

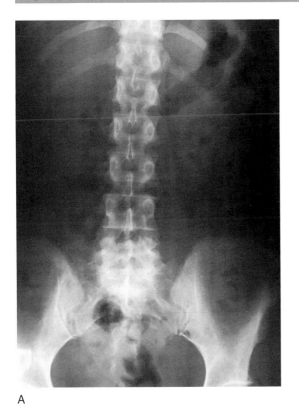

A

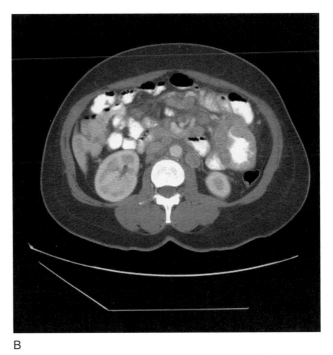

B

C

1. What is the abnormality shown on the plain film of the abdomen?

2. What conditions might give such an appearance?

3. On a prone film of the abdomen, what part of the stomach is most dependent?

4. Why are fascial planes and abdominal structures such as liver, spleen, and kidneys visible on plain film?

Linitis Plastica of the Stomach

1. Abnormal contours of the air-filled stomach.

2. The appearance of a rigid narrowed stomach (linitis plastica) can be caused by a variety of conditions both malignant and benign, with adenocarcinoma of the stomach being the most common malignant cause.

3. The fundus, being most posterior, would be the most dependent part when the patient is prone. Air configuration within the stomach can often indicate whether the image was obtained prone or supine.

4. Fat along fascial planes and around abdominal viscera creates fat–soft tissue interfaces, which make structures visible on plain film images.

Cross-Reference

Gastrointestinal Imaging: THE REQUISITES, ed 3, p 58.

Comments

Close attention to the gas pattern of the stomach on plain film images can sometimes reveal diffuse abnormalities of the stomach, such as in this case. The gas pattern of the stomach in this patient suggests a narrow rigid stomach with loss of pliability which is confirmed by barium UGI study (Fig. 46C). A CT image shows diffuse thickening of the gastric wall (Fig. 46B). In this case the findings (linitis plastica) are a result of diffuse scirrhous adenocarcinoma of stomach. However, other conditions can also give a similar appearance. Metastatic disease involving the stomach (especially from breast and lung) can result in an identical appearance, as can Hodgkin's type desmoplastic lymphoma of the stomach and inflammatory diseases such as severe diffuse peptic gastritis, corrosive gastritis, radiation gastritis, sarcoidosis, and Crohn's disease (ram's horn stomach), as well as some reported cases of syphilis.

Notes

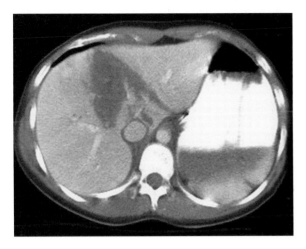

1. This patient was in a motorcycle accident. What is the CT finding?

2. What is the most common cause of this finding?

3. Where is this condition more likely to be located: anteriorly in the left lobe or posteriorly in the right lobe?

4. What percentage of patients require surgery for this condition?

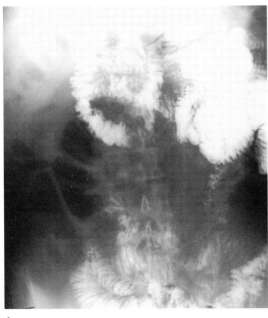

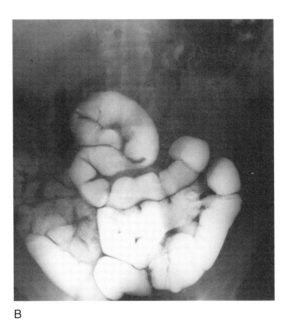

A   B

1. Describe the appearance of the small bowel on these images.

2. What does fold "effacement" mean?

3. What conditions might give this pattern?

4. What is the significance of "hypersecretion" on a small bowel study, and what is its appearance?

Liver Laceration

1. The CT image demonstrates an acute liver laceration; one very subtle in the posterior right lobe, the other very obvious.

2. Blunt trauma to the liver is the most common cause. Penetrating trauma would be the next most common cause.

3. Most liver lacerations occur in the right lobe, and most frequently in the posterior segments, probably due to compression against the posterior abdominal wall and spine.

4. The percentage varies, depending on extent of injury, amount of blood loss, and other associated intraabdominal injuries. It is generally accepted that 30% to 40% of these injuries can be treated without surgery.

Cross-Reference

Gastrointestinal Imaging: THE REQUISITES, ed 3, p 207.

Comments

After the spleen, the liver is the next most common solid organ injured in blunt trauma to the abdomen. Liver traumas can be solitary, but most often are seen with multiple injuries of the abdomen, abdominal wall, and thoracic wall as well as musculoskeleton and neurologic injuries elsewhere. By far the most common cause is trauma due to motor vehicle accidents. The injury to the liver is most serious when large blood vessels have been torn, such as the hepatic veins, the portal vessels, or the hepatic artery. Those with hepatic artery tears often do not make it to the ER.

Commonly what is seen in CT is a laceration with accompanying intrahepatic or subcapsular hematoma. Some degree of extrahepatic hematoma is seen in about 80% of cases. Such things as hepatic contusion may occur and can manifest as a focal area of diminished density. However, these injuries are almost always self-limiting conditions for which no treatment is required. Survival of patients with intra-abdominal solid organ trauma has increased over the last few decades with improved on-site patient care and rapid transport to a trauma center. Without doubt, a major contributing factor has been the availability of CT imaging in or adjacent to the trauma center.

Blunt liver trauma has been categorized by organ injury scale, ranging from contusion to hematoma and laceration at one end of the scale, and major vascular injuries and hepatic avulsion at the other.

Notes

Small Bowel Malabsorption

1. The images show moderately dilated small bowel (mostly ileum) with marked fold atrophy, effacement, and hypersecretion. This is the pattern of small bowel malabsorption.

2. Effacement is a term used by radiologists (and others) to describe a process whereby folds or structures become less distinct to the point of elimination. For example, the use and wear on a coin will eventually wear away, or "efface," the surface of the coin. Bowel folds that become atrophic, less distinct, or nonexistent are said to be "effaced." A diffuse infiltrating process can have the similar effect on bowel folds or any raised structure.

3. The commonest cause of fold effacement is fold atrophy in the small bowel secondary to malabsorption syndromes.

4. Hypersecretion is an important finding in malabsorption syndromes. The sign is indicative of failure of absorption and is characterized on barium examinations by dilution of the barium column and a gray instead of white appearance of the barium.

Cross-Reference

Gastrointestinal Imaging: THE REQUISITES, ed 3, p 112.

Comments

There can be degrees of malabsorption seen in patients with diarrhea and various food intolerances. The best known of these is celiac disease, a form of gluten intolerance (also known as nontropical sprue). There appear to be varying degrees of intolerance. The cases that come to medical attention are patients suffering from diarrhea, steatorrhea, and weight loss. The definitive diagnostic examination is small endoscopy with mucosal biopsy. Even with small ingested video capsules that can traverse the small bowel and provide video of the mucosal surface, the barium small bowel follow-through is the fastest and least expensive way of making a diagnosis. Patients with symptoms serious enough to seek medical attention will almost always have some or all of the findings of malabsorption on the barium examination. The classic appearance of flocculation, segmentation, and the famous "moulage" sign are infrequently seen due to the continued improvement of modern barium suspensions. What is seen is dilatation of bowel, atrophy and effacement of the fold pattern, particularly in the ileum, and hypersecretion (such as in this case).

Notes

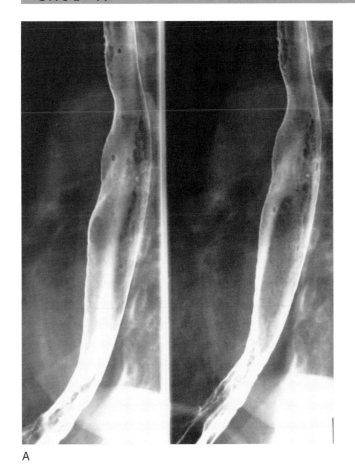

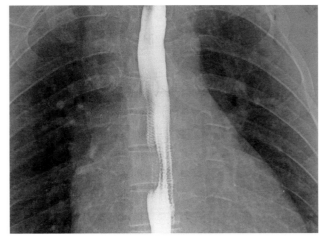

A

B

1. How would you describe the pattern seen in the esophagus on Figure 49B?

2. What might cause such a pattern?

3. What disease entities might be associated with this pattern?

4. The 16–year-old patient in image 49A complains of solid dysphagia, but there is little evidence of stricture or narrowing on the images. What should you do next?

The Feline Esophagus: Eosinophilic Esophagitis

1. This is the "feline" pattern seen in the esophagus, so named because of its similarity to the normal esophageal pattern of a cat.

2. It is thought that spasm and contraction of the longitudinal muscularis mucosa is responsible for the pattern.

3. A number of possibilities ranging from a response to gastric acid on the esophageal mucosa seen in GERD patients to the transient "corrugated" pattern described by endoscopists in patients with eosinophilic esophagitis (EOE).

4. Any patient who complains of solid dysphagia with a relatively normal-appearing barium esophagogram should immediately be given a 12.5-mm barium tablet with water, and its passage through the GE junction followed fluoroscopically. The GE junction can stretch to accommodate a much larger bolus than most people realize. In this case the barium tablet was held up at the GE junction for several minutes before dissolution and passage, confirming the diagnosis of occult stricture of the GE junction.

Cross-Reference
Gastrointestinal Imaging: THE REQUISITES, ed 3, p 31.

Comments
Most of the time the feline pattern of the esophagus has been associated with gastroesophageal reflux disease (GERD). It can be seen with or without other findings of GERD such as ulceration. It does not seem to have any connection to the presence of Barrett's metaplasia or esophageal carcinoma. However, in recent years the condition of eosinophilic esophagitis (EOE) has become widely recognized and discussed in the medical literature. Among the endoscopic findings associated with this condition is a transient corrugated pattern of the esophageal mucosa, which sounds suspiciously like the pattern radiologists have called the "feline" esophagus over the years. This condition, once consider a rarity, is now being recognized with some regularity. It seems to be a disease of Western industrialized nations, of younger patients (teens to 30s, although a case of EOE in a 56-year old patient was recently reported in the literature), with solid dysphagia being the most common symptom in older patients while chest pain and GERD-like symptoms prevail in younger patients. The condition (EOE) seems to exist independent of the other eosinophilic infiltrative conditions seen in the stomach and small bowel of atopic patients. There have been no cases of esophageal cancer reported in these patients at this time.

Notes

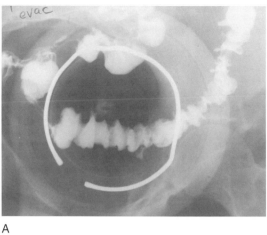

A

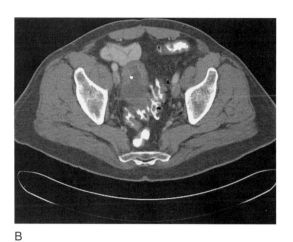

B

1. What is consistent on both the barium study and CT image?

2. What percentage of people in the United States over 60 years of age have colonic diverticula?

3. What percentage of these cases will result in painless rectal bleeding?

4. What percentage will go on to develop frank colonic diverticulitis?

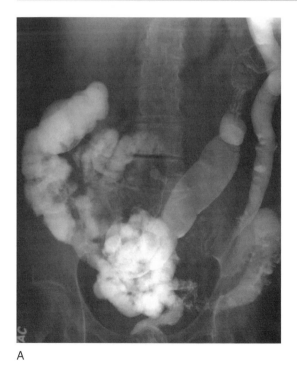

A

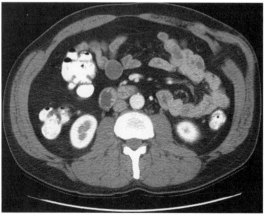

B

1. Through which anatomic area does this hernia pass?

2. What is meant by the term *Richter's hernia?*

3. What is the most common type of abdominal wall hernia in adults?

4. Name a type of hernia that contains a Meckel's diverticulum.

CASE 50

Sigmoid Diverticulitis

1. Both images demonstrate an extracolonic abscess.

2. Greater than 60%.

3. 15% to 30%.

4. About 15%.

Cross-Reference
Gastrointestinal Imaging: THE REQUISITES, ed 3, p 302.

Comments

Diverticular disease of the colon (diverticulosis coli) is a common disease of the Western world. The older the patient, the greater the likelihood. However, in the last three or four decades there appears to be an increased incidence in younger patients. Diverticula formation is probably related to increased intraluminal pressures, decreased bowel transit times, and diminishing quantities of fiber in the diet of Western industrialized countries. Most of these patients are asymptomatic or manifest vague abdominal discomfort. A small group will experience rectal bleeding, although a massive rectal bleed secondary to diverticulosis is uncommon (less than 5%). Very often the offending diverticulum is in the right colon.

About 15% of this population will go on to frank diverticulitis, such as shown in the images accompanying this case. The pathogenesis is thought to be infection secondary to impacted fecal matter within the diverticula, local peridiverticular inflammation, and finally, if untreated, frank diverticulitis with pericolonic abscess formation. Some of the abscesses will spontaneously drain via communication with the colonic lumen, such as shown in the barium enema image. Most will not, and will require surgical intervention or radiologic placement of an abscess drainage catheter. It is believed by some that the origin of the so-called "giant sigmoid diverticulum" is, in fact, the sequela of spontaneous drainage of a large diverticular abscess with the remaining cavity permanent, communicating with the sigmoid colon and epithelialized over time.

There is little doubt that CT of the abdomen is the best imaging method for diverticulitis. Not only can mild pericolic inflammatory changes be detected but a pericolic abscess is easily detected with positive contrast material in the colon. The lack of positive colonic contrast imaging is a potential pitfall.

Notes

CASE 51

Spigelian Hernia

1. Semilunar line (linea semilunaris).

2. Only a portion of the bowel wall is contained in the hernia.

3. Incisional.

4. Littre's hernia.

Cross-Reference
Gastrointestinal Imaging: THE REQUISITES, ed 3, p 329.

Comments

Numerous types of hernias can be identified along the anterior abdominal wall. With the increased use of CT, some hernias are identified in patients who have no symptoms. In the adult population, incisional hernias are by far the most common. These develop in up to 5% of patients who have abdominal operations and typically occur within the first 6 months after the surgery. Affected patients may remain asymptomatic, however. Even though laparoscopic surgery is becoming increasingly popular, hernias can still occur through those small defects in the abdominal wall because they are not surgically closed. Richter's hernia is an unusual type of hernia that contains only a portion of a loop of bowel wall and not the entire lumen (i.e., the tip of the cecum caught in a right inguinal hernia).

Spigelian hernias are unusual. They occur in the lower abdomen, either in the right or left lower quadrant. The area through which the bowel herniates, termed the *linea semilunaris*, consists of a fibrous band of tissue joining the rectus sheath muscles with the transverse abdominal and internal oblique abdominal muscle. The hernia is probably the result of a weakness or congenital defect in the union of these muscles and fibrous bands. The hernia courses obliquely between these groups of muscles and may reside between bands of muscles, making it difficult to identify on clinical examination. Often, patients with spigelian hernias have intermittent or constant pain in the lower quadrant. The hernias contain either small bowel (right) or sigmoid colon (left), depending on where they are situated. They can have a large orifice, in which case there is less likelihood of obstruction or strangulation than with other types of hernias. They also may spontaneously reduce. Because they do not fully herniate through the abdominal wall, they are difficult to clinically diagnose, especially in obese patients. These hernias occur with similar frequency in men and women. They may be bilateral or associated with other abdominal wall defects. Quite often the defect in the abdominal wall may contain fat and may be asymptomatic (such as in Fig. 51B).

Notes

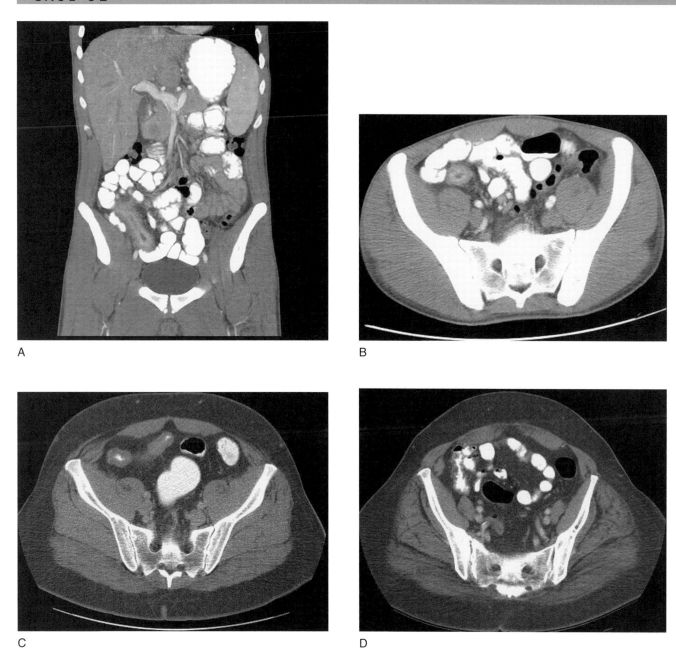

A

B

C

D

1. What is the abnormality shown in these images?

2. List some of the causes that might give these findings.

3. What percentage of Crohn's disease involves the terminal ileum?

4. What other parts of the gut can be involved with Crohn's disease?

Crohn's Disease of the Terminal Ileum

1. Thickening of the wall of the distal ileum with peri-ileal inflammatory changes.

2. Crohn's disease, *Yersinia* infection, and tuberculosis.

3. About 50% have disease involving the terminal ileum and cecum.

4. Esophagus, stomach, small bowel, and colorectum.

Cross-Reference

Gastrointestinal Imaging: THE REQUISITES, ed 3, p 126.

Comments

Crohn's disease (or regional enteritis), as seen in the distal ileum of this patient, is one of the major idiopathic IBDs (ulcerative colitis being the other). It is a transmural granulomatous inflammatory process and has been described in medical literature with various attached names for over 200 years. The cardinal clinical presentation includes diarrhea, abdominal pain, and weight loss. The incidence is higher in Europe and North America than in the Far East. The incidence has increased steadily in the West until about the mid-1980s when it began to stabilize. It tends to be a disease of young people (15–25 years old), although there is a second much smaller peak in the seventh decade. It has long been thought to be an immunologic response to some stimulating agent, although such an agent has never been identified. Barium studies can be helpful with colonic involvement by identifying the specific pattern, which is usually quite different from ulcerative colitis. However, when only the terminal ileum alone is involved (Fig. 52C, D) all imaging studies are much less specific. The presence of fistulous communication, perianal fissuring, and extragastrointestinal manifestation may be helpful.

Notes

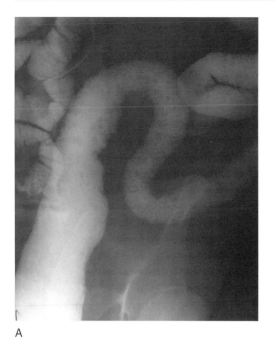

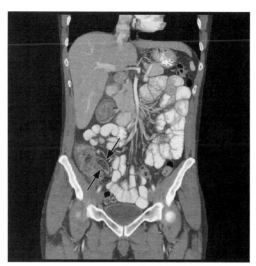

A   B

1. What findings does this film of the sigmoid colon in a 31-year-old man show?

2. What disease has this patient suffered from previously?

3. Would you expect this patient to have an enterovesicular fistula?

4. Does this patient have an increased risk for colorectal carcinoma?

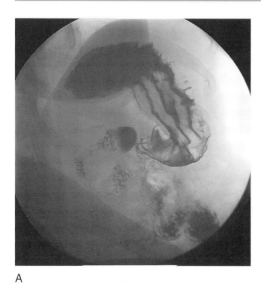

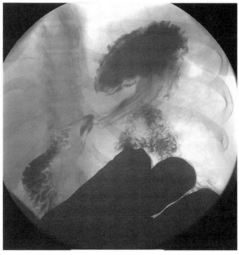

A   B

1. What neoplasm most commonly produces thickened gastric folds?

2. Name some infiltrative processes associated with thickened folds.

3. What is a cause of isolated fundal gastric varices?

4. What is the most common infectious cause of thickened folds?

Chronic Ulcerative Colitis

1. Multiple small filling defects of varying shape.

2. Acute severe ulcerative colitis.

3. No.

4. Yes.

Cross-Reference
Gastrointestinal Imaging: THE REQUISITES, ed 3, p 287.

Comments

Chronic or "burned out" ulcerative colitis can leave behind sequelae, such as the postinflammatory polyposis seen in this case. These defects are also known as filiform polyposis of the colon. In reality, they are not true polyps or even hyperplastic polyps (although a tiny number may be hyperplastic). They are, instead, mucosal tags, which have been left behind following the healing process. In the acute phase of severe ulcerative colitis there is marked ulcerative denouement of the colonic mucosal surface by the widespread ulcerative process. Not all the mucosa is ulcerated, and small islands of residual edematous mucosa remain (pseudopolyps). In the healing process, re-epithelization of the colonic surface occurs. The small islands of residual mucosa that have survived the inflammatory process are re-epithelized up to the base of the residual mucosal tags and in some cases beneath the tags, leaving them dangling in the bowel lumen and giving us the picture of filiform or postinflammatory polyposis. Although UC patients who have suffered pancolitis continuously over 10 years have a 10% chance of malignancy, patients who have had limited involvement and healing will have a much lesser, but still increased risk. The patient shown in Figure 53B has pancolitis. Note the normal appearance of the terminal ileum (*arrows*).

Notes

Gastric Fold Thickening

1. Lymphoma.

2. Eosinophilic gastritis, sarcoidosis, Crohn's disease, Ménétrier's disease, amyloidosis, alcoholic gastritis.

3. Thrombosis of the splenic vein.

4. *Helicobacter pylori*.

Cross-Reference
Gastrointestinal Imaging: THE REQUISITES, ed 3, p 64.

Comments

It is extremely common to find thickened gastric folds on upper gastrointestinal examinations. The width of the gastric folds is usually about 3 to 5 mm in the distal prepyloric stomach and 8 to 10 mm proximally in the fundus. When the stomach is fully distended, normal gastric folds tend to run parallel to the lumen, whereas folds that are irregularly thickened, nodular, or serpiginous in appearance are usually considered abnormal. Associated gastric wall thickening also may be visible on CT examination.

The presence of thickened rugal folds, gastric wall thickening, or both is a nonspecific finding. A variety of diseases may produce this radiologic finding, which can even be seen in healthy patients. The most common cause is some type of gastritis, such as alcoholic gastritis. *H. pylori* infection of the stomach is now recognized as an extremely common cause of inflammatory disease of the stomach and is by far the most common infectious process of the upper gastrointestinal tract. Zollinger-Ellison syndrome (gastrinoma) should always be considered, although it is rare. Numerous benign infiltrating processes, including eosinophilic gastritis, sarcoidosis, amyloidosis, Crohn's disease, and Ménétrier's disease, also may produce fold thickening. Of the neoplastic processes, lymphoma most typically presents as thickened folds. Adenocarcinoma and even metastases also must be considered but are less common.

Varices of the stomach usually have associated esophageal varices and are related to increased portal venous pressure resulting from a variety of causes. Isolated fundal gastric varices, however, are a specific condition associated with splenic vein occlusion. The spleen normally drains via the splenic vein, but if it occludes, there are short gastric veins that act as collateral circulation in the funal region of the stomach. These veins course over the proximal stomach and connect to the coronary vein, which then flows into the portal circulation. Splenic vein thrombosis is usually the sequela of pancreatitis or pancreatic carcinoma and less commonly the result of retroperitoneal processes, surgery, or hypercoagulability state.

Notes

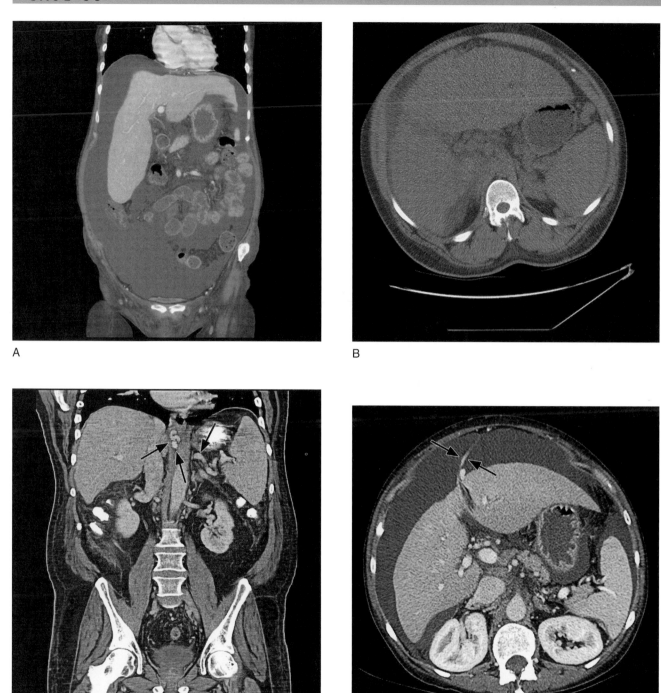

A

B

C

D

1. What do the images of this patient reveal?

2. Name the leading cause for this condition in North America.

3. What are some of the complications seen with this condition?

4. With widespread involvement of the liver, what areas may be spared or less affected? Why?

Portal Hypertension

1. Liver cirrhosis, ascites, portal hypertension, and varices.

2. Chronic alcoholism and irreversible alcoholic toxic hepatitis.

3. Hepatocellular carcinoma, esophageal varices, and in some patients portal vein thrombus and occlusion and possible cavernous transformation of the portal vein in chronic disease.

4. The caudate lobe, because it has its own blood supply.

Cross-Reference

Gastrointestinal Imaging: THE REQUISITES, ed 3, p 184.

Comments

Cirrhosis of the liver is the result of chronic liver hepatocyte toxicity resulting in fibrous tissue formation throughout the liver with resultant in tissue distortion and a smaller shrunken liver. The changes may initially be focal. However, when the entire liver is involved the classic CT appearance of a small liver with nodular or irregular margins is seen. The caudate lobe may be partially spared. Although most of the liver blood supply comes from the portal vein, the caudate lobe has a direct connection with the inferior vena cava in most patients. In the United States most cirrhosis is alcohol induced (Laennec's cirrhosis) and is seen with splenomegaly, ascites, and esophageal varices (Fig. 55C). The falciform ligament may also be seen if there is sufficient ascites (Fig. 55D).

Other causes of cirrhosis include Wilson's disease and hemochromatosis. Portal vein hypertension is a form of relative occlusion of the portal vein. In some cases of cirrhosis a true portal vein thrombus may be seen. However, there also may be other causes of portal vein thrombosis apart from cirrhosis, and they will be discussed elsewhere.

Notes

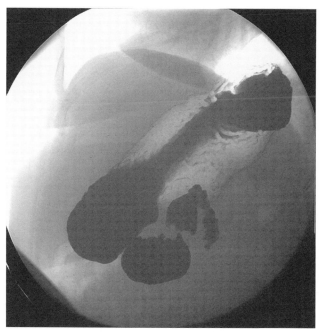

A

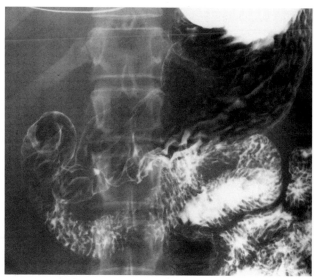

B

1. What is the most common location for a benign gastric ulcer?

2. What produces a so-called Hampton's line? What does it mean?

3. What do radiating folds that stop before the ulcer crater indicate?

4. Do all benign ulcers extend beyond the expected lumen of the stomach?

Benign Gastric Ulcer

1. The lesser curvature of the stomach.

2. Symmetrical and uniform undermining of the ulcer crater, giving a lucent circular base to the ulcer. Such ulcers are benign.

3. Generally folds that converge on an ulcer crater but appear to stop short of the crater are almost always malignant. However, it must be remembered that a small number of benign ulcers may have folds that stop short of the crater.

4. No. Benign greater curve ulcers and those with a great deal of edema do not. However, again, this sign is not infallable. Chronic benign ulcers, due to transient healing and cicatrixation, can project within the lumen of the stomach.

Cross-Reference

Gastrointestinal Imaging: THE REQUISITES, ed 3, p 82.

Comments

Benign ulcers may occur anywhere in the stomach, although they do have a propensity to occur in the lesser curvature, particularly in the middle of the body. This type of ulcer is often seen in the older patient, but the cause for this is uncertain. As a corollary, the majority of ulcers found in the fundus are malignant. The size of an ulcer has no bearing on its malignant potential, and giant gastric ulcers often represent a penetrating, walled-off, benign gastric ulcer. Also, the shape of the ulcer is usually round and well defined but this is not always the case.

Much has been said about the gastric ulcer as seen in profile. Most benign gastric ulcers project outside the expected lumen of the stomach. However, if there is a great deal of edema or the ulcer is chronic in nature, this may not be the case. Another common sign of a benign gastric ulcer is Hampton's line, which is a thin lucent line at the neck or base of the ulcer as it passes through the mucosal layer where undermining of the submucosa occurs. However, a very thick "ulcer collar," particularly if it is asymmetrical, at the neck of the ulcer is not a Hampton's line and may be seen in both benign and malignant ulcers.

Often, radiating folds are seen extending toward an ulcer. If these folds pass all the way to the edge of the crater, the process is most likely benign. Infrequently, folds may stop short as a result of a large collar of edema (in benign ulcers) or as a result of neoplastic tissue (in malignant ulcers); therefore, folds that stop short are a good but not absolute differential diagnostic feature. Also, the folds tend to be smooth and symmetrical in benign ulcers and more irregular, thickened, and fused in malignant ulcers. It has long been a part of gastric ulcer lore that malignant ulcers may show signs of healing. The veracity of this is dubious.

Notes

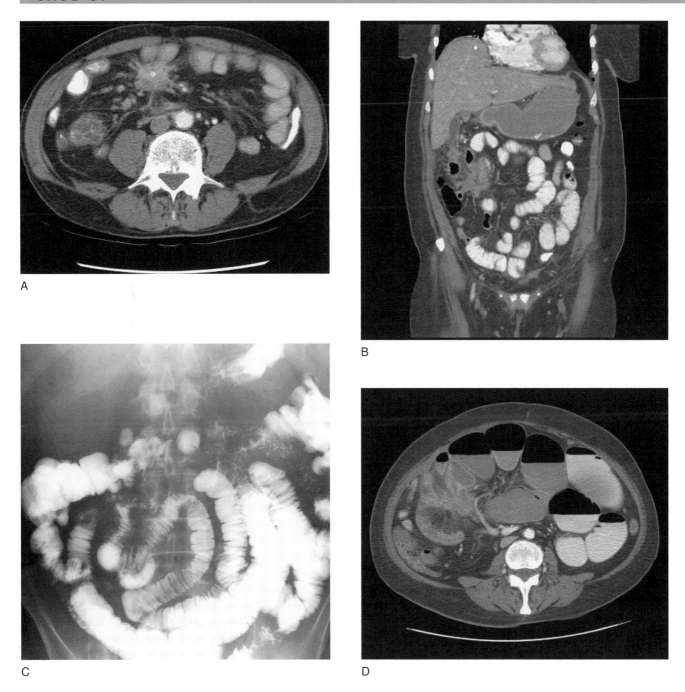

A

B

C

D

1. Given the unusual appearance of this lesion, what is the most likely diagnosis?

2. What is the most common site where this lesion occurs?

3. What nonimaging test can confirm the diagnosis?

4. What is the substance produced by this lesion that accounts for many of the symptoms?

Carcinoid of the Small Bowel

1. The "spoke-wheel" configuration of the lesion makes it most likely a small bowel–mesenteric carcinoid tumor.

2. The appendix.

3. Serotonin, kallikrein.

4. The presence of 5-HIAA (5-hydroxindoleacetic acid) in the urine.

Cross-Reference

Gastrointestinal Imaging: THE REQUISITES, ed 3, p 140.

Comments

Carcinoid tumors are unusual neoplasms that can arise in various structures of the intestinal tract and even the bronchi. The most common location in which carcinoids occur is the appendix. However, most symptomatic tumors arise in the small bowel, typically in the ileum. Rarely they are found in other parts of the intestinal tract, the abdominal cavity, and even the bronchi, which is an embryologic bud of the intestinal tract. Carcinoids are slow-growing tumors that invade little by little. They are multiple in about 20% of the cases. All carcinoids are considered premalignant, but those of the small bowel are most likely to metastasize and those of the appendix rarely do so. These tumors belong to the group of lesions termed *APUD* (*a*mine *p*recursor *u*ptake and *d*ecarboxylation cell) lesions. They are hormonally active, and the major by-product they release is serotonin. Secretion of histamine, 5-hydroxytryptophan, and other hormones also has been described. Serotonin is converted in the liver and lungs to 5-hydroxyindoleacetic acid (5-HIAA), which is excreted in the urine and easily detected.

On barium studies of the small bowel the findings are usually irregularity, "kinking" of the bowel secondary to the desmoplastic nature of the tumor, which accounts for the spoke-wheel effect seen on CT (Fig. 57C). Also seen on some cases are mass effect and small bowel obstruction.

Carcinoid syndrome occurs when liver metastases (it rarely occurs without liver metastases) excrete hormonally active substances, which cannot be metabolized by the liver, directly into the venous circulation. This action produces vasomotor changes of flushing and vasodilation. Bronchospasm and wheezing may occur. Intestinal hypermotility, with diarrhea and cramping, is another symptom. With time, right-sided endocardial fibrosis and valve problems occur in the heart.

The primary tumor may appear as a small mass on conventional barium studies. However, the serotonin secreted by the tumor incites an intense desmoplastic response in the mesentery, producing the fibrotic response evident in this patient. There is marked fibrosis of the mesentery, with tethering of the small bowel loops. Bowel obstruction and even vascular obstruction are possible complications of this fibrosis (Fig. 57D).

Notes

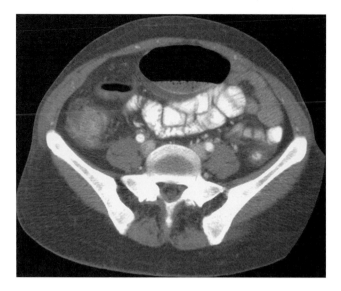

1. An immunocompromised young woman presents with pain, rectal bleeding, and diarrhea. From the given CT image, what are the findings?

2. Viral infections of the gastrointestinal tract tend to affect what part of the gut most frequently?

3. What viral infection of the colon is known to cause large deep ulceration?

4. Could pseudomembranous colitis account for the findings in the image?

AIDS Colitis

1. Cross-sectional image shows a severe inflammatory process involving the descending and ascending regions of the colon. Other images showed pancolitis.

2. The colon.

3. Cytomegalovirus infection.

4. Yes.

Cross-Reference

Gastrointestinal Imaging: THE REQUISITES, ed 3, p 297.

Comments

Cytomegalovirus (CMV) colitis is a type of colitis seen in AIDS patients and other immunocompromised patients. Both CT and barium studies can be quite helpful and suggestive. The discovery of large ulcers has been associated with CMV infection in AIDS patients. Ultimately the diagnosis is usually made when the virus is isolated in tissue specimens. Although CMV is probably the most common viral colonic infection seen today, other opportunistic infections are also seen, including *Cryptosporidium* infection and pseuodmembranous colitis, both of which are more common in AIDS patients. Bacterial infection colitis must be included in the diagnosis; *Salmonella*, *Shigella*, and *Campylobacter* and even tuberculosis must be considered, although TB tends to affect the ileocecal area, as it would in patients without an impaired immune system.

Notes

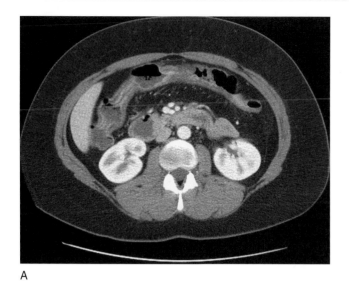

A

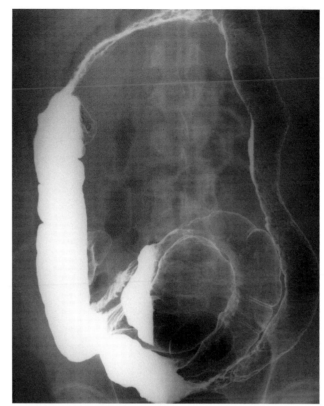

B

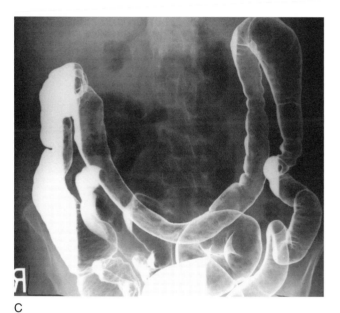

C

1. What inflammatory conditions produce collar-button ulcers?

2. What conditions produce aphthous ulcers?

3. What conditions produce long, fissuring ulcers?

4. What inflammatory bowel diseases result in fistula formation?

Crohn's Disease of the Colon

1. Most can produce collar-button ulcers, but by far the commonest cause of "collar-button" ulcers is ulcerative colitis, in which small superficial ulcers undermine the surrounding submucosa, giving the collar-button appearance.

2. Crohn's disease most frequently but occasionally some infectious colitides.

3. Crohn's disease, in which a number of long serpiginous ulcers in the same area produce a "cobblestone" effect.

4. Crohn's disease and tuberculosis.

Cross-Reference
Gastrointestinal Imaging: THE REQUISITES, ed 3, p 294.

Comments

Several types of ulcers are encountered with inflammation of the colon, and these ulcers can also affect all portions of the gastrointestinal tract because the bowel has only a limited number of ways to respond to inflammation of the mucosa. When ulceration extends through the mucosa and muscularis propria, it reaches the submucosa. The epithelium is relatively resistant, but the submucosa has difficulty containing the inflammatory process. Thus, ulcers tend to spread laterally when they reach the submucosa. With their thin necks and wide bases, the ulcers resemble collar buttons, hence the terminology.

Aphthous ulceration occurs in the colon as lymphoid follicles enlarge from inflammation and their overlying mucosa ulcerates. In other parts of the gastrointestinal tract, aphthous ulcers occur as focal ulcers, with surrounding edema. Either way, they produce a characteristic tiny ulcer surrounded by edema appearance. These ulcers were initially described in association with Crohn's disease (Fig. 59C) but can be found in a variety of infectious processes, particularly viral infections. Amebiasis, salmonellosis, and even ischemia have also been known to produce aphthous ulcers.

Long, linear ulcers are rare and much more specific to Crohn's disease. Rarely do other inflammatory conditions cause this type of ulceration, although tuberculosis is also a consideration. Fistulas between bowel loops are a sequela of inflammation of the bowel, occurring with Crohn's disease or tuberculosis. Fistulas are never seen in patients with ulcerative colitis. The possibility of malignancy and the sequelae of radiation or surgery are other considerations when fistulas are encountered. Diverticulitis also can produce fistulas and is the most common cause of enterovesicular fistulas. CT is fast becoming a valuable tool in the workup of Crohn's disease (Fig. 59A). Only about 25% of Crohn's disease is limited to the colon. The classic findings of discontinuous disease (skip lesions), and asymmetrical involvement are usually evident.

Notes

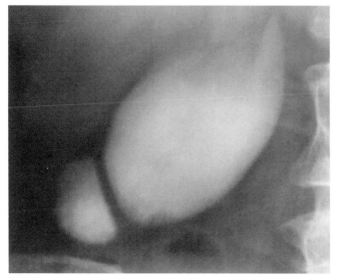
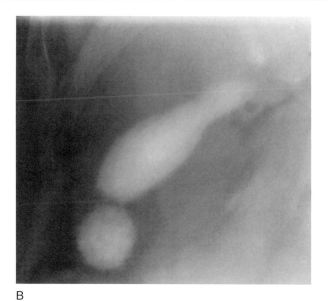

A   B

1. What is this unusual condition of the gallbladder?

2. What are the underlying pathologic processes?

3. Are there any long-term complications of this condition?

4. Name other conditions that may have a similar appearance on ultrasound or CT.

Adenomyomatosis of the Gallbladder

1. Adenomyomatosis of the gallbladder.

2. Proliferation of the smooth muscle and infolding of the mucosa.

3. No.

4. Chronic cholecystitis, cholesterolosis, and gallbladder carcinoma.

Cross-Reference

Gastrointestinal Imaging: THE REQUISITES, ed 3, p 252.

Comments

Two conditions—adenomyomatosis and cholesterolosis—are grouped together as the hyperplastic cholecystoses. These conditions are not pathologically or physiologically related in any way, but both produce an abnormal thickening of the gallbladder wall. In adenomyomatosis there is abnormal thickening of the smooth muscle layer of the gallbladder, which results in exaggerated infolding of the mucosal folds and epithelium. Sometimes the epithelium becomes surrounded by the muscle layers and forms cysts. The exact reason that this condition develops is uncertain. Adenomyomatosis is unusual in that frequently only portions of the gallbladder wall become involved; other gallbladder conditions usually involve the entire gallbladder.

On contrast examinations of the gallbladder, these infoldings of the mucosal surface trap contrast material and appear as tiny diverticula-like projections in the wall (called Rokitansky-Aschoff sinuses). They become particularly pronounced when there is contraction of the gallbladder wall. If the proliferation is severe, there can be narrowing or deformity of the gallbladder lumen. A thickened gallbladder wall can be demonstrated on CT examination. If this thickening is focal, it may be impossible to distinguish the condition from gallbladder carcinoma. Thickening of the wall of the gallbladder also is apparent on ultrasound examination. Ring-down artifacts may be evident on the nondependent wall of the gallbladder. The wall of the gallbladder also may appear nodular or may appear to contain small polyps. Unlike other gallbladder conditions, there is little associated morbidity with adenomyomatosis, and there are no known long-term complications. Adenomyomatosis is not a precancerous condition.

Notes

Fair Game

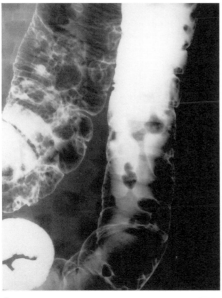
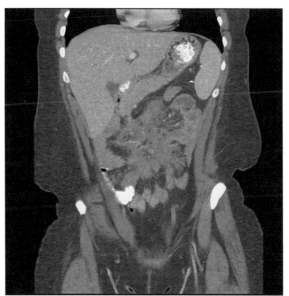

A   B

1. What conditions can give rise to fibrotic changes in the mesentery?

2. What polyposis syndrome is associated with mesenteric fibrosis?

3. What tumors may cause this appearance?

4. When this occurs in a round mass, what is it called?

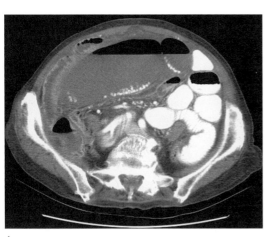
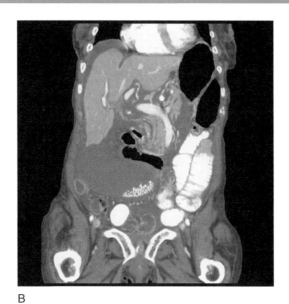

A   B

1. What is the large fluid-filled structure in the mid-abdomen?

2. What is the likely state of the cystic duct?

3. What was the origin (preceding pathology) of the condition?

4. What are the possible complications associated with acute cholecystis?

CASE 61

Gardner's Syndrome

1. Retractile mesenteritis, mesenteric panniculitis or lipodystrophy, and mesenteric fibromatosis.

2. Gardner's syndrome (familial adenomatous polyposis syndrome [FAPS]).

3. Lymphoma, carcinoid tumors, and peritoneal carcinomatosis.

4. Desmoid.

Cross-Reference

Gastrointestinal Imaging: THE REQUISITES, ed 3, p 284.

Comments

Various fibrous conditions, which represent a combination of fibrosis, inflammation, and fatty replacement, can affect the mesentery (Fig. 61B). These conditions have been given several names, which are somewhat dependent on which component of the disease predominates. Terms used for this condition include *retractile mesenteritis, fibrosing mesenteritis, mesenteric panniculitis, mesenteric lipodystrophy,* and *desmoids.* Many use the broad category of fibrosing mesenteritis to describe this condition. Most often this condition occurs in patients without any predisposing factors. Patients with FAPS (Gardner's syndrome) (Fig. 61A) are known to develop fibrotic lesions of the mesentery. The lesion may be an ill-defined fibrotic reaction, as in fibrosing mesenteritis, or it may be a more focal, rounded mass, which may be termed a *desmoid.*

The modality that allows the best visualization of these changes is CT. The tissue is denser than the mesenteric fat, although areas of fat may be seen within it. The fibrous tissue travels along the tissue planes and tends to surround structures, such as vessels or bowel, and may encase them to some degree. It also may be a more localized, ovoid mass that appears well defined, which is what some tend to refer to as a *desmoid.* This infiltrating fibrous reaction also mimics neoplastic processes, and it may be difficult to distinguish the two. Lymphoma, serosal spread of tumor, and even carcinoid tumors can resemble fibrosing mesenteritis. On barium studies of the bowel, the loops of bowel may be displaced or fixed in position.

Notes

CASE 62

Gallbladder Hydrops and Perforation

1. A massively enlarged gallbladder. Note the gallstones.

2. Most likely obstructed.

3. Acute cholecystitis.

4. Gallbladder hydrops, perforation, bile peritonitis.

Cross-Reference

Gastrointestinal Imaging: THE REQUISITES, ed 3, p 245.

Comments

Patients with clinical findings of acute cholecytitis can be imaged either by ultrasound or CT. Ultrasound is very good at making the findings to confirm the diagnosis. However, CT provides additional information about what is happening not only in the RUQ but throughout the abdomen. In this case the patient has developed a huge gallbladder (hydrops) with gallstones in the dependent position (Fig. 62B) as well as some extra some fluid in the pouch of Douglas and other places in the abdomen. Dilated loops of bowel secondary to bile peritonitis are seen nearby and a small amount of air is seen in the common bile duct. This patient started as a case of acute cholecystitis which, owing to delay in seeking treatment, went on to develop a gangrenous gallbladder wall, perforation, and bile peritonitis.

Chronic cholecystis is relatively common and is seen on many abdominal CT studies, mostly as an incidental finding. Small contracted gallbladder with wall thickening and possibly increased enhancement and occasionally wall calcification are the usual signs. Acute cholecystitis is usually a surgical emergency. CT findings include wall thickening (> 3–4 mm) and wall enhancement. There may be fluid in the gallbladder fossa and gallstones are usually present. High-resolution CT can often demonstrate the offending stone obstructing the cystic duct. One does have to remember that a small percentage of cases of acute cholecystitis are the acalculus type with all the above findings and no obvious stones.

Notes

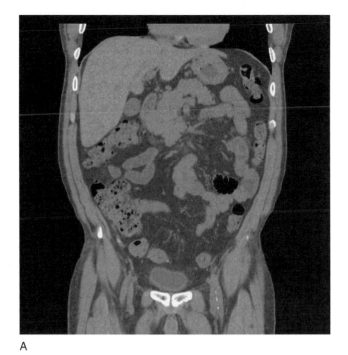

A

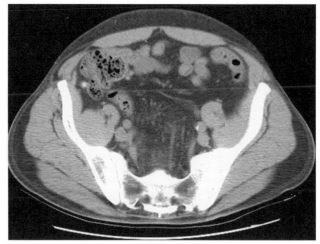

B

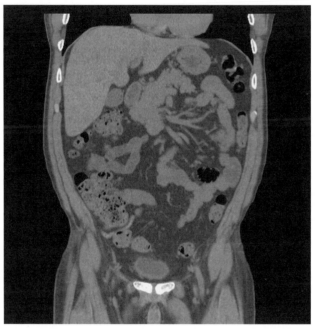

C

1. What is the tiny density seen in the RLQ of this patient complaining of back pain?

2. In what percentage of cases of appendicitis are appendoliths seen?

3. Is the presence of an appendolith pathognomonic of appendicitis?

4. What findings are most important in the CT diagnosis of acute uncomplicated appendicitis?

CASE 63

Appendolith with Appendicitis

1. A tiny calcified appendolith.

2. About 10% of cases.

3. No. In the presence of other CT findings and a positive clinical examination, the finding of an appendolith may be said to be pathognomonic.

4. Appendiceal wall thickening (> 6 mm) and periappendiceal stranding.

Cross-Reference

Gastrointestinal Imaging: THE REQUISITES, ed 3, p 318.

Comments

The advent of multidetector CT scanning (MDCT) in recent years has resulted in an enormous increase in anatomic and pathologic information available to the radiologist, with little change in the radiation dosage to patients. With the improved quality of multiplanar imaging we are seeing the body with breath-taking clarity compared to previous years. The "double duct" sign seen with pancreatic head masses is virtually passé, as we see both ducts (normal diameter) with relative ease on almost every patient these days.

The same may be said of appendoliths. We can now see small calcifications within an otherwise normal appendix, as in this case (in Figure 63C note the normal appendix at a different level). These small calcifications must begin at some time, and it is possible to image the normal appendix with a small appendolith within it. Is it a harbinger of impending appendicitis? That is not known with certainty, but it seems reasonable to assume that these patients are at a higher risk for appendicitis in the future. Currently MDCT has an accuracy rate approaching 100% in the imaging diagnosis of appendicitis. Ultrasound ranges between 70% and 90% in the current literature. Physical examination should be the primary examination of choice, and its role should not be diminished even as imaging becomes more important in the patient workup. It would be presumptuous to think that everywhere a patient presents with abdominal pain, there will be sophisticated imaging available to make primary diagnosis.

Notes

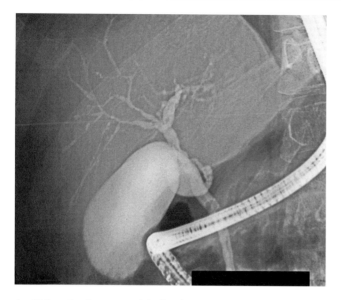

1. What is the most likely diagnosis?

2. What is the usual presentation of this entity?

3. In what group does this condition most commonly occur?

4. Is there any risk of malignancy associated with this lesion?

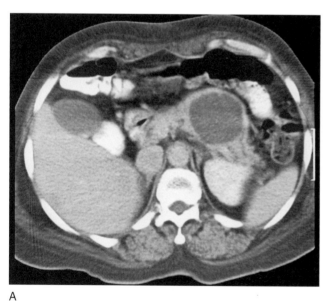
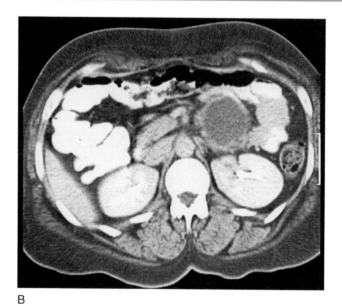

A   B

1. Name possible cystic tumors of the pancreas.

2. How do cysts appear in microcystic adenoma?

3. Describe the appearance of cysts in mucinous neoplasm.

4. What is the malignant potential of mucinous cystic tumors of the pancreas?

Sclerosing Cholangitis

1. Sclerosing cholangitis of the biliary system.

2. Inflammatory bowel disease (usually ulcerative colitis), retroperitoneal fibrosis, ascending cholangitis (often after biliary tract surgery), acquired immunodeficiency syndrome (AIDS), and parasitic infections.

3. Recurrent bacterial infection, particularly after biliary-enteric bypasses; AIDS-related cholangitis caused by either cryptosporidiosis or cytomegalovirus; and parasites, including *Ascaris lumbricoides* (roundworm) and *Clonorchis sinensis* (flatworm).

4. Yes, cholangiocarcinoma.

Cross-Reference

Gastrointestinal Imaging: THE REQUISITES, ed 3, p 228.

Comments

Primary sclerosing cholangitis is a chronic biliary disease of unknown etiology. The majority (70% or more) of cases are related to underlying inflammatory bowel disease, particularly ulcerative colitis. It is estimated that anywhere from 3% to 10% of patients with ulcerative colitis will develop sclerosing cholangitis. It is a disease of young people (third and fourth decades), with male predominance. Pathologically the condition is caused by multifocal areas of periductal fibrosis, which produce the narrowing, with intervening normal areas developing ductal ectasia.

Similar radiologic changes are apparent in patients with recurrent biliary tract infections. The groups that typically develop this condition are postoperative patients with complications and the AIDS population. Worldwide, the most likely cause is intestinal parasites, particularly *A. lumbricoides.* This roundworm migrates into the ducts from the small bowel and causes recurrent cholangitis.

The usual course of disease is one of secondary biliary cirrhosis, recurrent sepsis, and eventual hepatic failure. The time between the appearance of the initial symptoms and death is usually 5 to 10 years. Total colectomy (in cases of ulcerative colitis) may sometimes halt or diminish the course of the disease. Approximately 10% to 20% of patients with sclerosing cholangitis secondary to ulcerative colitis develop cholangiocarcinoma. Interestingly this condition does not develop in patients with Crohn's disease. Sometimes, total colectomy arrests the liver disease, but this effect is not predictable. If the disease progresses, the only treatment is liver transplantation.

Notes

Cystic Tumor of the Pancreas

1. Microcystic adenoma, mucinous cystic neoplasms, papillary epithelial neoplasm, rarely islet cell tumors, and cystic teratoma.

2. Multiple small cysts of varying size.

3. Large, either single or just a few septated cysts.

4. All are potentially malignant.

Cross-Reference

Gastrointestinal Imaging: THE REQUISITES, ed 3, p 166.

Comments

Several neoplasms of the pancreas present as cystic lesions, although all are fairly rare compared with ductal adenocarcinoma, which almost never has a cystic component. Central necrosis is usually easily distinguishable from a cystic component. One of the most common cystic tumors is microcystic adenoma, which has multiple small cysts of varying size. If the cysts are too numerous to count, the diagnosis should be considered microcystic adenoma. This condition occurs in older patients, mostly female. This tumor is associated with von Hippel–Lindau disease. It is a hypervascular tumor that develops central necrosis and scarring, often with calcification.

The term *mucinous cystic neoplasms* describes what has been termed *mucinous cystadenoma* and *mucinous cystadenocarcinoma*. These tumors are difficult to distinguish, and because cystadenomas have malignant potential, they are now classified together, and all are considered malignant or potentially malignant. The cysts in the patient shown with this case are large. Often the cyst is unilocular, resembling a pseudocyst, or cysts can be large, with multiple distinct septations. These tumors are hypovascular, and if they calcify, they do so in a peripheral location.

Another tumor that may resemble a mucinous cystic neoplasm is a cystic teratoma, although this tumor is rare. This tumor also has multiple large cysts and dystrophic calcification. Papillary epithelial neoplasms can be cystic. The cyst is usually thick walled, with mural tumor projections. This tumor occurs in young women and is considered a low-grade malignancy. Also, islet cell tumors that undergo necrosis may show cystic changes.

Notes

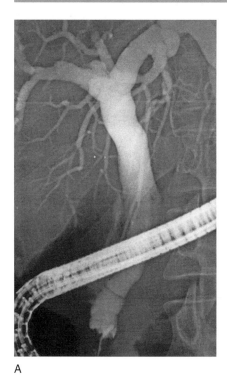

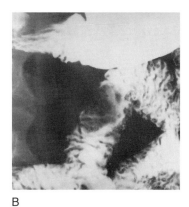

A   B

1. Histologically, of what tissue type are most duodenal polyps?

2. Where do most villous adenomas of the duodenum occur?

3. What is the most common cause of polypoid-like filling defects at the base of the duodenal bulb?

4. What is the incidence of duodenal polyps in patients with familial polyposis coli?

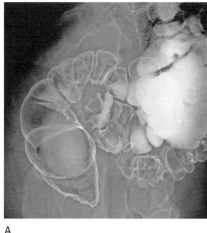

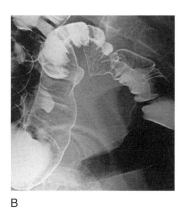

A   B

1. Name some malignancies that may affect this portion of the rectum.

2. What inflammatory conditions may occur in this area?

3. If this patient were a young woman, what would be a likely diagnosis?

4. What other imaging modalities may be helpful?

CASE 66

Villous Adenoma of the Duodenum Obstructing Papillae

1. Adenomatous polyps.

2. Periampullary region.

3. Prolapse of gastric mucosa.

4. More then 50% of these patients will develop small bowel (including duodenum) polyps.

Cross-Reference

Gastrointestinal Imaging: THE REQUISITES, ed 3, p 94.

Comments

Once thought to be rare, in recent decades the occurrence of solitary polyps in the duodenum has been found to be more common than once thought. In contrast to the stomach, where most polyps are hyperplastic, in the duodenum, solitary polyps are most frequently adenomas and dangerous. Hyperplastic polyps of the duodenum are rare, despite the inflammatory changes that occur there. As is true of colonic polyps, the larger the adenoma, the more likely it is to be malignant. However, unlike the colon, any adenomatous polyp in the duodenum has a greater risk for malignancy.

The location of the polyp may be a helpful distinguishing feature. A polypoid filling defect in the bulb may be a gastric polyp, prolapsing through the pylorus along with gastric mucosa, a Brunner's gland adenoma (not a true adenomatous polyp), another type of tumor (GIST, metastasis, etc.), an adenoma, or an ectopic pancreatic rest. The more distal the polyp is in the duodenum, the more likely it is to be an adenoma or villous adenoma. Villous adenomas are particularly common in the periampullary region and can result in biliary and pancreatic duct obstruction such as in this case. GIST tumors and ectopic pancreatic rest can occur anywhere but are more common in the proximal half of the duodenum. As a general rule of thumb, the more distal the lesion is in the duodenum, the more likely it is to be clinically important.

Duodenal polyps are seen with increased frequency in the patient with virtually any of the polyposis syndromes. In the patient with familial polyposis coli, the growths may be either adenomas or hyperplastic polyps. Patients with Gardner's syndrome or familial polyposis coli have a high incidence of periampullary malignancies, particularly those with Gardner's syndrome.

Notes

CASE 67

Endometriosis Involving the Rectum

1. Serosal metastases to the cul-de-sac region from ovarian, gastric, and pancreatic malignancies.

2. Tubo-ovarian abscess, appendicitis, and diverticulitis.

3. Endometriosis.

4. Ultrasound and MRI.

Cross-Reference

Gastrointestinal Imaging: THE REQUISITES, ed 3, p 307.

Comments

The anterior wall of the rectum abuts some major structures and can be involved by disease processes arising from these organs. Most important, however, the lowermost portion of the peritoneal cavity, the cul-de-sac, overlies the anterior portion of the upper rectum. Typically this abuts the rectum above the first or second valve of Houston. In this location, any peritoneal process may reside and secondarily involve the rectum.

Inflammatory processes or bleeding from above can result in fluid or pus in the pouch of Douglas (cul-de-sac), but malignancy is the most important factor, and any abdominal tumor may seed the peritoneal cavity with metastatic disease involving the cul-de sac and the contiguous rectal wall. The most important consideration in a female patient is ovarian carcinoma. Endometrial carcinoma is another possibility. In both sexes, gastric, pancreatic, or colon cancer can produce peritoneal metastases. The appearance of all these tumors is identical. Inflammatory processes include appendicitis, diverticulitis, and pelvic inflammatory disease. Because the region is the most dependent portion of the peritoneum, all pelvic inflammatory processes may spread to it, either before or after surgery.

Endometriosis is a condition produced when there are extrauterine deposits of endometrial tissue. The etiology is uncertain. When endometrial tissue becomes implanted on intra-abdominal structures, it is typically on the ovaries (chocolate cysts) or the serosal surface of the bowel. The tissue is able to maintain viability, and it also responds to the monthly hormonal cycles. The tissue undergoes its normal cyclic changes, including proliferation and then desquamation, just as if it were in the uterine cavity. It is this recurrent shedding of tissue that can lead to complications, including fibrosis. The changes apparent on barium enema relate to fibrotic changes occurring in the wall of the bowel, with some mass effect produced by the tissue. In addition to the anterior rectum, the sigmoid colon, distal small bowel, cecum, appendix, and other pelvic structures may be involved. Very rarely the condition may spread to the upper abdominal cavity.

Notes

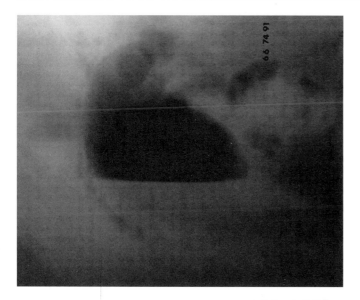

1. What organism typically produces the process shown in this image of the right upper quadrant?

2. What underlying condition does this patient probably have?

3. What is the major complication leading to a high mortality rate?

4. What other problem is often present when this condition occurs?

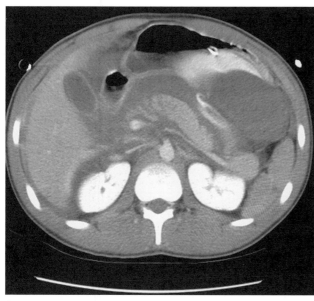

A

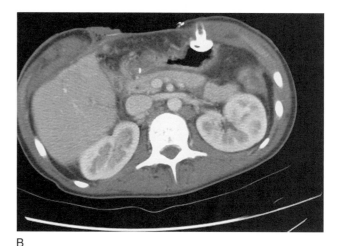

B

1. What is the most common cause of this abnormality in adults?

2. What is the most common cause of this injury in children?

3. What structure must be assessed to determine definitive treatment?

4. What is the most common treatment for this condition?

CASE 68

Emphysematous Cholecystitis

1. *Clostridium* species (*Clostridium welchii* or *Clostridium perfringens*).

2. Diabetes mellitus.

3. Perforation.

4. Cystic duct obstruction.

Cross-Reference
Gastrointestinal Imaging: THE REQUISITES, ed 3, p 255.

Comments
The appearance of air in the lumen or the wall of the gallbladder is diagnostic of a condition known as *emphysematous cholecystitis.* The air is the result of the gasforming organism that is causing the cholecystitis. Most commonly, clostridial organisms are to blame. Patients who develop this condition are typically diabetic; rarely does emphysematous cholecystitis occur in individuals without diabetes as an underlying condition. Often the patient is older and has had diabetes for many years, resulting in vascular insufficiency to the gallbladder, which is probably a major underlying cause for the development of emphysematous cholecystitis. Usually, cystic duct obstruction is also present. Although air is present in the gallbladder lumen, air is rarely encountered in the rest of the biliary system. The risk of perforation in patients with emphysematous cholecystitis is five times higher than that in patients with ordinary acute cholecystitis.

Emphysematous cholecystitis is one of the few diagnoses that can be readily made based on conventional radiographs. When the patient is experiencing severe abdominal pain and there is air in the gallbladder lumen, particularly if the patient is diabetic, the diagnosis of emphysematous cholecystitis must be a primary consideration. Many conditions can result in the accumulation of air in the lumen of the gallbladder, but there is usually an abnormal connection of the biliary tract to the bowel lumen allowing this to occur. Also, in some instances air is visible in the wall of the gallbladder, indicating necrosis of the gallbladder wall. On CT the abnormalities are shown quite well and pericholecystic complications of inflammation and abscess are demonstrated. This condition may not be readily diagnosed on ultrasound, however, because the air may mimic gallstones and produce acoustic shadowing.

Notes

CASE 69

Pancreatic Trauma

1. Motor vehicle accident.

2. Child abuse or sports injury.

3. Integrity of the pancreatic duct.

4. Usually requires surgery.

Cross-Reference
Gastrointestinal Imaging: THE REQUISITES, ed 3, p 174.

Comments
The pancreas is not often injured by blunt abdominal trauma. (It is injured in fewer than 12% of cases of blunt abdominal trauma.) The spleen and liver are much more commonly injured. However, the pancreas extends rather far anteriorly in the abdomen and crosses the spine, and both factors contribute to its risk of injury during blunt trauma. Motor vehicle accidents and deceleration injuries are the leading causes of pancreatic injury in adults, whereas child abuse or sports-related or bicycle injuries more typically produce the damage in children. Penetrating trauma is another frequent cause of pancreatic injury.

When pancreatic injury occurs, there is a high incidence of associated injuries to the bowel, spleen, liver, and blood vessels. The mortality rate for this injury approaches 20% because of both the pancreatic injury and all the other associated injuries. Patients with pancreatic injury have pain, leukocytosis, and elevated amylase levels. The injury may be just a contusion, a laceration, or a complete transection. The integrity of the pancreatic duct is important; if the duct is compromised or transected, surgical resection is required.

For this type of injury, CT is the imaging modality of choice. The appearance of the injury can be quite variable. Sometimes little or nothing can be seen. Changes related to pancreatitis, involving fluid, inflammation, or both, can be evident in the region. A contusion may produce a low density area in the parenchyma or an area of higher density if there is hemorrhage. The actual laceration or tear of the pancreatic tissue may be evident, particularly on high-resolution scans through the pancreas. Surgery is frequently indicated for patients with this injury to at least drain the peripancreatic tissues of fluid that may accumulate. If the pancreatic duct is injured, the treatment usually requires surgical resection of the pancreas proximal to the injury. Ductal patency may have to be determined by endoscopic retrograde cholangiopancreatography.

Notes

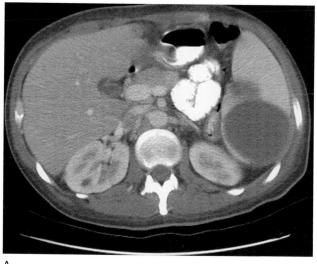

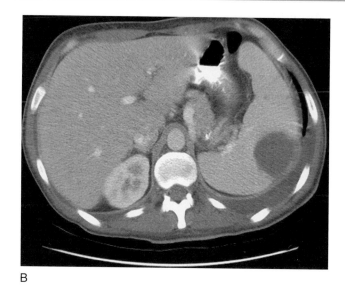

A

B

1. What are the diagnostic possibilities?

2. What clinical conditions might lead this findng?

3. What cardiac condition produces the finding?

4. What local conditions are associated with the development of this abnormailty?

Splenic Abscess

1. Hematoma, abscess, infarction, lymphoma, and cyst.

2. Immunosuppression.

3. Endocarditis.

4. Pancreatitis and pyelonephritis.

Cross-Reference
Gastrointestinal Imaging: THE REQUISITES, ed 3, p 218.

Comments
Pancreatic abscesses are being encountered more frequently as a result of better diagnostic studies, such as CT and ultrasound, and the increased number of patients with immunosuppression (e.g., patients with acquired immunodeficiency syndrome, transplant recipients, and those undergoing chemotherapy). Splenic abscesses can develop in several ways, including as a result of metastatic infection from septic emboli (endocarditis), as a result of contiguous infection (pyelonephritis or pancreatitis), as a sequela of an infarct or trauma with secondary infection, and as a result of generalized immunosuppression with sepsis. A small portion of splenic abscesses develop in the absence of any underlying condition. Most infectious organisms, such as staphylococci, streptococci, and *Escherichia coli,* are aerobic. There is often a high incidence of fungal abscesses, no doubt because many of these patients are immunosuppressed.

The most common finding on plain radiography is a left pleural effusion. CT is the best modality for detecting splenic abscesses, although they also may be demonstrated by ultrasound or even MRI. The problem with CT is that many other conditions have an appearance similar to that of an abscess, and from an imaging perspective it might be impossible to differentiate an epithelial or a post-traumatic splenic cyst from an abcess. Clinical history is as important to the radiologist as it is to the clinician. Those who do not understand this have a poor grasp on the role of imaging in patient care.

Abscesses are areas of low density caused by necrotic or infected tissue. Air is rarely demonstrated but is pathognomonic of an abscess if present. A hematoma or an infarct may appear like an abscess, as would a neoplastic process, such as lymphoma. The wall of an abscess is usually thick and somewhat irregular, which may help to differentiate it from a splenic cyst. The rim of a splenic cyst enhances only when a well-defined capsule develops about the edge of the cyst, which occurs only later in the inflammatory process. Nuclear imaging may be helpful if there is concern about the nature of a splenic mass. Gallium scans and labeled white blood cell studies are active in areas of an abscess; however, lymphoma is also gallium positive. Labeled leukocyte studies always show splenic activity and may obscure an abscess.

Notes

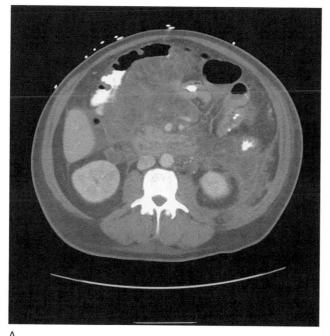

A

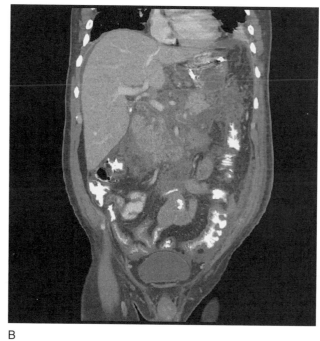

B

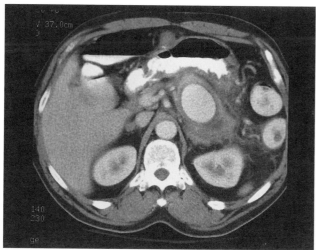

C

1. Given the images shown, what is your diagnosis?

2. How can inflammation of such a small organ as the pancreas have such a widespread impact?

3. What is the condition called when blood vessels are eroded and significant bleeding occurs?

4. What is the major cause of this condition?

C A S E 7 1

Hemorrhagic Pancreatitis

1. Severe pancreatitis.

2. Pancreatic inflammation is inflammation in which pancreatic enzymes autodigest the gland. Because the pancreas is a retroperitoneal organ and has no capsule, it cannot be contained and can have a widespread effect involving the abdomen and even the thorax.

3. Hemorrhagic pancreatitis.

4. In the West, usually alcoholism.

Cross-Reference

Gastrointestinal Imaging: THE REQUISITES, ed 3, p 155.

Comments

Pancreatitis is a relatively common inflammatory condition in which, for various reasons, autodigestion of the gland occurs, resulting in edema and fluid around the gland, swelling and loss of the normal planes around the gland, and in the acute phase, almost invarably changes at the left lung base secondary to diminished diaphragmatic excursion, hypoventilation, and resultant atelectasis and effusion. If the vessel is eroded, significant bleeding can occur, such as in this case. The incidence ranges from 20 to 30 cases per 100,000. The usual presentation is epigastric pain, sometimes radiating to the back, nausea, tachycardia, tachypnea, and often fever. Occasionally the patient may be hypotensive, especially in severe hemorrhagic pancreatitis. The swollen head of the gland may impress the common bile duct, causing some degree of biliary obstruction.

The most common cause is alcohol abuse. However, other causes include ERCP, trauma, gallstones, certain medications, penetrating peptic ulcers, and pancreatic divisum. One of the more interesting complications is splenic artery pseudoaneurysm (Fig. 71C). These pseudoaneurysms develop as a result of inflammation and enzymatic activity weakening a point in the splenic artery wall. Although this complication is unusual, if found it constitutes a danger to the patient of sudden life-threatening bleeding.

Notes

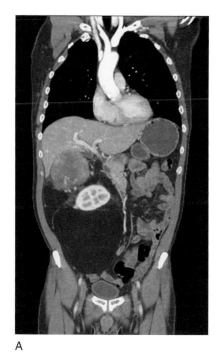

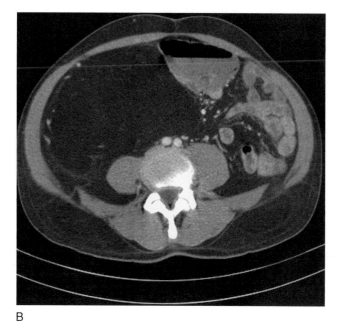

A   B

1. Describe the findings on these images.

2. What type of lesion might give these mixed findings?

3. In adults what is the most common soft tissue sarcoma?

4. What is the 5-year survival rate for these lesions?

Liposarcoma of the Abdomen

1. A large mixed density lesion made up of fat and soft tissue taking up most of the right abdomen.

2. Liposarcoma.

3. Liposarcoma.

4. Less than 50%.

Cross-Reference

Gastrointestinal Imaging: THE REQUISITES, ed 3, p 279.

Comments

Liposarcomas are relatively uncommon lesions seen in approximately 5000 patients in the United States annually. They are lipogenic tumors that can become widespread in the abdomen and extremely difficult to remove surgically. They are seen more commonly in adults, as opposed to the small, well-contained lipomas of the gut seen in children and young adults. Liposarcomas are rare in children. They can be mostly lipomatous in nature with some soft tissue component, such as in this case, or almost purely lipomatous. They occur slightly more so in males, and the less well differentiated the lesion, the poorer the outlook. Most patients will have few or no symptoms until the tumor reaches a very large size. Eventually the patients become aware of swelling or pain and consult a physician. The imaging modality of choice is CT, in which the size, nature, and extent of involvement can be well described. CT diagnosis is usually quite accurate. Plain film can be helpful in determining the presence of a mass.

Notes

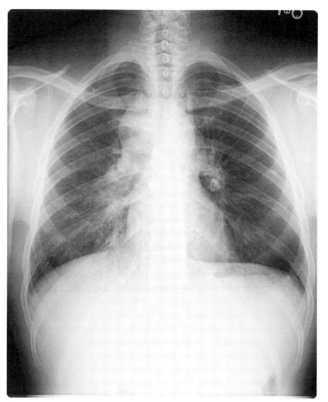

A

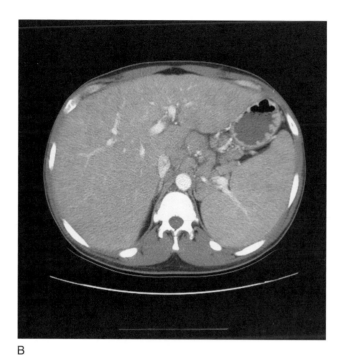

B

1. What disease processes might have manifestations above and below the diaphragm?

2. How common is hepatic involvement with this condition?

3. Can this process result in portal hypertention?

4. What places in the gut are most frequently involved?

Sarcoidosis with Hepatosplenomegaly

1. Many diseases can have lesions above and below the diaphragm. The most common would be metastatic disease, lymphoma, and a number of inflammatory conditions such as, in this case, pulmonary and hepatosplenic sarcoidosis.

2. From an imaging perspective hepatic involvment is not common. However, biopsy and postmortem examinations show much greater involvement than we are able to image. Some reports have placed hepatic involvment as high as 80%.

3. Yes, rarely.

4. Sarcoid of the hollow viscera seems to be found most commonly in the stomach.

Cross-Reference

Gastrointestinal Imaging: THE REQUISITES, ed 3, p 61.

Comments

Sarcoidosis is a disease generally seen involving the thorax, skin, or eyes, but it is also seen, on occasion, involving both solid and hollow viscera of the abdomen. The disease is of unknown etiology but at times correlation with some microorganism has been suggested but never proved. It is a noncaseating granulomatous disease. Most involvement of the liver is not a serious issue and usually goes unnoticed. However, about a third of patients with liver involvement will have some abnormalities of liver enzymes. Most of these patients will show no clinical symptoms. However, in a very small subset of that third (less than 2%) sarcoid involvement of the liver can lead to significant and serious hepatic disease. This ranges clinically from jaundice and pruritus as a result of chronic progressive disease. Hepatic enlargement may be seen radiologically. In some patients there might be diffuse involvement with the spleen. Most sarcoid involvement of the spleen does not result in splenomegaly, but infrequently it may be seen, such as in this patient. Patients with diffuse severe involvement of both spleen and liver may go on to develop portal hypertension.

Notes

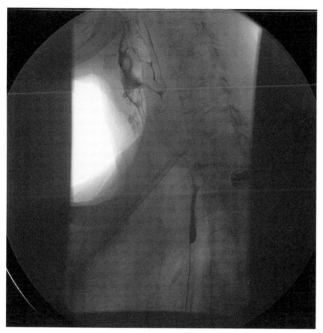

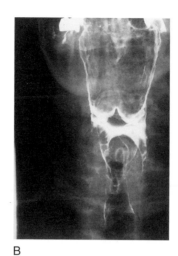

A   B

1. What is the most common tumor of the pharynx?

2. What is the second most common tumor of the pharynx?

3. Name some other tumors that may metastasize to the pharynx.

4. What is the significance of Plummer-Vinson syndrome?

Squamous Carcinoma of the Hypopharynx

1. Squamous carcinoma.

2. Lymphoma.

3. Although rare, pharyngeal metastases are seen with breast cancer, lung cancer, melanoma, and Kaposi sarcoma.

4. Increased incidence of pharyngeal or esophageal carcinoma.

Cross-Reference

Gastrointestinal Imaging: THE REQUISITES, ed 3, p 5.

Comments

The majority of tumors involving the pharynx are squamous in origin. These tumors are seen radiologically as small nodules or masses or sometimes as a thickening or obliteration of the normal structures. Laryngoscopy is the method of choice for identification, but with the increase in swallowing studies being performed to diagnose conditions causing dysphagia, the radiologist may be the first to encounter these tumors.

The pharynx and hypopharynx are repositories of a substantial amount of lymph tissue. Thus it is to be expected that patients with lymphoma may develop neoplastic infiltration of these structures. In patients with lymphoma and dysphagia the hypopharynx must be studied closely. Squamous tumors of the hypopharynx typically arise in the vallecula, piriform sinuses, or epiglottis. Lymphomas more frequently involve the posterior or lateral wall and may be submucosal in location, producing subtle changes. If a tumor is substantially posterior in location, lymphoma must be strongly considered. Potentially, all tumors may metastasize to this region. However, it is a rare event, given the number of patients with malignancies. Two common cancers—breast and lung—are known to metastasize to the pharynx on occasion. Also, cancers of the skin, such as melanoma and Kaposi sarcoma, seem to metastasize to the hypopharynx relatively frequently. Patients with Plummer-Vinson syndrome have anemia associated with cervical esophageal webs. Although it is controversial, some authors believe that the syndrome is a premalignant condition and that affected patients have a higher incidence of pharyngeal and esophageal carcinoma.

Notes

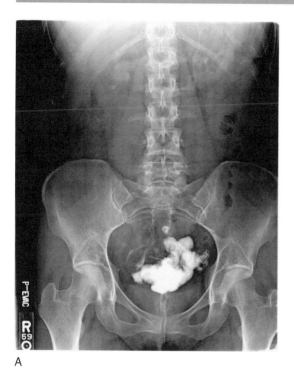

A

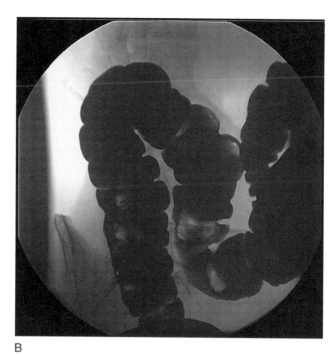

B

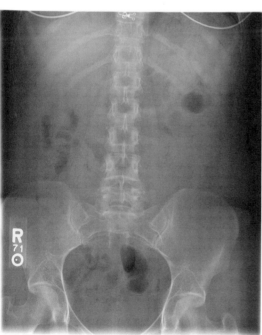

C

1. A postevacuation film from a water-soluble enema shows what findings?

2. How common is this phenomenon?

3. Are there contributing factors that might increase the incidence?

4. Where else can this be seen?

Renal Vicarious Excretion Following GG Enema

1. Vicarious excretion of the water-soluble contrast agent from the kidneys. Note the contrast material in the collecting systems of the kidneys.

2. 10% to 20% of water-soluble enemas.

3. Yes. IBD, radiation enteritis, ischemic changes, bowel lymphoma, and serum protein azotemia have all been implicated.

4. Vicarious excretion can also be seen in the gallbladder.

Cross-Reference

Gastrointestinal Imaging: THE REQUISITES, ed 3, p 267.

Comments

The use of iodinated water-soluble contrast agent is common in radiologic practice. Occasionally vicarious excretion, usually following an enema study, can be seen in the kidneys. In this case the contrast agent was not present prior to the examination, as the scout film shows (Fig. 75C). Vicarious excretion has also been reported in post-ERCP patients. When used as a contrast agent for the colon, vicarious excretion has been seen in as many as 20% of normal subjects in at least one study. Thus, its appearance in the kidneys is not necessarily indicative of diseased colon. However, it is very likely that inflamed or ischemic bowel mucosa may allow the contrast agent to cross the mucosal barrier at such a rate that it may be detected in the kidneys. Indeed, the main function of the colon, apart from storage, is water absorption, which it does quite efficiently under normal circumstances.

Notes

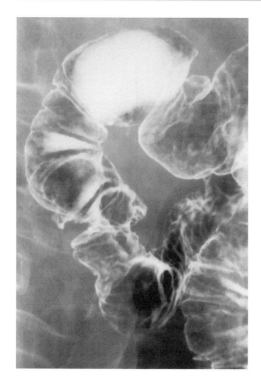

1. What is the size of a normal papilla?

2. What is the most common cause of benign enlargement of the papilla?

3. What biliary anomaly may produce an enlarged papilla?

4. Name the polyposis syndrome associated with tumors of the papilla.

Enlarged Papilla of the Duodenum

1. 1.5 cm is considered the upper limit of normal.

2. Edema caused by stones in the distal bile duct.

3. Choledochocele.

4. Familial polyposis has an association with tumors developing near the papilla.

Cross-Reference

Gastrointestinal Imaging: THE REQUISITES, ed 3, p 98.

Comments

On normal upper gastrointestinal tract examinations the papilla and associated structures may be identified along the medial wall of the second portion of the duodenum. The papilla is an elevated mound of tissue that is typically smaller than 1 cm. It is considered abnormal when larger than 1.5 cm, although healthy patients have been known to have papillae enlarged up to 3 cm. Inferior to the papilla, folds may be visible, extending up to 3 cm in length.

The papilla is usually enlarged as a result of benign disease. The most common cause of edema of the papilla is the presence of stones in the distal common bile duct. Other causes include pancreatitis (either short- or long-term), which may produce swelling (Poppel's sign). Typically the enlargement of the papilla with edema produces a smooth and symmetrical enlargement. Rarely, acute duodenal ulcer disease produces papillary enlargement but is usually associated with duodenal fold thickening. A choledochocele, an abnormal enlargement of the most distal end of the common bile duct and ampullary region, also causes enlargement of the papilla.

Tumors arising in or about the papilla are called perivaterian malignancies. Carcinoma of the papilla is the most common tumor. Polyps or mesenchymal tumors, such as leiomyoma, may also arise in the region and produce enlargement. Certain polyposis syndromes—familial polyposis coli and the associated Gardner's syndrome—predispose patients to tumor development in the perivaterian region. Such a patient may require routine screening of the upper gastrointestinal tract throughout his or her life because of this association.

Notes

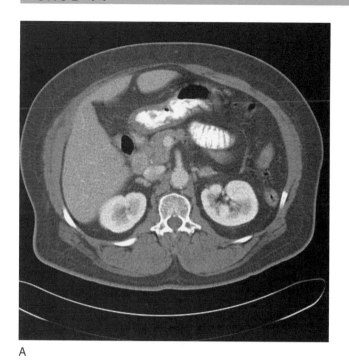

A

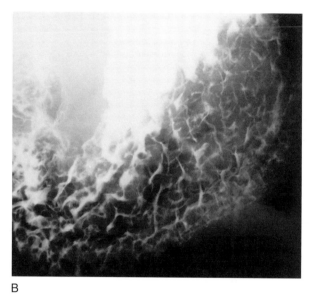

B

1. What is the leading cause of gastric ulcer disease in industrialized societies?

2. What is the leading cause of duodenal ulcer disease?

3. What substance does the breath test for bacterial infection in the upper gastrointestinal tract detect?

4. What is the treatment of choice for this infection?

Helicobacter Gastritis

1. *Helicobacter pylori* infection (causes at least 50% of gastric ulcers).

2. *H. pylori* infection (causes at least 90% of duodenal ulcers).

3. Urease. It is a by-product of bacterial infection in the stomach.

4. Triple therapy (usually two antibiotics and bismuth).

Cross-Reference

Gastrointestinal Imaging: THE REQUISITES, ed 3, p 57.

Comments

The presence of *H. pylori* in the upper gastrointestinal tract is now believed to be the major cause of peptic ulcer disease among individuals who live in industrialized countries. The majority of gastric ulcers also are attributed to this organism, which is considered a major cause of chronic gastritis as well. Almost all duodenal ulcer patients also have *H. pylori* infection.

The radiologic abnormalities in these patients can be quite variable, and many patients have normal radiologic studies. By far the most common radiologic abnormality seen in patients with *H. pylori* infection is thickened gastric folds. The abnormality may vary from mild thickening of the folds in either the proximal stomach or antral region to bizarrely nodular folds involving a large portion of the stomach. These folds may become so thickened that they can resemble a neoplastic process, such as lymphoma. Often these fold abnormalities can be detected on CT examination. Polyps of varying sizes also have been described. Typically these are small hyperplastic polyps, although rarely a large focal polypoid mass is encountered. In many of these patients, endoscopy may be necessary to exclude malignancy. Of course, ulcers and erosions can be identified in the stomach, but this finding is less common than are the fold abnormalities. Enlarged areae gastricae also have been described, although this finding is subtle. In the duodenum, radiologic findings include ulcers, thickened folds, and narrowing or deformity.

Noninvasive techniques for detecting *H. pylori* include a breath test that detects urease activity within the upper gastrointestinal tract. Serologic tests may detect antibodies to the *H. pylori* antigen. Endoscopic studies are considered the mainstay for detection because the bacteria can be diagnosed on biopsy specimens. However, the infection itself is patchy, and multiple biopsies are often necessary to detect the organism. Treatment includes antibiotic therapy, usually involving a combination of agents, including metronidazole, tetracycline, or amoxicillin. Also, oral bismuth therapy is recommended, and histamine blockers are given to reduce acid levels.

Notes

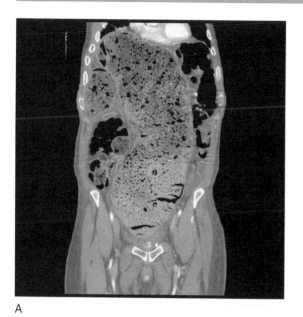

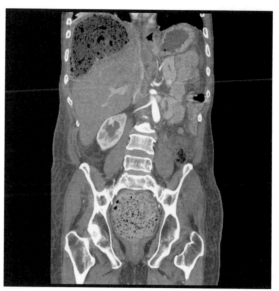

A   B

1. What is the pathologic basis of the process shown in these images?

2. At what age is this condition most commonly seen?

3. In which sex is this condition most commonly seen?

4. What other conditions may be seen with this condition?

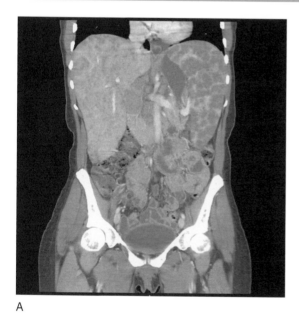

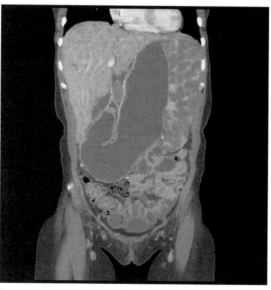

A   B

1. What is the commonest cause of gastric outlet obstruction (GOO)?

2. In which is gastric outlet obstruction more common: benign or malignant disease?

3. Which is more likely to cause GOO: gastric adenocarcinoma, lymphoma, or pancreatic cancer?

4. What significance does the duration of GOO symptoms have?

CASE 78

Adult Hirschsprung's Disease

1. Congenital aganglionosis of the distal colon, Hirschsprung's disease.

2. 90% are diagnosed in the first years of life.

3. In females; there is a 4:1 female-male ratio.

4. Trisomy 21 as well cardiac malformations may be seen in Hirschsprung's disease.

Cross-Reference

Gastrointestinal Imaging: THE REQUISITES, ed 3, p 304.

Comments

Hirschsprung's disease is a congenital disorder of the gut characterized by a segment of absent ganglion cells in the distal colon. The degree of involvement can vary, but most cases are diagnosed in the neonatal stage with the failure to pass meconium. However, lesser degrees of aganglionosis may result in a delayed diagnosis such as in this case. The massive enlargement of the colon is obvious. However, the aganglionic segment is also visible in the rectum. The disease is more common in girls and has no racial predilection. Patients who have delayed diagnosis (this one in the teens) are much affected by the disease. They suffer from chronic severe debilitating constipation, abdominal distention, some with encopresis and an overall life-altering health state.

Plain films and CT studies are usually diagnostic or suggestive in most cases. Rectal biopsy is the definitive diagnostic procedure. Surgery aimed at the removal of the aganglionic segment and some excess colon is usually the treatment of choice. Laparoscopic surgery for Hirschsprung's disease in newborns has been recently reported with some initial success.

Notes

CASE 79

Gastric Outlet Obstruction

1. Peptic ulcer disease is the most common cause of GOO.

2. Malignant disease is more likely to result in GOO than benign disease.

3. Pancreatic cancer (by contiguous invasion) is probably the leading cause of outlet obstruction.

4. Chronic GOO is almost always a result of peptic ulcer disease, and symptoms of a short duration are more ominous.

Cross-Reference

Gastrointestinal Imaging: THE REQUISITES, ed 3, p 49.

Comments

With newer and more effective medications inhibiting acid secretion, gastric outlet obstruction (GOO) is not as common as it was 20 years ago. However, peptic ulcer disease (PUD) is still the most common cause. Malignancy is becoming a larger and more dangerous issue as a cause for GOO in the 21st century. Patient with a long history of PUD and who have ineffective treatment or are incompliant in the medications regimes (e.g., alcoholics) who present with pain and gastric distention are probably going to have ulceration and inflammation as the cause of their GOO. Alternatively, severe pancreatitis that causes inflammation and spasm of the second portion of the duodenum can also result in GOO. Patients who have little or no history of PUD who present with GOO present more ominous possibilities, such as carcinoma of the distal antrum or pylorus, as well as pancreatic carcinoma invading and obstructing the duodenum. In this case widespread metastatic disease involving liver and spleen with duodenal invasion or compression is the cause of the outlet obstruction.

Notes

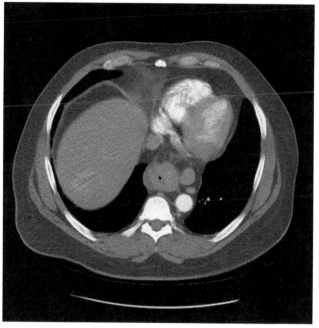
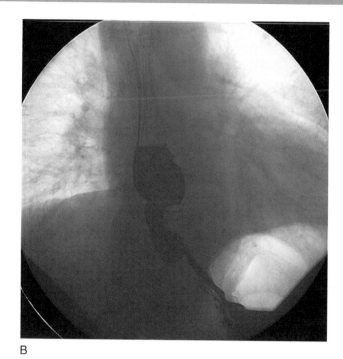

A

B

1. What is the most common cause of hematogenous metastases to the esophagus?

2. What tumor most frequently invades the esophagus through direct extension?

3. What hematologic neoplasms can involve the esophagus?

4. What is the most common site of secondary esophageal involvement by tumor?

Metastatic Disease to Esophagus

1. Breast cancer.

2. Gastric carcinoma.

3. Lymphoma and leukemia.

4. Middle of the esophagus, secondary to direct extension from lymph nodes.

Cross-Reference

Gastrointestinal Imaging: THE REQUISITES, ed 3, p 11.

Comments

Metastases to the esophagus are not uncommon findings on autopsy studies. However, it is somewhat more rare for them to be encountered in radiologic practice. The most common cause of secondary tumor involvement of the esophagus is direct invasion or extension of an adjacent neoplasm. The most likely of these neoplasms is gastric carcinoma, which extends into the distal esophagus. However, with new knowledge about Barrett's metaplasia and its progression toward adenocarcinoma of the distal esophagus and GE junction, direct spread from stomach to esophagus is much less common than previously thought. Carcinoma of the lung also involves the esophagus either by direct extension or by secondary involvement of the mediastinal adenopathy. Breast cancer is the most likely distant tumor to secondarily involve the esophagus. It usually involves the esophagus by first spreading to mediastinal lymph nodes and then invading into the esophagus. However, it is also the most common cancer to have direct hematogenous metastases to the esophagus. Hematogenous metastases are quite rare. Although all tumors may metastasize to the esophagus, the hematogenous metastases are more commonly associated with breast cancer, Kaposi sarcoma, melanoma, and renal cell carcinoma.

Notes

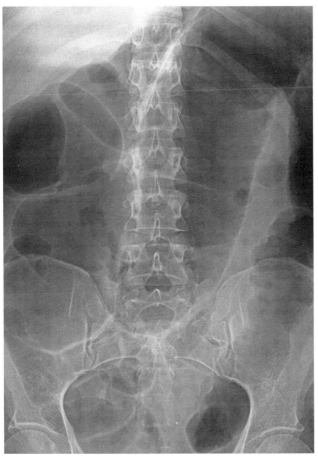

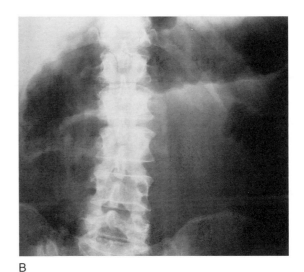

A

B

1. Name some diseases that might produce this condition.

2. What measurements would indicate the seriousness of the disease?

3. What is the causal factor for the development of this condition?

4. What is the long-term outcome in this condition?

Toxic Megacolon

1. Ulcerative colitis, Crohn's disease, infectious colitis, ischemia, and pseudomembranous colitis.

2. None. Measurements do not always indicate severity.

3. Transmural inflammation damaging the ganglion cells.

4. Usually poor. Surgery is often required, even at a later date.

Cross-Reference

Gastrointestinal Imaging: THE REQUISITES, ed 3, p 312.

Comments

Toxic megacolon is a relatively uncommon complication of colitis but is one of the most life-threatening as well. Its incidence varies, but it probably affects fewer than 10% of ulcerative colitis patients. It has also been described in Crohn's disease, pseudomembranous colitis, ischemia, and infectious colitis (particularly in AIDS patients).

Toxic megacolon occurs when there is severe transmural inflammation extending into the muscularis propria. There is accompanying vasculitis of the arterioles and destruction of the ganglion cells in the myenteric plexuses. Inflammation can extend all the way to the serosa, producing peritoneal inflammation and clinical changes of peritonitis, even without perforation. The bowel wall becomes quite thin because the mucosa and submucosa are often sloughed as a result of the inflammation. There is an associated loss of muscle tone caused by the inflammation of the muscle layers and the ganglion cell destruction. Adding to this problem are the effects of the narcotic drugs and steroids that may be given to the patient for treatment, as well as possible electrolyte disturbances. These problems all lead to an atony of the bowel, with subsequent dilation. Some authors have stated that, if the transverse colon exceeds 8 cm, it is an indication of impending megacolon. The transverse colon usually dilates the most because it is in the least dependent portion of the colon and air accumulates in it. However, other parts of the colon may be involved as well. It may be better to disregard measurements because a large colon may be present without severe disease and perforation may occur without significant dilation.

Perforation is the most serious complication, with an associated high mortality rate. Often it is clinically occult because the high-dose steroids used to treat toxic megacolon mask the symptoms of peritonitis, which accompanies the perforation. The diagnosis can be made only on plain abdominal radiographs or CT scans. Patients who are successfully medically treated for toxic megacolon still do poorly in the future and are often at risk for recurrence or require colectomy at a later date.

Notes

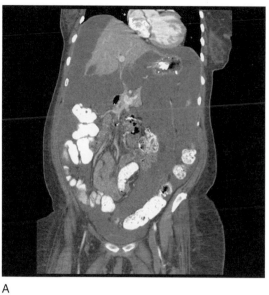

A

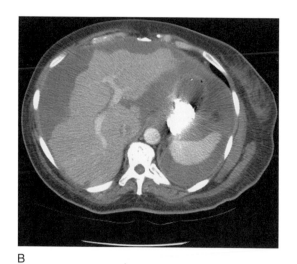

B

1. What benign tumor may produce this condition?

2. What other intestinal tumors cause this condition?

3. Can malignant tumors produce this condition?

4. What is the definitive treatment for this condition?

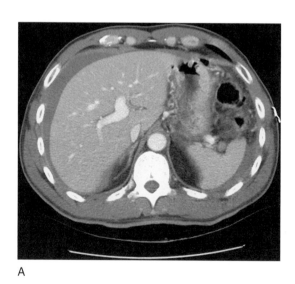

A

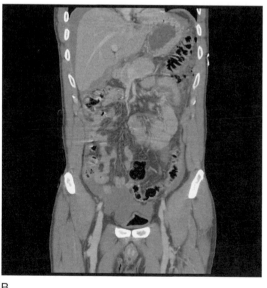

B

1. The CT images on this young man show what findings?

2. What might be the etiologic basis of these findings?

3. How often is the colon involved in this condition?

4. If the patient is hemodynamically stable, what is the imaging procedure of choice?

CASE 82

Pseudomyxoma Peritonei

1. Mucocele of the appendix.

2. Rarely, mucinous pancreatic or gastric tumors.

3. Yes.

4. There is no definitive treatment.

Cross-Reference

Gastrointestinal Imaging: THE REQUISITES, ed 3, p 138.

Comments

These CT images demonstrate large collections of low-density material throughout the abdominal cavity, resembling ascites. However, in this instance the material appears loculated or cystic in the lower abdominal cavity. Scalloping of the liver edge also is present. Finally, areas of fine calcification are evident within the peritoneal cavity on some of the images. All these findings make this case atypical for conventional ascites and suggest the possibility of pseudomyxoma peritonei.

Pseudomyxoma peritonei is the presence of gelatinous or mucinous material in the peritoneal cavity. It is produced by the rupture of a mucin-producing neoplasm into the peritoneal cavity. It can be either a malignant process, such as a mucinous adenocarcinoma, or a benign process, such as a mucocele of the appendix. Once the tumor ruptures, the cellular debris continues to produce mucin within the peritoneum, and the process tends to be progressive whether it is the result of a benign or a malignant cause.

In women by far the most common cause of pseudomyxoma peritonei is a mucinous neoplasm of the ovary, typically mucinous cystadenocarcinoma. In men the usual origin of the process is an appendiceal tumor, such as a mucocele of the appendix or a mucinous cystadenocarcinoma. Mucinous cystic tumors of the pancreas also may cause this condition. Mucinous tumors of the stomach, intestines, or bile ducts are even more rare. In this patient the scalloping of the liver and the calcification favor the diagnosis of a malignant mucinous process. Treatment is typically supportive because the material cannot be successfully removed surgically, and the remaining cells within the peritoneum will continue to produce the material.

Notes

CASE 83

Splenic Flexure Trauma—Stab Wound

1. The transaxial and coronal CT images show fluid in the peritoneum and small collections of air around the splenic flexure of the colon.

2. Stab wound in the left upper abdomen penetrating the splenic flexure.

3. When the peritoneal envelope is penetrated, the incidence of colonic involvement can be almost as high as that of liver, 20% to 25%.

4. CT imaging.

Cross-Reference

Gastrointestinal Imaging: THE REQUISITES, ed 3, p 300.

Comments

CT imaging, especially MDCT imaging, is the examination of choice in penetrating abdominal trauma when the patient is hemodynamically stable. Penetrating wounds are mostly stab wounds and bullet wounds. When the hollow viscus is penetrated, not only blood can be spilled into the peritoneal cavity (such as in this case) but also the content of the hollow viscus. Small collections of air or bubbles must be accounted for. If it is determined that the air collections or bubbles are outside the bowel, and there has been no other cause for such a finding (recent surgery or peritoneal lavage), then a breeching injury of the bowel must be presumed. It is possible for bowel to be injured but not necessarily penetrated. This is usually seen as blood in the bowel wall. Some small amount of bleeding into the peritoneal cavity may occur even in this situation. Penetration of the colon will lead to widespread peritonitis, sepsis, and death within a few days. The morbidity and mortality rates for stab wounds depend entirely on how early diagnosis and surgical intervention occur. In urban trauma centers penetrating trauma to the abdomen accounts for about 30% of patients and less than half that in suburban centers.

Notes

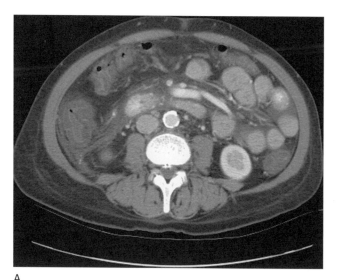

A

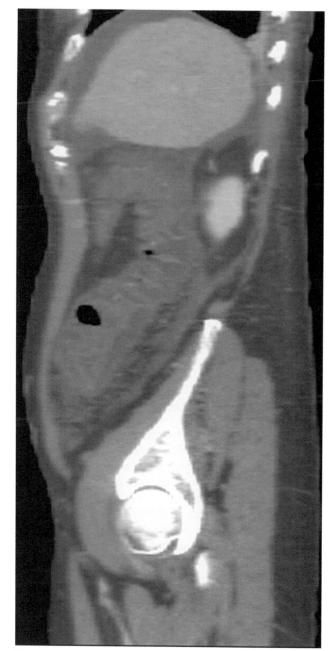

B

1. What is the predisposing factor for the development of this condition?

2. What organism is responsible?

3. How often is there rectal sparing in this condition?

4. What is the treatment?

Pseudomembranous Colitis

1. Use of antibiotics, often multiple.

2. Clostridium difficile.

3. Often (in 20% to 70% of cases).

4. Discontinuation of antibiotics; sometimes vancomycin is prescribed.

Cross-Reference
Gastrointestinal Imaging: THE REQUISITES, ed 3, p 313.

Comments
Pseudomembranous colitis is frequently encountered. It actually represents an infection with the *Clostridium difficile* bacillus, although the relationship is variable. *C. difficile* can be found in many healthy patients (20% of the population), in whom it does not produce extensive colonization. Under certain circumstances (e.g., during the course of antibiotic therapy or chemotherapy), an overgrowth of this bacterium may develop, which is why this condition is often called *antibiotic-associated colitis*. However, many episodes of diarrhea associated with antibiotic use are not caused by *C. difficile* infection; probably only the most severe cases are caused by this bacterium. The relationship is even more difficult to establish in that the onset of symptoms may occur anywhere from a few days to 8 weeks after antibiotics have been initiated, although typically it takes fewer than 2 weeks.

C. difficile produces several endotoxins, some of which are detectable with laboratory assays. These toxins produce an inflammatory and necrotic change in the mucosa, with subsequent loss of fluid through the wall of the bowel. On sigmoidoscopy there are small, raised, yellowish plaques; cellular debris; and mucus, hence the term *pseudomembranous colitis*. The inflammatory process may involve the whole colon, but in a substantial number of patients the rectum is spared or only segments of the colon are involved.

Radiologically, in severe cases the abnormalities may be apparent on plain abdominal images. The findings include thickening of the haustral folds, thickening of the bowel wall, and a shaggy appearance of the mucosa. The changes may mimic ischemia. Barium studies are usually not indicated but show the thickened folds and irregular margins to the barium. Toxic megacolon can occur in patients with this condition. CT is probably the best modality for evaluation of severe cases because the thickened bowel is readily apparent and the study does not precipitate any complications. Treatment is discontinuation of the antibiotics, sometimes use of vancomycin, and supportive therapy.

Notes

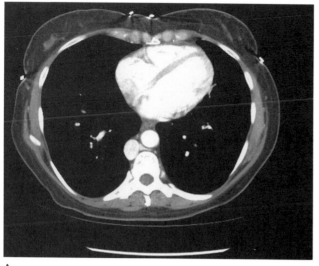

A

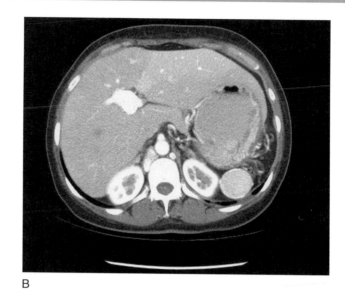

B

1. What is the abnormality in these images called?

2. What is the physical cause?

3. Can this be a congenital anomaly?

4. What is clinical significance of this finding?

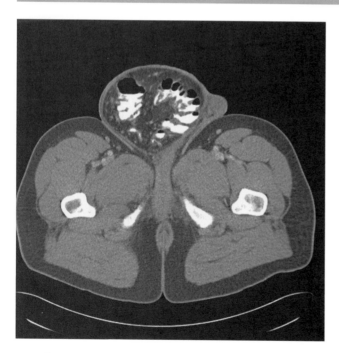

1. What would be the clinical presentation of appendicitis in this patient?

2. What is the most common cause of small bowel obstruction?

3. What are the clinical implications of this finding?

4. What is the fastest method for demonstrating mechanical obstruction?

CASE 85

Azygous Continuation

1. Azygous continuation.

2. Occlusion, or failure of development of the inferior vena cava.

3. Yes. Many are discovered incidentally and are asymptomatic.

4. There is an association of congenital inferior vena cava (IVC) interruption with congenital heart disease.

Cross-Reference

Gastrointestinal Imaging: THE REQUISITES, ed 3, p 183.

Comments

Azygous continuation can be seen in a variety of settings. It can be a congenital failure of the development of the inferior vena cava or it can be chronic disease that slowly occludes the hepatic vein or the IVC over time. Any condition that results in hepatic venous occlusion can result in hepatomegaly, and if chronic, distention of the azygous-hemiazygous system as an alternative collateral route to return venous blood from the lower body to the heart. Such conditions would include hepatoma and other indolent neoplasms as well as blood dyscrasias, such as sickle cell anemia and leukemia. In this case the reason for the unusually large size of the azygous vein is failure of development of the inferior vena cava. Hepatic veins are visible but no IVC is identifiable. The finding was incidental. Other incidental CT findings in this vein would include duplication of the IVC, persistent cardinal vein, and commonly retroaortic left renal vein.

Notes

CASE 86

Inguinal Hernia

1. Scrotal pain. The cecum and appendix can be seen in the scrotum in this severe inguinal hernia.

2. Fibrous adhesions.

3. Possible incarceration, vascular occlusion, and bowel necrosis.

4. CT.

Cross-Reference

Gastrointestinal Imaging: THE REQUISITES, ed 3, p 314.

Comments

Although the main cause of small bowel obstruction is surgical adhesions, other important causes include hernias, either in the abdominal wall or internally. Inguinal hernias are very common. Only ventral hernias are seen with more frequency. Both can lead to obstructive pathology with inguinal hernia being more likely to incarcerate and obstruct as well as threaten the bowel blood supply (strangulated bowel).

For decades, contrast examination of the small bowel, along with plain film radiography, has been the standard for evaluation of the patient with suspected obstruction. Enteroclysis or a dedicated small bowel follow-through have been shown to be of benefit, but are often impractical for the postoperative patient, time–consuming, and very uncomfortable for patients. Most now advocate the use of CT, which can assess the site of obstruction and possible underlying causes of the problem. It is as sensitive as the other modalities and can be quite specific for determining the cause of the problem, which is most helpful for clinicians. In this case, despite the size of the herniation, it was shown to be nonobstructive in a very short period.

Notes

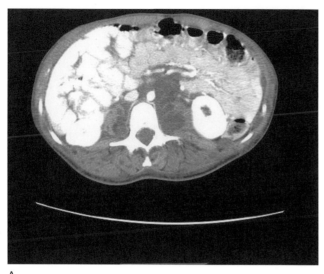

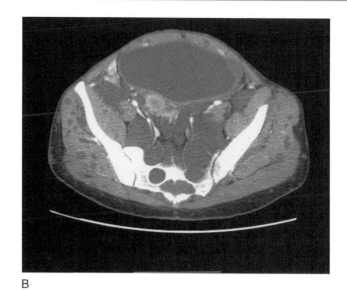

A   B

1. Describe the findings in these images.

2. What is the hereditary description of this condition?

3. What parts of the body can it affect?

4. Is the appearance of the neural foramina significant?

Neurofibromatosis of the Abdomen

1. Large soft tissue masses that seem to have a paraspinal origin with extension into the mesentary.

2. This is an autosomal dominal disorder.

3. It affects multiple organ systems: skin, GI tract, CNS, musculoskeletal system, etc.

4. Yes, growth along the paraspinal neural roots can cause expansion and erosion of the foramen, suggesting the diagnosis of neurofibromatosis.

Cross-Reference

Gastrointestinal Imaging: THE REQUISITES, ed 3, p 131.

Comments

Neurofibromatosis is an autosomal dominant disease that can affect multiple organ systems. The best known area affected is the skin. However, the process can be much more far ranging and dangerous. The disease has been divided into two types, neurofibromatosis type 1 (von Recklinghausen disease), which accounts for almost 90% of cases, and type 2, which involves the acoustic nerves.

Neurofibromatosis type 1 is one of the more common autosomal hereditary disorders (1 in 4000). Involvement of the abdomen and GI tract can be extensive, as seen in this patient. Tumors may be found within the liver or mesentery as well as in the bowel itself. It can result in GI bleeding, obstruction, or intusucception, chronic abdominal pain, and distention. There is thought to be an increased incidence of adenocarcinoma of the small bowel when the gut is involved.

Notes

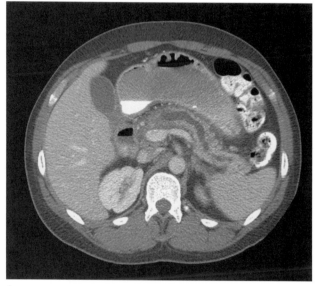

A

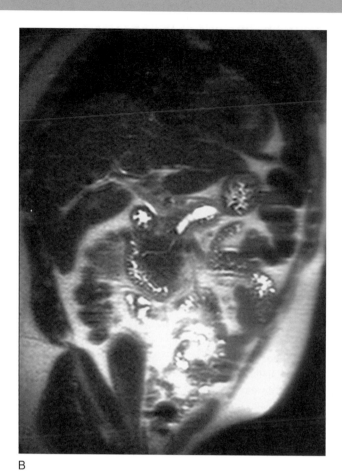

B

1. Describe the findings in these images.

2. What might be the etiologic basis for this finding?

3. Does the absence of a mass in the images exclude malignancy?

4. What is the role of the radiologist in this case?

Benign Stricture of Chronic Pancreatitis

1. On both CT and MR cholangiography a pancreatic duct stricture is seen in the body of the pancreas.

2. Usually chronic pancreatitis. Benign or malignant neoplasm and trauma are also considerations.

3. Very unlikely, but it can never be excluded as a possibility.

4. Diagnosis only. As of this time, radiologic therapeutic intervention in pancreatic duct disease has not been developed.

Cross-Reference

Gastrointestinal Imaging: THE REQUISITES, ed 3, p 227.

Comments

Unlike the biliary duct stone formation, pancreatic stones (which usually form in the pancreatic ductal system rather than the acinar tissue) are not a major factor in pancreatic duct obstruction. In cases of benign stricture of the pancreas the cause is usually chronic pancreatitis. When the stricture is located directly over the spine and there has been a prior history of blunt trauma to the abdomen, such as in this case, trauma should be included in the etiologic considerations.

Pancreatic strictures present a difficult therapeutic problem. The surgical approach, which includes the Puestow procedure (longitudinal pancreaticojejunostomy) and Whipple procedure, involves long and highly invasive surgery, especially if there is no demonstrable mass on imaging. In recent years placement of stents across a benign pancreatic duct has become more common, but there are also problems associated with this as well. Although there have been reports of pain relief with stent placement, there is a question of whether a chronically dilated pancreatic duct can generate intrinsic drainage despite surgical intervention or stent placement. Moreover, pancreatic duct stents have an increased incidence of occlusion and are suspected by many investigators of causing chronic pancreatitis by their presence.

Notes

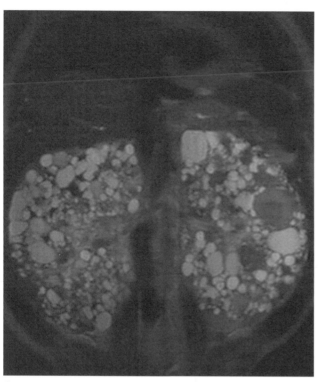

A

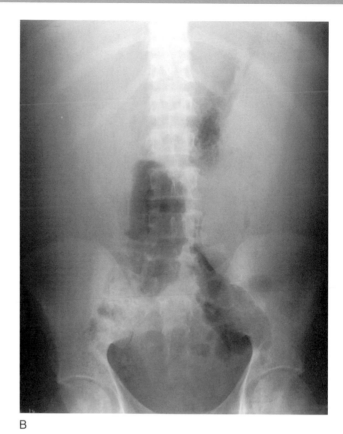

B

1. What can cause air-filled loops of bowel to collect centrally in the abdomen?

2. The ascending and descending colon occupy the paracolic gutters. What might displace them away from the properitoneal fat line?

3. In the supine patient what is the lowest, most dependent part of the abdomen?

4. Can retroperitoneal adenopathy affect bowel position?

Bilateral Abdominal Masses Displacing Bowel

1. Large fluid collections.

2. Fluid.

3. Lower pelvic recesses.

4. Generally no.

Cross-Reference

Gastrointestinal Imaging: THE REQUISITES, ed 3, p 132.

Comments

Bowel can be displaced by a number of processes in the abdomen. One of the more dramatic is the case shown here of huge adult polycystic kidneys that force bowel into a narrow "hour-glass" shape in the central abdomen. It is also possible to get the exact same appearance with massive hepatosplenomegaly.

Fluid in the peritoneal cavity, ascites, and blood can also displace bowel. Large amounts will cause air-filled loops of bowel to rise as the fluid level increases. Because the abdomen is dome-shaped in most of us, when the bowel reaches the top of the dome, it will appear as if the bowel (with air in it) has collected in a circle in the middle of the abdomen. This is called centralization of bowel loops and is a wonderful sign for a large amount of fluid in the abdomen on plain films of the abdomen. Lesser degrees of fluid in the abdomen may be suspected when there is separation (more than 2 cm) of the properitoneal fat stripe from air in the ascending or descending colon. A less specific sign is loss of the inferior margin of the liver. This is usually a fat–soft tissue interface. However, when fluid occupies the Morrison pouch it becomes a soft tissue–soft tissue interface, which is an invisible interface on plain film. This sign does require the patient to have some intraperitoneal fat, and the extremely thin patient may be an exception. Another sign of fluid in the abdomen is fluid in the lateral pelvic recesses giving the so called "dog ears" sign. This is also a soft sign and can be reproduced by fluid in bowel and even loops of collapsed bowel.

Notes

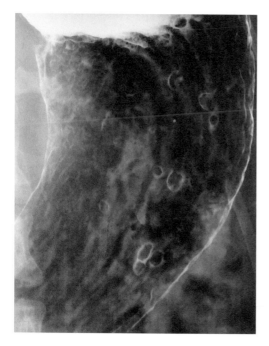

1. What is the most common cause of multiple gastric polyps?

2. What type of polyposis may produce gastric polyps?

3. What histologic type of tissue composes the polyps in Cronkhite-Canada syndrome?

4. What other lesions are found in patients with Cowden disease?

Multiple Gastric Polyps

1. Inflammation producing hyperplastic polyps.

2. Familial polyposis, including Gardner's syndrome, Peutz-Jeghers syndrome, Cronkhite-Canada syndrome, Cowden disease, and juvenile polyposis.

3. Inflammatory or juvenile hamartomatous type.

4. Circumoral papillomatosis, skeletal malformations, and tumors of the gastrointestinal tract, skin, breast, and thyroid.

Cross-Reference

Gastrointestinal Imaging: THE REQUISITES, ed 3, p 72.

Comments

With the increased use of biphasic upper gastrointestinal examination, it is not uncommon to encounter multiple small polyps within the gastric lumen. These growths are often found throughout the body and in the proximal stomach. For the most part these small polyps are the sequela of previous inflammation of the stomach and histologically are hyperplastic or inflammatory polyps. On occasion, they are due to metastases, and rarely they indicate the presence of a polyposis syndrome of the gastrointestinal tract.

Almost all polyposis syndromes may cause polyps to develop in the stomach. Patients with familial polyposis (or Gardner's syndrome) have a high incidence of gastric polyps. Unlike their adenomatous counterparts in the colon, gastric polyps can be either adenomatous or hyperplastic. Patients with Peutz-Jeghers syndrome develop hamartomatous lesions in the stomach with no malignant potential. Juvenile polyps also are hamartomas and may occur sporadically or as part of a diffuse juvenile polyposis syndrome.

Cronkhite-Canada syndrome is a nonfamilial polyposis syndrome. It is associated with a group of skin abnormalities, including alopecia, onychodystrophy, and hyperpigmentation. Clinically these patients also have weight loss and protein and electrolyte depletion. It is this last group of symptoms that may be life-threatening. The condition usually occurs in middle-aged patients and sometimes in the elderly. Patients with Peutz-Jeghers syndrome develop hamartomatous lesions in the stomach with no malignant potential. Juvenile polyps also are hamartomas and may occur sporadically or as part of a diffuse juvenile polyposis syndrome. The polyps are inflammatory or hamartomatous and have no malignant potential. Typically the growths are quite small. Cowden disease is a rare cause of hamartomatous polyps in the stomach; this disorder is hereditary and results in formation of diffuse hamartomatous and ectodermal abnormalities throughout the body.

Occasionally one will encounter what appear to be multiple small bead-like polyps lined up on folds in the body and antrum of the stomach. Erosions occurring in the stomach evoke a edematous response around the erosions that are sometimes mistaken for multiple small polyps. Careful barium coating of the stomach will often show the erosion (a tiny barium collection) on a raised edematous mound.

Notes

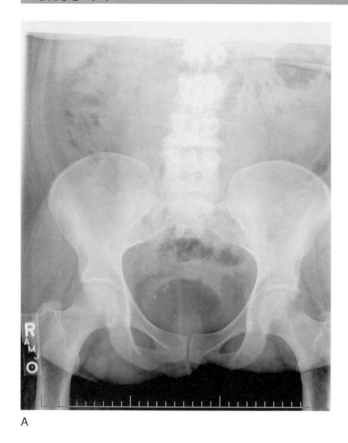

A

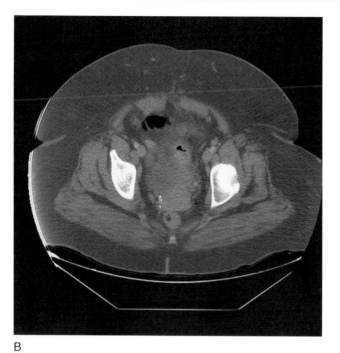

B

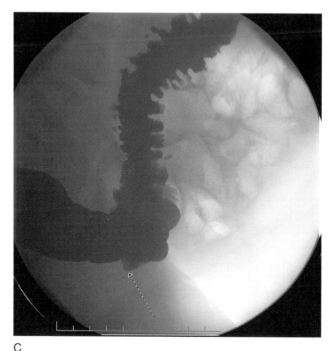

C

1. What is the significant finding on the plain film?

2. Apart from iatrogenic causes, what is the most pathologic etiology?

3. What other diseases can cause this complication?

4. What would be the best method for evaluating this finding?

Colovesicular Fistula

1. Air in the urinary bladder.

2. Diverticulitis.

3. Crohn's disease, radiation treatment, malignacies.

4. Cystogram.

Cross-Reference

Gastrointestinal Imaging: THE REQUISITES, ed 3, p 283.

Comments

A fistula is defined as an abnormal tract extending from one mucosa-lined organ into the mucosal surface of another organ. The possible types include enteroenteric (between two loops of bowel), enterovesical (bowel to bladder), enterovaginal, and enterocutaneous, among others. A sinus tract is also a small communication with bowel, but it ends blindly or in a cavity that is not normally lined with mucosa.

Diverticulitis is by far the most common cause of enterovesicular fistulas, such as seen in this case; Figure 91C shows a tract developing from inflamed sigmoid colon directing toward the urinary bladder. Crohn's disease is a relatively common causes of fistula formation in the gastrointestinal tract. Malignancy can also result in fistulous formation, especially if it is fairly extensive or is already being treated (leading to necrosis) before the fistula occurs. Inflammatory conditions also lead to the formation of numerous fistulas. In the colon, diverticulitis is the most common cause of fistulas in industrialized society. Crohn's disease is a well-known cause of fistula formation between adjacent loops of bowel, as well as other structures. Other infections that may produce fistulization are tuberculosis and actinomycosis. This chronic inflammatory process ulcerates and produces a variety of unusual fistulas. Fistulas may form as a complication of surgery, typically at an anastomotic site that dehisces. Radiation is a well-known cause of fistula development; this complication results from microvascular ischemic changes and fibrosis and "matting together" of organs.

Evaluation of fistulas can be quite difficult. Often, contrast material will travel in only one direction through a fistula. Also, the fistula must be open at the time of the study, or it cannot be demonstrated. CT is often considered a good modality for revealing the presence of a fistula, its complex communications, and the underlying cause of the complication. However, because some fistulas originate in the small bowel a cystogram should be considered first. In the Bourne test a sample of urine is taken after the study, the material is centrifuged, and then the spun material is radiographed to detect barium.

The presence of barium is believed to be indicative of an enterovesical fistula.

Notes

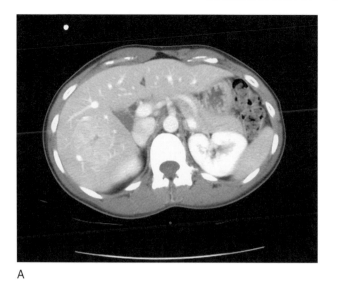

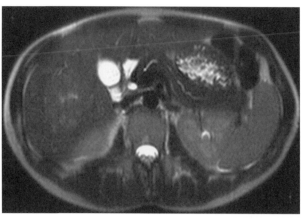

A   B

1. What do both these images have in common?

2. Why do these lesions take up sulfur colloid?

3. In what demographic group is this lesion most commonly seen?

4. What is the vascular supply usually serving this lesion?

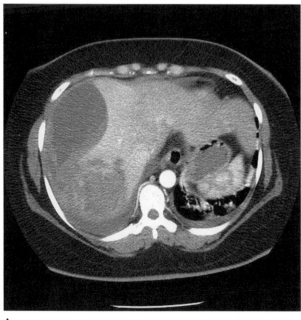

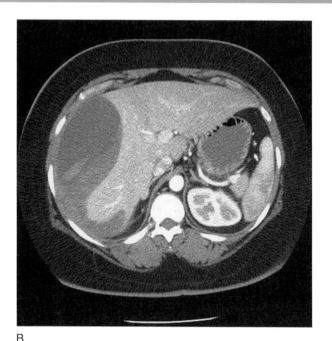

A   B

1. In which gender does this lesion predominantly occur?

2. Consumption of what drug predisposes to the development of this abnormality?

3. How does this lesion appear on a sulfur colloid liver scan?

4. Name the most common clinical presentation of this lesion.

CASE 92

Focal Nodular Hyperplasia

1. They both show an hepatic lesion with a central scar.

2. The lesion contain Kupffer cells.

3. Young women. In this case, a 25–year-old woman.

4. Centrally.

Cross-Reference

Gastrointestinal Imaging: THE REQUISITES, ed 3, p 189.

Comments

Focal nodular hyperplasia (FNH) of the liver is the second most common benign tumor of the liver after hemangiomas. The tumor is a hyperplasia of normal, non-neoplastic liver tissue that has an abnormal arrangement and is similar to a hamartomatous type of lesion. It is believed to develop as some type of response to a congenital vascular abnormality in the region, and there is a slight association between hemangiomas and FNH. Histologically the liver tissue is arranged in small nodules, with septa in between. Arterial vessels feed the nodules from a centrally located artery that is often within a central scar or septum. They do not have a portal venous supply. FNH contains Kupffer cells in most instances.

Adenomas and FNH are similar in that they both occur in young women, although FNH also occurs in children and older patients. Unlike adenomas, FNH is not associated with oral contraceptive use. This tumor is rarely found in men. FNH must be differentiated from other hepatic tumors, such as adenomas, fibrolamellar hepatomas, and giant cavernous hemangiomas. All these tumors are large vascular tumors that affect young women and often have a central scar.

Focal nodular hyperplasia is easily detected on ultrasound as a well-defined lesion with echogenicity different from that of the normal liver. A large central vessel may be detectable on Doppler scanning. On CT scanning the lesion may be of similar density as the liver and difficult to distinguish from the normal liver parenchyma. A central scar or low-density area may be visible. Because of the functional reticuloendothelial cells, FNH may be detectable on sulfur colloid scanning as an area of increased uptake. On MRI, FNH is slightly hyperintense on T_2-weighted images, but the central scar is often markedly hyperintense.

Notes

CASE 93

Hepatic Adenoma with Bleed

1. Women.

2. Oral contraceptives.

3. Cold defect.

4. Bleeding with right upper quadrant pain.

Cross-Reference

Gastrointestinal Imaging: THE REQUISITES, ed 3, p 196.

Comments

Hepatic adenomas are composed of hepatocytes that are loosely arranged, have no portal tracts, and have poorly formed hepatic veins. They form bile to a slight extent. These tumors tend to be large and solitary, often exceeding 10 cm in diameter. They are also quite vascular and because of their poorly developed venous system have a propensity for spontaneous hemorrhage, which is the major clinical presentation. Usually the hemorrhage is internal within the adenoma and liver produces pain by heptic capsular distention, such as in this case, but if the hemorrhage spreads into the peritoneal cavity, it could be fatal. Adenomas occur predominantly in women, usually younger women. They are believed to be estrogen-associated tumors, and their incidence is increased in women taking oral contraceptives. Cessation of oral contraceptive use causes the tumors to shrink. Rarely the tumor occurs spontaneously in men. Men taking anabolic steroids are at increased risk of developing a tumor that is similar to both an adenoma and a hepatocellular carcinoma. Patients with glycogen storage disease also are at greater risk of developing adenomas.

Hepatic adenomas are usually easily identifiable on cross-sectional imaging, but their differentiation from other hepatic tumors is the major concern. Ultrasound typically reveals a large hyperechoic lesion, which may have central areas of low density caused by hemorrhage or necrosis. On CT the lesion may be hypodense because of glycogen, which is often within the tumor. After contrast material injection, the tumor enhances and may become isodense. At the periphery of the tumor are large vessels, which are feeding vessels for the tumor. This finding is apparent on angiography; large peripheral arteries can be seen draped around the tumor and feeding into the center of the mass. Adenomas are visible as cold defects on sulfur colloid scans; this point is important in differentiating the tumor from focal nodular hyperplasia, which appears "hot" on sulfur colloid scan. On MRI, adenomas may be hyperintense on T_1-weighted images because of the presence of glycogen and fat in the tumors.

Notes

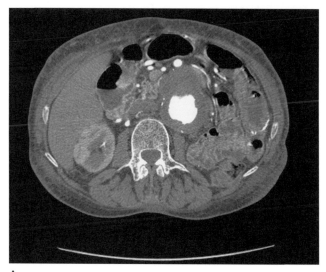

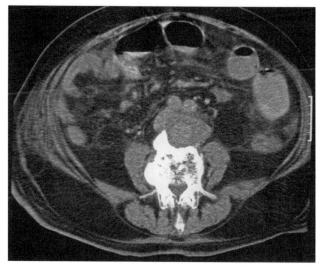

A

B

1. What do these two patients (both in their 70s) have in common?

2. What size must the abdominal aorta be to qualify as an aneurysm?

3. How might these patients present clinically?

4. What complications are associated with this condition shown in these images that can be demonstrated on MDCT?

Abdominal Pain Due to Abdominal Aortic Aneurysm

1. They both have abdominal aortic aneurysms (AAA).

2. In excess of 3 cm.

3. Multiple clinical presentations, from abdominal pain and palpable mass (Fig. 94A) to back pain (Fig. 94B).

4. One of these patients presented with a uncommon but known complication, erosion of the AAA into the adjacent vertebral body. More commonly, the complications relate to AAA leakage of blood with pain, hypotension, and hypovolemic shock. Sudden, unconfined ruptures will result in death within minutes.

Cross-Reference

Gastrointestinal Imaging: THE REQUISITES, ed 3, p 138.

Comments

Abdominal aneurysms are relatively common in elderly patients. Whites are more likely to have it and men are affected seven times more often than women. The aorta comprises three layers: intima, media, and adventitia. Abdominal aortic aneurysms (AAAs) occur over long periods of time during which medial degeneration takes place, resulting in a gradual dilatation of the vessel. However, not all AAAs are caused by degenerative disease. In a small percentage of cases (3–5%), the mycotic aneurysm results from the hematogenous spread of bacteria. Most AAAs are fusiform in shape and are located below the renal arteries and the bifurcation. Some may extend into the iliac vessels.

Most AAAs are asymptomatic until sudden expansion, leakage, rupture, or compromise of renal or enteric vessels. Almost two thirds of patients with sudden rupture will expire from rapid cardiovascular collapse before reaching the hospital. CT will usually reveal a large dilated abdominal aorta with varying degrees of intramural thrombus. Care should be taken to evaluate for dissection, blood leakage, and quality of renal and bowel perfusion. Pain associated with AAA can be misdiagnosed, as the classic presentation of tachycardia, hypotension, and a pulsatile mass on physical diagnosis is, as most classical presentations, not the most common. Often these patients will present with flank pain and renal stone. MDCT protocols are performed looking for the offending calculi. In the event of an elderly patient presenting with flank pain with no obvious urologic source, with or without an AAA, the possibility of dissection should not be overlooked.

Uncommon causes of AAA include Marfan syndrome and Ehlers-Danlos disease.

Notes

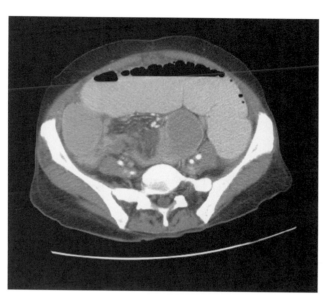
A

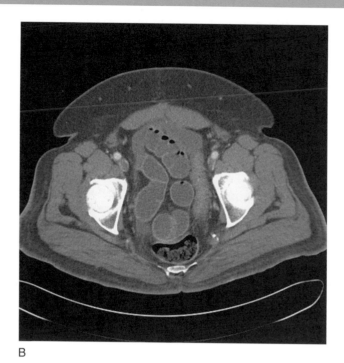
B

1. What is the origin of air in dilated bowel in a patient with obstruction?

2. What is the most common cause of small bowel obstruction?

3. What is the definition of a "differential air-fluid level"?

4. What is the most specific modality for demonstrating mechanical obstruction?

Grossly Dilated Small Bowel

1. Swallowed air.

2. Fibrous adhesions.

3. Differing air-fluid levels seen within the *same* loop of bowel.

4. CT.

Cross-Reference

Gastrointestinal Imaging: THE REQUISITES, ed 3, p 106.

Comments

One of the problems most frequently evaluated by the radiologist (and surgeon) is dilated loops of small bowel. This evaluation is particularly difficult in the patient who develops distention after a surgical procedure. The main differential diagnostic concern is whether a true mechanical obstruction has developed or whether the bowel dilation is secondary to an adynamic ileus.

Most mechanical obstructions occur as the result of fibrous adhesions, which develop within days after surgery. However, mechanical obstruction within the first few days after abdominal surgery is quite rare. Usually it takes months or years before obstructions from adhesions become symptomatic (if they become symptomatic). When symptomatic, most are treated successfully with nasogastric decompression. The CT images in this case show high-grade small bowel obstruction and *collapsed distal small bowel.* The transition point is visible with no evidence of mass, and with a history of prior surgery, the radiologist will be correct, in almost every case, assuming this is a postoperative adhesion.

However, in the postoperative patient the radiologist should be wary of diagnosing a mechanical obstruction when the colon is dilated up to the level of the anatomic splenic flexure (that point where the descending colon passes behind the phrenicocolic ligament and becomes retroperitoneal). Spasm at that site is relatively common in the immediate postoperative abdominal surgery patient, and the radiologist should consider this before deciding it is a mechanical obstruction.

Other causes of grossly dilated small bowel include hernias, either in the abdominal wall or internally. Fibrous bands also may lead to volvulus or closed loop obstructions. For decades, contrast examination of the small bowel, along with plain film radiography, has been the standard for evaluation of the patient with suspected obstruction. Enteroclysis has been shown to be of somewhat greater benefit but is impractical for the postoperative patient. Many now advocate the use of CT, which can assess the site of obstruction and possible underlying causes of the problem. It is as sensitive as the other modalities and can be quite specific for determining the cause of the problem, which is most helpful for clinicians.

Notes

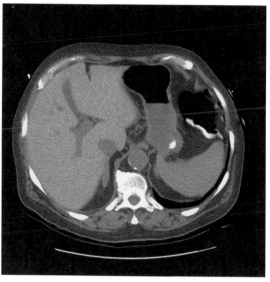
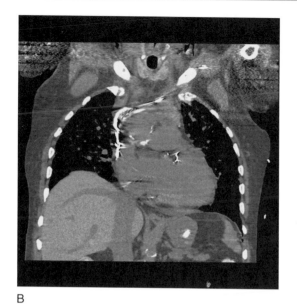

A   B

1. What cardiac dysfunction does this patient suffer from?

2. How does the relative density of the liver indicate this problem?

3. What other conditions can cause increased liver density?

4. What is the most serious side effect of the drug this patient is being treated with?

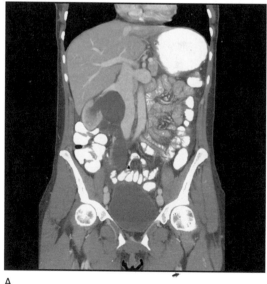
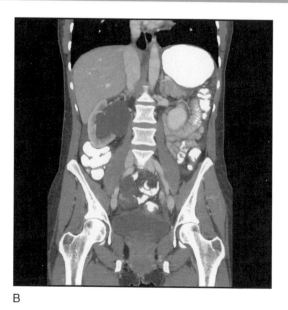

A   B

1. This 47-year-old woman presented with lower abdominal pain. What are the differential diagnostic considerations?

2. Which is more likely to obstruct both ureters: cervical, endometrial, or ovarian carcinoma?

3. How does cervical carcinoma affect the gut?

4. How often does endometriosis cause ureteral obstruction?

CASE 96

Patient on Amiodarone and Dense Liver

1. Acute and chronic cardiac arrhythmias.

2. Relatively increased density of the liver can be due to the iodine content of amiodarone.

3. Hemosiderosis, hemochromatosis, chronic cirrhosis, Wilson's disease.

4. The most serious side effect of amiodarone is idiopathic pulmonary fibrosis.

Cross-Reference

Gastrointestinal Imaging: THE REQUISITES, ed 3, p 209.

Comments

The antiarrhythmic drug amiodarone causes the liver to increase in density due to its accumulation and metabolism in the liver and the fact that amiodarone contains iodine. Increased liver density may be common in this useful medication, but actual heptotoxicity is uncommon. Relative density on an unenhanced scan of the liver should raise the question of the use of amiodarone. In addition, other considerations should include hemochromatosis and hemosiderosis in a patient who has received multiple blood transfusions over the course of hospitalization. Wilson's disease, a disease of copper metabolism malfunction is rare but can result in a dense liver. Older patients who received Thorotrast in the 1960s and who are still surviving (there are very few today) would have increased density of liver and spleen. Patients treated with IM gold for rheumatoid arthritis might have such a finding as well as those with some of the glycogen storage diseases.

Notes

CASE 97

Ovarian Carcinoma with Ureteral Obstruction

1. Any pelvic mass causing compression or invasion of the ureters or primary ureteral processes.

2. Cervical carcinoma (10–12%).

3. Often it does not affect the gut. In a small percentage of patients there may be contiguous spread to the rectum.

4. Uncommon; less than 1% of cases.

Cross-Reference

Gastrointestinal Imaging: THE REQUISITES, ed 3, p 315.

Comments

Ovarian carcinoma as seen in this case is a disease of middle-aged and older women (although ovarian carcinoma in younger women is not infrequently seen). The incidence is thought to be higher in women who have had no children. There is also a peculiar relationship between this disease and breast cancer, with patients with ovarian cancer having a higher risk for breast cancer and vice versa.

Ovarian cancer can commonly affect the gut. This is usually in the later stages when interperitoneal, intermesenteric spread can cause narrowing and invasion and obstruction of the bowel, especially the small bowel and sigmoid colon. CT is the examination of choice, capable of showing the lesion as well as its spread to the peritoneal cavity and other findings such as ureteral obstruction and small bowel involvment. Tiny metastatic nodules studding the mesentery and without ascites at that point will be invisible on CT, and if very early mesenteric spread is suspected, laparoscopy is indicated. Early in the disease transvaginal ultrasound can be quite helpful in the evaluation of the ovaries when the exmination is undertaken with an empty bladder.

Notes

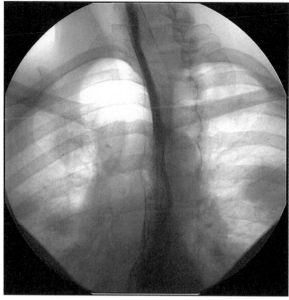

A

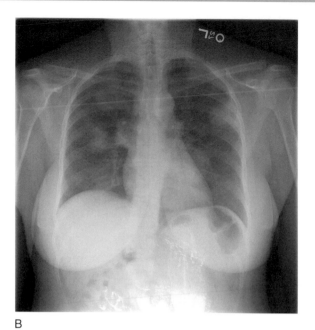

B

1. What is the finding on this patient being worked up for GERD?

2. Would the characteristics of the finding lead you to think benign or malignant?

3. When doing an UGI, should the radiologist have a "quick" look over the lungs to check for pulmonary lesions?

4. What responsibility does the radiologist have regarding lung findings?

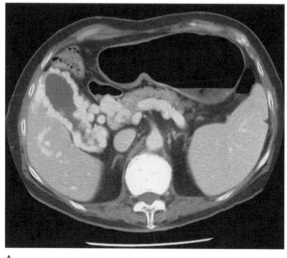

A

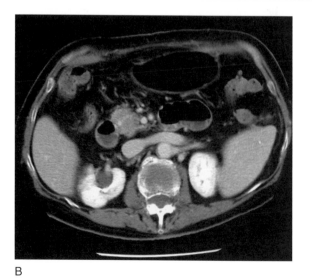

B

1. What is the likely underlying abnormality resulting in these images?

2. What is the name given to a chronically occluded or congenitally absent portal vein?

3. Why is this finding important for future reference?

4. What percentage of patients with portal hypertension might show these findings?

Incidental Finding of Pulmonary Lesion on UGI

1. Rounded areas of density are seen in both lungs. The esophagus is normal.

2. Because the margins of the density are hazy, one would think of focal areas of infiltrate, more likely to be benign.

3. No.

4. Everything on the image is the responsibility of the radiologist.

Cross-Reference
Gastrointestinal Imaging: THE REQUISITES, ed 3, pp 2-3.

Comments
This incidental finding of pulmonary lesions during a UGI examination (in this case blastomycosis), better seen on a chest film taken immediately after the completion of the UGI study, is a good example of an incidental but important finding. When doing the esophageal part of the examination, the patient should be rotated to the left to get the esophagus off the spine, and tight collimation should routinely be utilized to limit ionizing radiation exposure to the lungs and breasts. In fact, considerably more collimation could have been used on the fluoroscopic spot image included in this case (see pages 2 and 3 in *Gastrointestinal Imaging: REQUISITES*). The main reason to avoid doing a check of the lungs during an esophagogram or UGI is to limit radiation exposure and the fact that it is less than an ideal screening method. If the situation warrants it, such as in this case, it may be a consideration. But because a PA and lateral chest were planned to immediately follow the UGI examination, it is of questionable value and contributes yet more to radiation exposure. Even when evaluating the diaphragms for the possibility of diaphragmatic paralysis, transverse collimation should be employed with the patient in a steep oblique position (so both diaphragms are included in the image). Radiation safety should be a major consideration for every radiologist, resident, and nonradiologist using ionizing radiation.

Notes

Gallbladder Varices

1. Gallbladder varices are the result of portal hypertension or portal vein occlusion.

2. Cavernous transformation (multiple collateralization along the course of the portal vein).

3. Cholecystectomies are one of the most common surgeries performed. To know the gallbladder is surrounded by distended veins would be helpful to the surgeon, especially in patients with known portal hypertension.

4. In some of the literature the presence of gallbladder varices is given as high as 20% in portal hypertension (mostly with ultrasound). Other authors consider it a rare finding.

Cross-Reference
Gastrointestinal Imaging: THE REQUISITES, ed 3, p 211.

Comments
Gallbladder varices are a rare finding in patients with portal hypertension. In the West the most common cause of portal hypertension is alcoholic cirrhosis of the liver. Smaller numbers of patients may develop cirrhosis and portal hypertension as a result of portal or splenic vein thrombosis, parasitic infection involving the portal system (schistosomiasis), chronic hepatitis or liver injury secondary to hypervitaminosis A, congenital diseases such as congenital absence of portal vein or congenital hepatic fibrosis, as well as a host of relatively uncommon prehepatic, hepatic, and posthepatic causes.

All these conditions can result in either occulsion or increased pressures in the portal vein causing collateralization of veins in the splenic circulation. Although the incidence of varices in portal hypertension secondary to hepatic cirrhosis is high (up to 75–80%), the most common manifestation is distention of the coronary veins that ascend to the gastroesophageal junction and give rise to uphill varices. Other manifestations of varices are dilated veins in the abdominal wall, around the umbilicus (caput medusa sign) and splenorenal shunting. Duplex doppler ultrasound can gauge the flow in the portal vein, collateralization, and the texture of the liver. CT, in patients who are able to have IV contrast material, is an excellent way to demonstrate collateralizations without flow quantification, such as obtained in ultrasound, and to evaluate the liver.

Notes

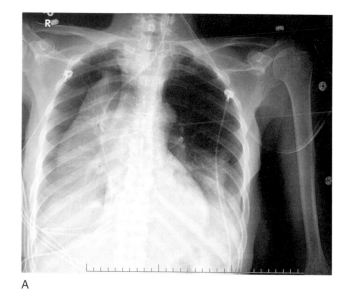

A

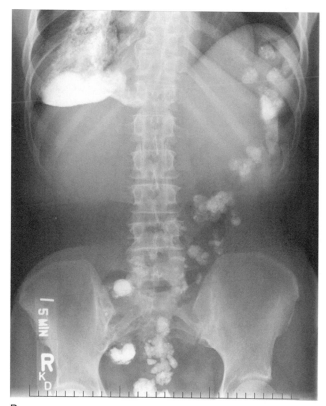

B

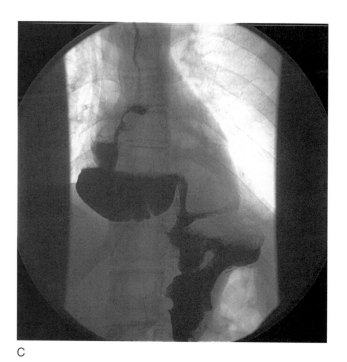

C

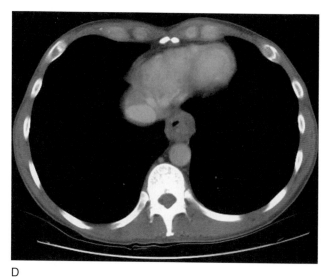

D

1. What are the findings on the PA view of the chest of this man?

2. What are some conditions that will result in a widened mediastinum?

3. What is the difference between primary and secondary achalasia?

4. What is the etiologic basis for primary achalasia?

Long-standing Achalasia

1. The PA chest shows a widened mediastinum on the left with well-defined margins.

2. A number of conditions ranging from vascular lesions, tumor, large cysts, achalasia, secondary achalasia, scleroderma, dermatomyocytis, and polymyositis, to some rare cases of diffuse esophageal spasm.

3. Primary achalasia results from degenerative changes involving the myenteric plexuses of the esophagus, and secondary achalasia most commonly results from the destruction of the plexuses by tumor infiltration at the GE junction.

4. Not known. Theories range from central CNS causes to local neurodegeneration to a self-limiting occult microorganism infection that leave the neuroplexuses destroyed.

Comments

Achalasia is a fairly common, but poorly understood disorder of the myenteric plexuses of the esophagus resulting in dilatation, absence of peristaltic activity, and spasm at the gastroesophageal junction. It is more common in men and is usually seen in the third or fourth decade of life. In the images accompanying this case, a barium esophagogram demonstrates a dilated esophagus with a sigmoid configuration and the classic area of tapered narrowing and spasm in the distal esophagus at the GE junction. The PA chest film with barium retained in the esophagus shows how chronic achalasia will affect the esophagus over time. Take care not to confuse it with esophageal resection and colonic interposition (Fig. 100C).

Other conditions, such as scleroderma and other collagen vascular disorders, may mimic achalasia. There have been reports of patients with Diffuse Esophageal Spasm (DES) with dilated esophagus, minimal peristaltic activity, and spasm at the GE junction. In fact, some investigators feel that achalasia and diffuse esophageal spasm may be part of the same spectrum of diseases. Although this is occasionally seen, it is not the usual pattern of presentation seen in most cases of achalasia. Primary and secondary achalasia may be identical in appearance and presentation. However, secondary achalasia is usually seen in an older age group, and the underlying condition is esophageal or gastric cardiac carcinoma (Fig. 100D), which has infiltrated the wall of the lower esophagus or GE junction and destroyed the myenteric plexuses, giving an achalasia-like apperance. Dysphagia and a dilated esophagus in an older individual should arouse suspicion. The only differentiating feature on a barium swallow may be some mucosal irregularity at the site of spasm and narrowing. Endoscopic ultrasound and in many cases CT will be more sensitive methods for making the diagnosis of secondary achalasia.

Notes

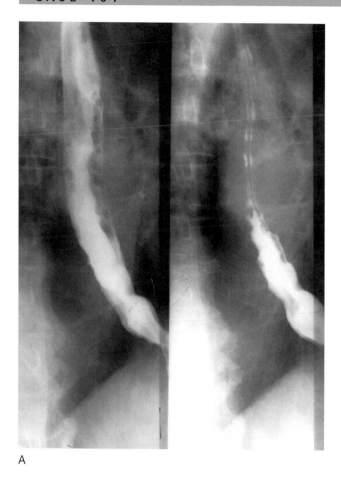

A

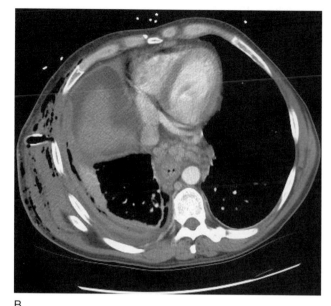

B

C

1. What are the findings on this barium esophagogram and CT image?

2. What are some diagnoses that can cause serpiginous filling defects in the esophagus?

3. What is the physiologic basis for these findings?

4. What is the difference between "downhill" and "uphill" varces?

Esophageal Varices

1. Wave-like serpiginous filling defects in the mid- and distal esophagus and blood-filled structures surrounding the GE junction on the CT image.

2. The most common cause would be dilated veins in the esophageal submucosa (varices). Other considerations would include "varicoid" infiltration with tumor and some cases of leukemia affecting the esophagus.

3. Varices (as demonstrated in this case) are the result of portal hypertension and collateralization of the left gastric veins in an effort to get blood around the portal occlusion or hypertension into the azygos veins and thus back into the right side of the heart.

4. Most cases of varices are related to portal hypertension and are referred to as "uphill" varices. However, in cases of superior vena cava obstruction (usually the result of tumor in the upper mediastinum) "downhill" varices can form in the upper esophagus as the body forms collateral pathways to get blood past the SVC obstruction into the right side of the heart.

Cross-Reference
Gastrointestinal Imaging: THE REQUISITES, ed 3, p 9.

Comments

In Western society the most common cause for portal hypertension and the formation of esophageal varices is hepatic cirrhosis. This is usually the result of chronic alcoholism. However, many other causes can lead to liver cirrhosis, especially chronic hepatocellular disease (such as hepatitis), chronic portal vein occlusion by thrombus, or parasitic infection. Chronic portal vein occlusion can also result in some patients in cavernous transformation of the portal vein in which collateralization along the entire route of the former portal vein is seen. This results in less evident esophageal varices, and indeed, the patient may be asymptomatic. Cavernous transformation in portal hypertension related to liver cirrhosis is uncommon. Esophageal varcices can bleed (as seen in Fig.101B, in which the entire esophagus is filled with blood due to bleeding varices). This most alarming complication of the condition carries a high morbidity rate.

At the other end of the esophagus, obstruction of the superior vena cava can result in "downhill" varices (Fig. 101C) seen in the upper esophagus and representing prominent collaterization of the venous system in an attempt to bypass an occluded superior vena cava, usually secondary to marked adenopathy resulting from adjacent malignancy, most commonly small cell carcinoma of the lung. Lymphoma can also be the underlying condition. The patients are usually not difficult to diagnose because of their physical appearance of having congested facial features and engorged neck veins.

Notes

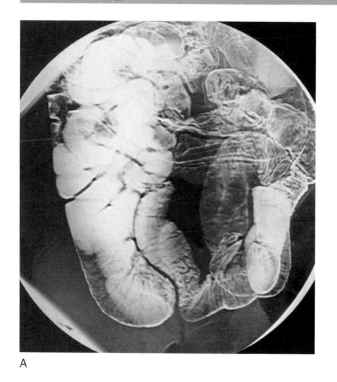

A

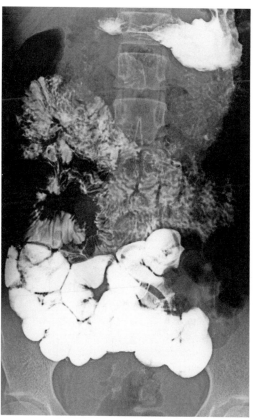

C

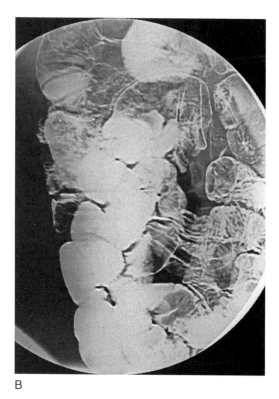

B

1. What is this parasitic infection called?

2. What is its prevalence?

3. What is a common complication of this parasitic infection?

4. What changes can it produce in the chest?

Ascariasis of the Small Bowel

1. Ascariasis.

2. It is the most common intestinal parasitic infection, affecting up to a quarter of the world's population.

3. Migration into the biliary system.

4. Pulmonary hypersensitivity with bronchospasm, infiltrates, and eosinophilia.

Cross-Reference

Gastrointestinal Imaging: THE REQUISITES, ed 3, p 135.

Comments

One of the most common parasitic infections is produced by the nematode *Ascaris lumbricoides.* It infects a major proportion of the world's population. With the ease of worldwide travel, as well as immigration, this parasite is encountered in all areas of the world. The pathway of infection is quite complicated. The eggs of this parasite are ingested when infected water or food is consumed. In the gastrointestinal tract (small bowel) the larvae hatch and burrow through the intestinal wall. From there, they reach the portal venous system and travel to the liver and the lungs. The larvae then reach the bronchial system, where they can be found in the sputum, and reach the intestines by being swallowed in the sputum. Once they again reach the intestines, they grow into adult worms, which can be quite large.

The parasite produces diseases in many ways. The larvae may produce a local hypersensitivity reaction, which is particularly evident when they are in the lungs. When they are in the intestines, the worms cause nutritional deficiencies. As the worms grow, the large mass of the worms can produce obstruction and even appendicitis. Perforation of the intestines with peritonitis can even occur. Often the patient's symptoms are quite vague, with occasional pain and diarrhea. The worms can also migrate into the biliary system, where they can produce cholangitis or pancreatitis because of their size as well as a local inflammatory response.

Radiologically the worms are visible on barium studies because they are so large. There may be a single worm, or they may occur in large masses. A hallmark of these worms is that they ingest the barium during the examination, and then barium outlines the intestinal tract of the worms, as is evident in this images.

Notes

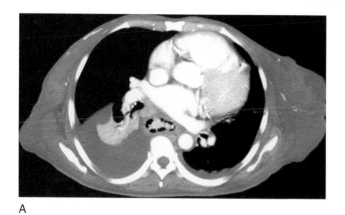

A

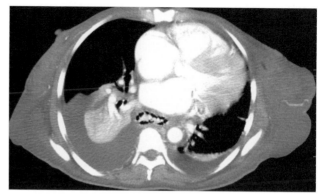

B

1. What is the important finding in these images?

2. What might be some of the etiologic explanations of these findings?

3. Can GERD or Barrett's metaplasia lead to this appearance of the esophagus?

4. What is the Mallory-Weiss syndrome?

Mallory-Weiss Tear and Pneumatosis of the Esophagus

1. Air (pneumatosis) in the wall of the distal esophagus.

2. Anything that can lacerate the mucosa or wall of the esophagus might conceivably result in air in the esophageal wall. Such things would include penetrating trauma, severe retching resulting in a tear of the esophageal mucosa (Mallory-Weiss syndrome), or a full-thickness tear (Boerhaave syndrome). Iatrogenic causes, such as instrumentation or endoscopic treatment of Barrett's metaplasia must also be considered.

3. No.

4. The Mallory-Weiss syndrome is bleeding associated with a mucosal tear in the distal esophagus or GE junction. It is generally associated with episodes of severe retching.

Cross-Reference
Gastrointestinal Imaging: THE REQUISITES, ed 3, p 19.

Comments

Air is the esophageal wall is an uncommon finding. It is extremely difficult to see on plain film or even on barium esophagograms. However, the finding is easily identified on CT. The Mallory-Weiss patient can have air in the esophageal wall if an open mucosal tear exists. These patients usually are alcoholics (but not always). The condition has also been described in a few patients with severe hiccups. They present with blood-tinged vomiting and chest pain. They are almost always treated conservatively and about 95% will spontaneously heal. Patients with portal hypertension and a Mallory-Weiss tear are a more serious problem. Patients experiencing a full-thickness tear of the distal esophagus (Boerhaave syndrome) are a surgical emergency and require immediate intervention. The morbidity rate is high. Endoscopic instrumentation may also infrequently be the cause of mucosal tears. However, the risk of iatrogenic injury to the mucosa will probably increase as newer methods of endoscopic ablation of Barrett's metaplasia are being tried with varying degrees of success and associated complications (including pneumatosis). Some of these procedures include photo-dynamic therapy, laser therapy, electrocoagulation, argon plasma coagulation therapy, and mucosal surface resection. In addition, radiofrequency and cryotherapy are being evaluated.

Notes

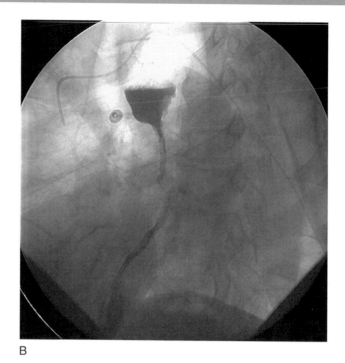

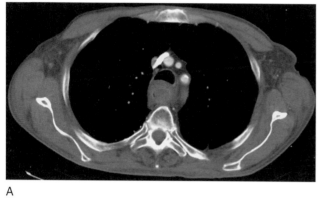

A

B

1. What are the most common radiologic findings in patients with acute caustic esophagitis?

2. Does acid ingestion affect the esophagus in a manner similar to caustic ingestion?

3. Ingestion of which product—acid or lye—involves the stomach?

4. What important complication is seen with this condition?

Lye Ingestion

1. Motility disorders and superficial mucosal irregularity.

2. Ingestion of either product may involve the esophagus, but acid damage is often less severe.

3. Acid ingestion tends to cause more severe damage to the stomach.

4. Squamous cell carcinoma of the esophagus.

Cross-Reference

Gastrointestinal Imaging: THE REQUISITES, ed 3, p 17.

Comments

Ingestion of alkaline (lye) or acid substances may be either intentional or, in rare cases, accidental. Many household cleansers contain alkali or caustic substances. The degree of injury that occurs in the gastrointestinal tract is related to both the concentration and the volume of the ingested substances. The immediacy of treatment also has a significant impact regarding the sequela of this injury. Alkaline substances produce coagulative necrosis and tend to cause a more deeply penetrating injury to the bowel.

Radiologic studies may be performed (but are not recommended in known cases of caustic ingestion) as long as there are no signs of perforation, such as a widened mediastinum, soft tissue emphysema, or intraperitoneal air. Initial radiologic assessment may be performed before endoscopy is attempted and should be done with water-soluble contrast agent followed by thin barium. In the early stages (fewer than 12 hours after the ingestion) the only apparent problem may be a motility disorder, ranging from spasm to atony and even dilation. If there has been a severe caustic burn, superficial ulceration may be apparent in the mucosa. Over the ensuing days, the damaged mucosa sloughs and becomes edematous, with the most severe changes subsiding after several days. Radiologic examination typically is not performed during this time unless there is suspected perforation. A water soluble study may show the location and size of the leak. The final phase of scarring, fibrosis, and stricture formation takes several weeks to months to develop. Not all patients develop esophageal stricturing, but it is more common in patients who ingested lye than in those who ingested acid. The strictures that are apparent can be either long and diffuse or weblike areas of narrowing. A significant number of these patients have developed, over time, squamous cell carcinoma of the esophagus, a well-known complication of lye ingestion.

Ingestion of both alkaline and acid substances may involve the stomach, usually in the distal antrum along the greater curvature, which is where the ingested substance often comes to rest when the patient is upright. The degree of gastric injury is usually worse with ingestion of acids. The appearance has an almost identical look as a malignancy: a large ulcerated mass on the greater curve of the stomach. Alkaline substances may be neutralized by the gastric acidity. However, up to 20% of patients who ingested lye develop gastric injury.

Notes

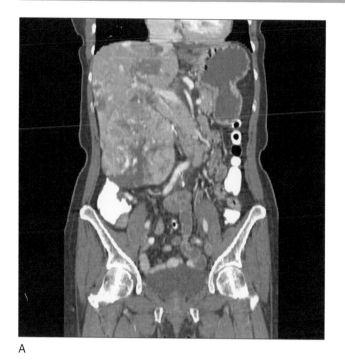

A

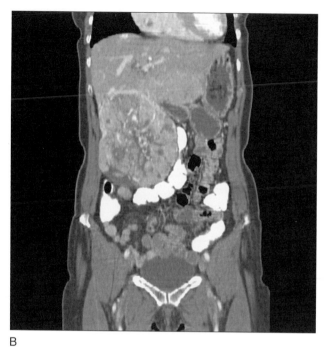

B

C

1. Name some diagnostic possibilities for this radiologic appearance of the liver.

2. What age group does this lesion affect?

3. What vascular tumors may involve the colon?

4. How does the appearance of cavernous hemangiomas differ from the appearance of capillary hemangiomas?

Cavernous Hemangioma of the Liver

1. Ischemia, focal nodular hyperplasia, hepatoma, hemorrhage, and hemangioma.

2. Typically, nonpediatric age group.

3. Hemangiomas and lymphangiomas.

4. Cavernous hemangiomas are more diffuse; capillary hemangiomas are localized.

Cross-Reference

Gastrointestinal Imaging: THE REQUISITES, ed 3, p 186.

Comments

Hemangiomas of the liver, unlike those of the rest of the GI tract, are a common finding. In the rest of the gastrointestinal tract, they are rare lesions. There is no malignant potential associated with this lesion. The problem is one of attempting to distinguish the harmless hemangioma from other lesions such hepatic metastatic disease. There are two different types of hemangiomas to consider: simple hemangiomas (by far the most common) and cavernous hemangiomas, such as seen in this case. Hemangiomas of the liver are the most common benign neoplastic tumors of the liver. It is thought that these tumors affect 2% to 5% of the population. They are more common in women and occur most frequently in the right lobe of the liver. Multiple hemangiomas occur in 10% to 15% of these patients. By themselves, hemangiomas are rarely symptomatic and are of no consequence to the patient. Their importance lies more in the fact that their appearance can mimic that of more sinister conditions of the liver, such as metastases or malignant tumors.

Most discussions regarding hemangiomas concern the diagnostic tests that may help distinguish them from other lesions. Dynamic scanning of the liver by CT is quite helpful. In this case, initial CT scans show the hemangioma to be a low attenuation lesion in the liver. Delayed images of the lesion over the next several minutes demonstrate increasing opacification of the hemangioma from the periphery toward the center, the so-called centripetal opacification. However, not all cavernous hemangiomas show the classic findings, and often other studies are required. Ultrasound often shows a well-defined echogenic lesion, although the findings are not always pathognomonic. MRI is often useful because hemangiomas have a high signal intensity on T_2-weighted images, but cysts and even some metastatic lesions may have a similar appearance. Radionuclide scanning is quite helpful for evaluating the liver hemangioma. On tagged red blood cell studies the hemangioma typically appears as a cold defect during the early scans, but in later images the lesion fills in and actually has increased activity on delayed images. With all these imaging studies, the greatest difficulty is encountered when the hemangioma has a central area of necrosis or fibrosis (Fig. 105C), which can mimic other lesions.

Notes

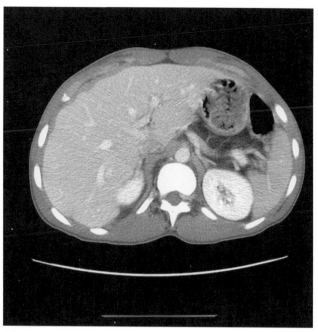

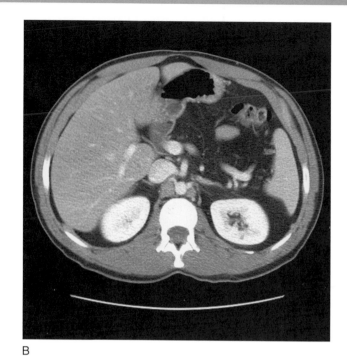

A   B

1. What is the genetic defect in this patient?

2. What is the result of the genetic defect involving the vas deferens?

3. What is the definitive treatment for this condition?

4. What percentage of these cases affect the pancreas?

Cystic Fibrosis and Atrophy of Pancreas

1. Cystic fibrosis (CF), a recessive genetic defect. The CT images show marked atrophy of the pancreas.

2. Almost all males with CF are sterile owing to defects in vas deferens formation.

3. There is no cure. All treatment of the lungs is aimed at diminishing and treating the complications of pulmonary function caused by CF. With pancreatic involvement treatment involves replacement of exocrine digestive pancreatic enzymes. If a cure is to be found, it will be at the genetic level.

4. 85% to 90% of CF patients will have pancreatic deficiency.

Cross-Reference

Gastrointestinal Imaging: THE REQUISITES, ed 3, p 158.

Comments

Cystic fibrosis is a recessive genetic disorder caused by the malfunction of a single gene on chromosome 7. The gene, cystic fibrous transmembrane conductance regulator (*CFTR*), has to do with transport of chlorine and, to a lesser extent, sodium ions from within the cell to outside the cell. There can be a variety of mutations of this gene, all resulting in the production of excessive, thick mucus within the glands of the cells of the glandular structures. This, in part, accounts for the "salty skin" of patients with CF. The thick mucus has its most deadly effect on the lungs, where it will provide a near perfect medium for chronic bacterial infections, which over time, distorts and destroys the lung and bronchial architecture and further decreases respiratory capability.

Pancreatic involvement resulting in marked pancreatic atrophy and deficiency (such as in this case: note the absence of pancreatic tissue in its expected anatomic location) is extremely common. Supplementation with pancreatic enzymes is the common treatment along with a careful diet. With the use of CT over the years, we have come to recognize pancreatic atrophy as a common finding in older patients, with fatty infiltration of the pancreas. It seems to be a senile atrophy of the pancreas. However, the pancreatic atrophy of CF is seen in younger patients and is striking in its absence of pancreatic tissue.

Notes

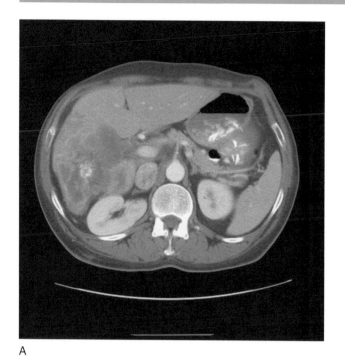

A

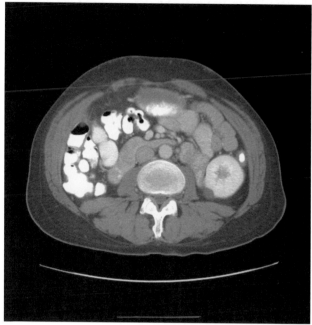

B

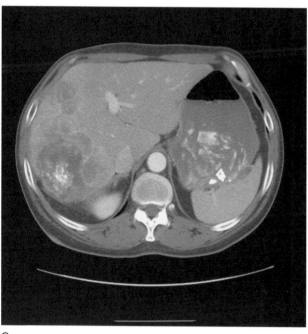

C

1. What is the most common cause of these liver lesions in adults?

2. What is the most common cause of these liver lesions in children?

3. What extra-abdominal tumors may produce these lesions?

4. Do treated metastases ever calcify?

Mucinous Metastatic Disease to Liver with Calcification

1. Mucinous adenocarcinoma of the colon.

2. Neuroblastoma.

3. Breast or lung carcinoma and melanoma.

4. Only rarely.

Cross-Reference
Gastrointestinal Imaging: THE REQUISITES, ed 3, p 172.

Comments
The CT image demonstrates calcified liver lesions. Primary liver tumors may calcify but typically are solitary. Infectious processes that have involved the liver, such as granulomatous infections, also may produce multiple liver calcifications. Parasitic diseases, such as echinococcal cysts, can cause calcification. However, the illustrated case shows several small lesions that are either partially or completely calcified, which is strongly suggestive of metastatic disease.

Metastases to the liver rarely calcify. In the adult population, calcification of liver metastases is typically the result of a mucinous adenocarcinoma, which produces a psammomatous type of calcification that is detectable on CT scans. Most often, mucinous adenocarcinoma is found in the colon. Other sites of mucinous carcinomas include the pancreas, stomach, and ovaries. Tumors such as osteogenic sarcoma and chondrosarcoma can produce calcification or ossification, and their metastases could have this appearance as well. In children the most likely cause is neuroblastoma; up to 25% of neuroblastoma metastases calcify. Tumors outside the abdominal cavity rarely produce calcified liver metastases, but lung tumors, breast tumors, melanomas, and testicular tumors produce these lesions on rare occasion. Tumors that have been treated with chemotherapy or radiation also may calcify, although admittedly this presentation is rare. Calcification has been reported in various treated tumors and in treated lymphoma of the liver.

Notes

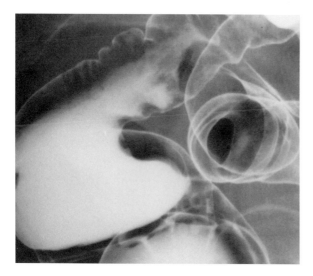

1. In a young woman with furrowed filling defects in the rectum what would be the most likely diagnosis?

2. The rectum is a good location for what type of metastases?

3. What type of abnormality is often the sequela of solitary rectal ulcer syndrome?

4. On defecography, what finding may be evident in this patient?

Colitis Cystica Profunda

1. Endometriosis.

2. Peritoneal seeding into the cul-de-sac.

3. Colitis cystica profunda.

4. Internal rectal prolapse.

Cross-Reference

Gastrointestinal Imaging: THE REQUISITES, ed 3, p 300.

Comments

The anterior wall of the rectum is a relatively common location for pathologic findings. Probably the most common abnormalities in this area are external diseases of the cul-de-sac, including endometriosis and numerous abdominal tumors (ovarian, gastric, pancreatic, and intestinal) that produce peritoneal seeding or drop metastases to this region. All these processes have a similar appearance on barium enema. Primary tumors of the colon, mainly adenocarcinoma, can also develop in this region.

However, the anterior mucosal wall of the rectum also is a location for abnormalities, which occur as the sequela of anorectal defecation disorders. Patients with defecation problems, primarily constipation or chronic straining, may suffer from prolapse of the rectal mucosa. The anterior wall of the rectum above the peritoneal reflection is not fixed; it is free to move. This form of prolapse (or intussusception) happens every time the patient attempts to defecate. This prolapse is usually internal and difficult to document. At times even external prolapse (beyond the anal sphincter) can occur and the diagnosis becomes self-evident. Either way the anterior wall of the rectum becomes a vulnerable structure prone to injury and induration. This, in turn, can lead to mucosal ulceration, leading to rectal bleeding. This condition, termed solitary rectal ulcer syndrome, affects all age groups but particularly younger patients and mostly females.

Colitis cystica profunda is a sequela of chronic prolapse and solitary rectal ulcer syndrome. With recurrent prolapse and ulceration, there are stages of ulceration and then healing of the rectal mucosa. Over time, the regenerating mucosa may trap mucus glands underneath the mucosa. These trapped mucus glands continue to secrete mucus but do not drain because of overlying mucosa. Thus, the glands become cystic structures filled with mucin, and hence the name. With time, the cysts produce one of several polypoid structures, typically along the anterior surface of the rectum because this segment is most susceptible to this trauma. This entity is difficult to diagnose in the absence of a history of long-standing defecation dysfunction. Biopsy confirms the diagnosis, and often defecography is helpful in identifying the patient's underlying defecation problems.

Notes

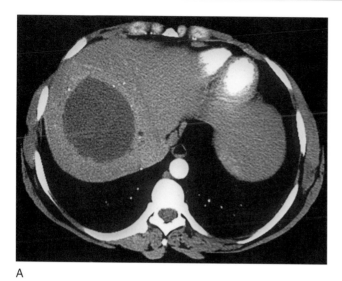

A

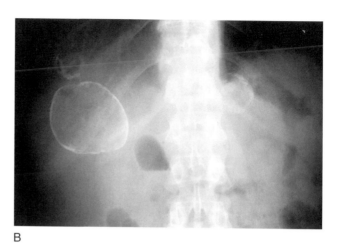

B

1. Which cystic structures of the liver calcify?

2. What organisms produce this disease?

3. Where do these cysts spontaneously drain?

4. Can these cysts be drained percutaneously?

Echinococcal Cyst

1. Echinococcal cysts and sometimes simple liver cysts.

2. *Echinococcus granulosus* and *Echinococcus multilocularis.*

3. Biliary system and rarely the peritoneal, pleural, or pericardial region.

4. Yes.

Cross-Reference

Gastrointestinal Imaging: THE REQUISITES, ed 3, p 202.

Comments

Echinococcal cysts are produced by two types of tapeworms—*E. granulosus* and *E. multilocularis.* *E. granulosus* is the species most commonly seen in North America. These tapeworms live in the intestinal tract in dogs. Humans, and more commonly, sheep are the intermediate hosts, harboring the parasite in its larval stage. Humans contract the parasite by eating contaminated food, such as unwashed vegetables, or through contact with an infected dog or sheep. When the eggs of the parasite are ingested, they penetrate the mucosa of the intestine and are then carried via the portal vein to the liver. Sometimes the lungs, spleen, and kidneys are involved as well. The embryos then develop in a hydatid stage in which they form cysts in the liver. The life cycle is completed when the intermediate host dies and is consumed by the final host.

Hydatid cysts consist of three layers. The outer pericyst is a rigid fibrous structure that is vascular and may enhance on CT. There is an intermediate layer, and finally the inner layer or endocyst is the living parasite. These cysts represent the larval stage, and there are often multiple small cysts seen within the larger cyst. Debris produced by brood capsules may be visible on the dependent portion of the cysts. Most cysts cause no symptoms until they are large enough to create pressure on adjacent structures. Approximately 20% to 30% of the cysts calcify, which is much higher than the percentage of simple hepatic cysts that calcify. Sometimes the cysts spontaneously rupture into the biliary system or the peritoneal, pleural, or pericardial surfaces. Symptoms vary, but this complication can produce cholangitis or inflammation of the structures it comes in contact with. A fatal anaphylactic reaction is also possible. The plain film shown with this case is an example of chronic disease, whereas the CT image is indicative of a more acute stage.

Hydatid cysts must be drained for treatment. Surgery was once considered necessary for treatment of this condition because of the possibility of anaphylactic reaction if the cyst drained into the peritoneum. However, it is now recognized that these cysts can be managed by percutaneous catheter drainage and instillation of scolecidal agents.

Notes

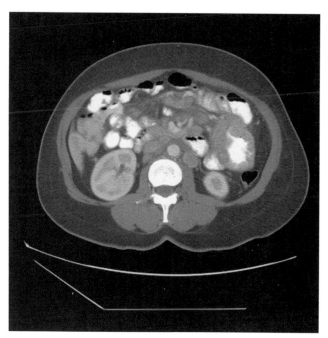

A

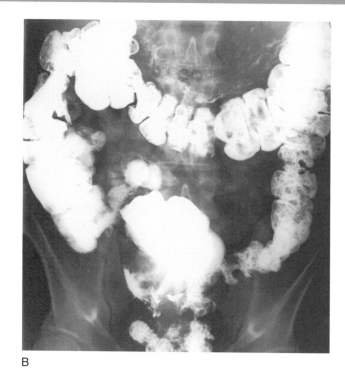

B

1. What is the finding in the images of this patient?

2. What conditions can give this appearance?

3. Can metastatic disease result in this finding?

4. What is the very important secondary finding in this case?

Aneurysmal Dilatation of the Small Bowel

1. Large dilated irregular luminal collection of barium surrounded by soft tissue mass. This is known as "aneurysmal dilatation" of the small bowel.

2. By far the most common cause is non-Hodgkin's lymphoma. However, it can infrequently be seen in malignant GISTs of the small bowel.

3. It is rarely seen in metastatic disease of the small bowel. The only exception is some cases of melanoma that spread to small bowel.

4. Please note that in the both the CT image and the delayed small bowel follow-through image, there is no evidence of obstruction despite the large mass. This is a hallmark of non-Hodgkin's lymphoma.

Cross-Reference

Gastrointestinal Imaging: THE REQUISITES, ed 3, p 129.

Comments

Lymphomas occur most commonly in the distal small bowel (compared with adenocarcinoma, which is proximal), but it may occur infrequently in other parts of the small bowel. A feature of lymphoma is that it may often be multicentric in location. The majority of small bowel lymphomas are the non-Hodgkin's type, with Hodgkin's disease of the small bowel being considered rare.

Lymphoma is difficult to characterize because of its variable morphologic appearance. Radiologic features include multiple nodules, solitary masses with an excavated cavity which acts as the bowel lumen, infiltrating tumors, and predominant mesenteric masses. The infiltrating or the endoexenteric mass is believed to be the most common type. The excavating form, or "aneurysmal dilation," is produced when lymphoma infiltrates, replaces the muscular layer, and destroys the nerves in the area. This results in bulging of the abdominal wall, with resultant dilation. The bowel wall may become completely replaced by tumor with a persistent irregular lumen. Because of this unusual scenario, large masses of the small bowel will show no evidence of bowel obstruction, such as in this case. However, perforation is a possibility. The bowel lumen and various layers of the bowel wall can grow back with therapy.

A variety of conditions may lead to the development of lymphoma. Any type of immunosuppression, such as that associated with AIDS, can lead to lymphoma. Perhaps at highest risk are transplant recipients, who are 50 to 100 times more likely to develop lymphoma compared with the general population. Many of these patients have an associated infection with the Epstein-Barr virus. Other conditions that increase the incidence of small bowel lymphoma include celiac disease (sprue) and systemic lupus erythematosus.

Notes

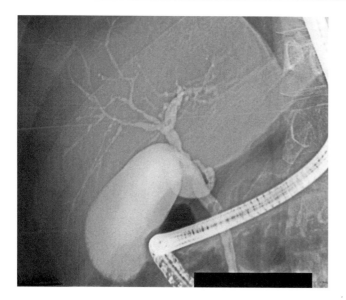

1. The pattern of the biliary tree suggests what diagnosis?

2. What underlying diseases are associated with this condition?

3. What infectious or parasitic conditions may produce this appearance?

4. What is the malignant potential associated with this condition?

Sclerosing Cholangitis

1. Sclerosing cholangitis of the biliary system.

2. Inflammatory bowel disease (usually ulcerative colitis), retroperitoneal fibrosis, ascending cholangitis (often after biliary tract surgery), acquired immunodeficiency syndrome (AIDS), and parasitic infections.

3. Recurrent bacterial infection, particularly after biliary-enteric bypasses; AIDS-related cholangitis caused by either cryptosporidiosis or cytomegalovirus infection; and parasites, including *Ascaris lumbricoides* (roundworm) and *Clonorchis sinensis* (flatworm).

4. 10% to 20% will develop cholangiocarcinoma.

Cross-Reference

Gastrointestinal Imaging: THE REQUISITES, ed 3, p 228.

Comments

Primary sclerosing cholangitis typically occurs in young men. In some instances the disease is considered primary or idiopathic, with no known underlying etiology. The majority (70% or more) of cases are related to underlying inflammatory bowel disease, particularly ulcerative colitis. Conversely, it is estimated that about 10% of patients with ulcerative colitis will develop sclerosing cholangitis. Pathologically the condition is caused by multifocal areas of periductal fibrosis, which produce the narrowing, with intervening normal areas developing ductal ectasia. Typically, ERCP (endoscopic retrograde cholangiopancreatography) has been the imaging modality of choice. However MR cholangiography is now being used considerably more frequency and provides a safer and less expensive alternative method of evaluating the biliary system.

Similar radiologic changes are apparent in patients with recurrent biliary tract infections. The groups that typically develop this condition are postoperative patients with complications and the AIDS population. Worldwide, the most likely cause is intestinal parasites, particularly *A. lumbricoides*. This roundworm migrates into the ducts from the small bowel and causes recurrent cholangitis.

The usual course of disease is one of secondary biliary cirrhosis, recurrent sepsis, and eventual hepatic failure. The time between the appearance of the initial symptoms and death is usually 5 to 10 years. Total colectomy may sometimes halt or diminish the course of the disease. Approximately 10% to 20% of patients with sclerosing cholangitis secondary to ulcerative colitis develop cholangiocarcinoma. Interestingly, this condition does not develop in patients with Crohn's disease. Sometimes, total colectomy arrests the liver disease, but this effect is not predictable. If the disease progresses, the only treatment is liver transplantation.

Notes

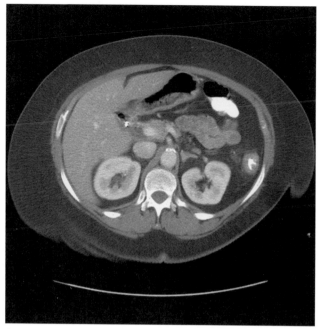

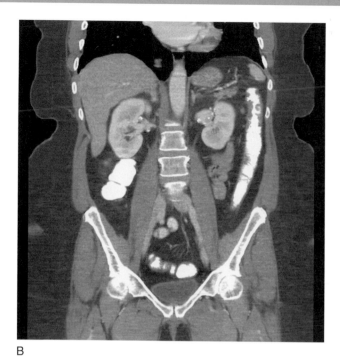

A   B

1. What percentage of colorectal cancers, such as shown in these images of the splenic flexure, can be attributed to the inherited predisposition of Lynch syndrome?

2. What is another name for the Lynch syndrome?

3. What other lesions are associated with inherited Lynch syndrome?

4. What is the molecular basis of the Lynch syndrome?

Colorectal Cancer: Inherited Lynch Syndrome

1. About 2% of all colorectal cancers are attributed to Lynch syndrome.

2. Also called hereditary nonpolyposis colorectal cancer (HNPCC).

3. There is increased risk for endometrial, ovarian, hepatobiliary, stomach, and small bowel cancers.

4. Defective DNA mismatch repair sequences that can be inherited.

Cross-Reference

Gastrointestinal Imaging: THE REQUISITES, ed 3, p 302.

Comments

Given that approximately 170,000 new cases of colorectal cancer will be diagnosed in 2007, we can assume that approximately 3000 will fall into the category of heredity nonpolyposis colorectal cancer. HNPCC as well as the familial adenomatous polyposis syndrome are considered to be in the high-risk category and should undergo regular screening. Although the air contrast barium enema (ACBE) has been shown to be a good screening tool, its impact in cancer screening has decreased to the point that it is not even discussed in most literature on the subject and its use has diminished. This is an unrelenting downward spiral for the ACBE. The examination must be done by competent radiologists with considerable experience and expertise in technique and diagnosis. The fewer ACBEs done, the less reliable the examination is likely to be, setting up a vicious circle. We are moving into the era of colonoscopy as the routine examination of choice. Radiologists, however, have begun to seriously evaluate CT colonography as a far safer option (and hopefully with respectable accuracy and sensitivity) than colonoscopy. Routine CT is proving to be a good diagnostic tool for picking up bowel lesions. These are usually incidental findings and except for some of the polyposis syndromes, high-risk or Lynch syndrome patients cannot be identified radiologically. DNA mismatch repair sequences are normal genetic processes that identify and repair replication errors during cell division. When the mismatch repair sequence is unstable or dysfunctional on certain of several genes, mutation can occur and the risk of cancer is increased.

Notes

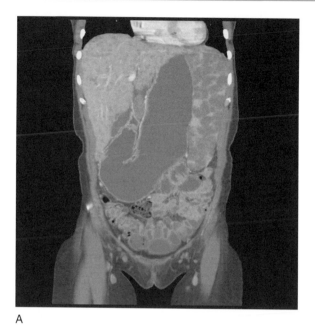
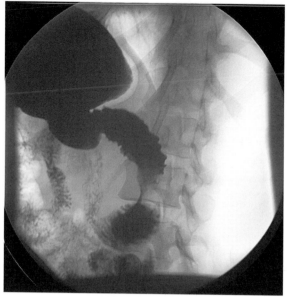

A

B

1. What are some of the common causes of the appearance of the stomach as seen in this case?

2. In the 1950s what was the most common cause?

3. What is the most common cause today?

4. What condition results in gastric obstruction due to a gallstone lodged in the pyloric channel?

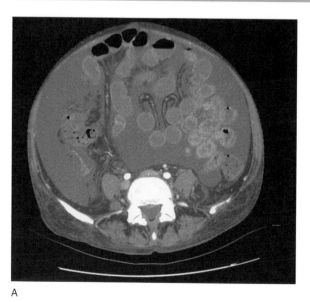
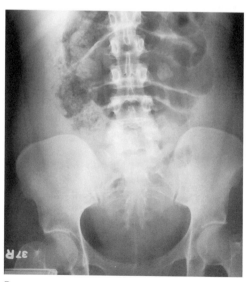

A

B

1. What does the centralization of air loops mean?

2. What solid organ is most commonly injured by blunt trauma?

3. If the patient has a positive pregnancy test, what is the diagnosis?

4. What renal abnormality could cause this appearance?

Gastric Outlet Obstruction Caused by Metastatic Disease

1. The causes of gastric outlet obstruction (GOO) are numerous. Mechanical obstruction such as in scarring in PUD or malignancy are among the most common.

2. By far the most common cause was PUD. With dramatic improvements in the treatment of hyperacidity disease of the upper GI tract, it is uncommon today.

3. Malignancy is now the most common cause.

4. Bouveret syndrome; a variant of "gallstone ileus" in which the gallstone erodes into the gastric antrum instead of the duodenum.

Cross-Reference
Gastrointestinal Imaging: THE REQUISITES, ed 3, p 49.

Comments
In the pediatric population, especially in males in the first year of life, pyloric hypertrophy with stenosis is not an uncommon cause of gastric outlet obstruction and is usually easily diagnosed using ultrasound imaging. However, in the older population pyloric hypertrophy is very rare. The most common cause of gastric outlet obstruction in adults today is probably malignancies, primary and secondary. The usual lesion is pancreatic or peripancreatic. In this case the lesion is widespread metastatic disease that has also invaded both liver and spleen and the duodenum itself. Primary carcinoma involving the head of the pancreas is often the obstructing lesion. Pancreatic carcinoma can also invade the stomach itself, but this seldom causes outlet obstruction. Primary duodenal lesions can result in outlet obstruction.

Simple single contrast UGI studies can establish the presence of a mechanical cause of gastric distention and may even suggest the cause. Upper GI endoscopy can do the same with the added benefit of biopsy, if called for. Multiplanar CT has become an outstanding tool in the workup of these patients and is being used with increasing frequency. CT evaluation also includes the surrounding structures and the entire peritoneal cavity. Whatever diagnostic pathway is utilized, multiplanar MDCT is usually the eventual imaging choice. MRI is being used with more frequency but is still far behind CT in terms of time, cost, and availability.

Notes

Hemoperitoneum and Ectopic Pregnancy

1. Fluid. Air-filled loops of bowel float up to the dome of the abdomen.

2. Spleen.

3. Ruptured ectopic pregnancy.

4. The kidneys being retroperitoneal would probably never result in this constellation of findings.

Cross-Reference
Gastrointestinal Imaging: THE REQUISITES, ed 3, p 132.

Comments
The radiograph shows evidence of free fluid within the abdominal cavity. Findings include increased density in the pelvis as well as fluid density in the paracolic gutters between the ascending and descending colon and the flank stripes. Fluid within the peritoneal cavity can represent ascites, inflammation, blood, or urine or bile. The appropriate history should be obtained in this situation. Ascites can be the result of a variety of causes and is by far the most common cause of long-standing fluid accumulation in the abdomen.

In the setting of severe symptomatology or trauma, all of the diagnostic possibilities must be considered. Hemoperitoneum is the most likely cause. In patients who have sustained blunt trauma, the fluid could be the result of laceration of the spleen or the liver. Laceration of bowel or mesentery is less common. Other acute but nontraumatic causes include a ruptured ectopic pregnancy and ruptured blood vessel. A perforated viscus caused by ulceration, inflammation, or trauma usually produces ascitic fluid with little hemorrhage. Urine is another consideration in the setting of trauma, but the only cause is rupture of the bladder. Injury to a retroperitoneal structure almost never causes intraperitoneal bleeding unless it is penetrating. Pancreatitis is the only condition affecting a retroperitoneal structure that produces free intraperitoneal fluid, and this finding occurs only in the setting of acute pancreatitis.

Notes

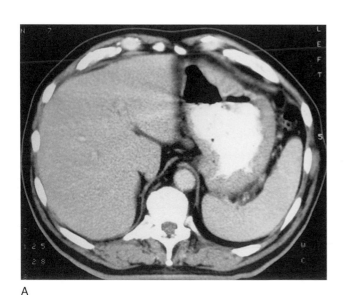

A

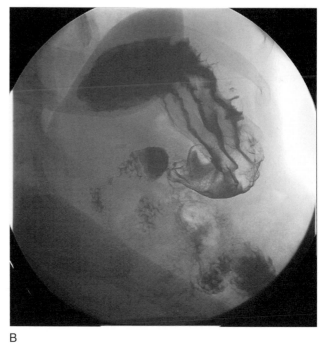

B

1. How often will patients with eosinophilic gastroenteritis develop a peripheral eosinophilia?

2. What portions of the stomach are involved by Ménétrier's disease?

3. What are the manifestations of sarcoidosis of the stomach?

4. Which of these conditions will respond to steroids?

Ménétrier's Disease of the Stomach

1. Nearly always, and typically the eosinophilia is 10% or greater.

2. Although classically described as "antrum-sparing process," the disease can also involve the antrum in up to one half of patients.

3. Slight nodularity to thickened folds. In advanced cases the thickening of the wall resembles a scirrhous process and linitus plastica

4. Eosinophilic gastritis and sarcoidosis respond well to steroids; Ménétrier's disease does not.

Cross-Reference
Gastrointestinal Imaging: THE REQUISITES, ed 3, p 70.

Comments
Thickened gastric folds are a common radiologic finding that can be produced by a number of unusual disorders. The imaging finding itself is so nonspecific that all of the various disorders cannot be distinguished by their radiologic appearance. In a patient with peripheral eosinophilia and thickened gastric folds, eosinophilic gastritis should be strongly considered. There is often associated small bowel disease in patients with fold thickening. Sarcoidosis of the stomach may be more common than first appreciated; according to some reports the condition can be identified in up to 10% of gastric biopsies. With sarcoidosis there is always associated pulmonary disease, and other portions of the gastrointestinal tract may be involved. Both of these conditions respond dramatically to steroids, as do a few other gastric conditions.

Ménétrier's disease is a rare condition in which marked glandular hypertrophy of the stomach develops without any underlying cause. There is associated enlargement of the gastric rugae, hypochloremia, and hypoproteinemia. Despite the fact that there is often increased mucus secretion in the stomach, gastric acid output is reduced, which differentiates the disease from other types of hypertrophic gastritis in which acid output is often elevated. Protein-losing enteropathy is another distinguishing characteristic of Ménétrier's disease. Patients often have pain, weight loss, vomiting, and diarrhea. According to the classic description of the disease the hypertrophic fold changes occur only in the proximal stomach, but it is now known that the thickened folds can be seen throughout the stomach, even the antrum. Spontaneous remission can occur, but often Ménétrier's disease is a chronic recurrent illness that responds poorly to various therapies (e.g., antibiotics and H_2 blockers). In severe instances, gastric resection may be required. Controversy remains regarding whether the condition is premalignant. The prevailing thought is that it is not.

Notes

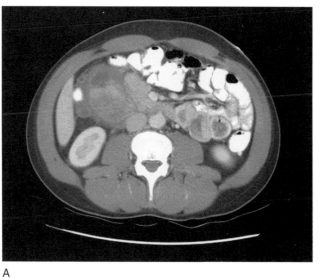

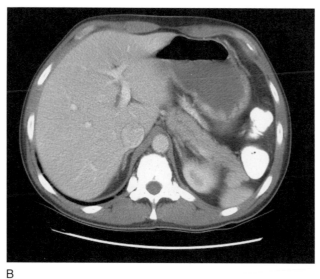

A   B

1. What diagnostic considerations are suggested in these images?

2. What specific findings will lessen the possibility of cancer?

3. What other masses might affect the pancreatic head?

4. If the CT examination was repeated in 6 weeks what might you expect to see?

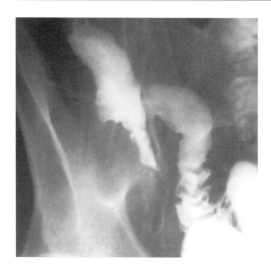

1. Name conditions that produce a "coned" cecum and terminal ileal disease.

2. What infectious condition in that region typically spares the terminal ileum?

3. Ulcerative colitis typically produces what change in the terminal ileum?

4. What fungal infection may produce this abnormality?

CASE 116

Unusual Presentation of Acute Pancreatitis

1. Without a clinical history, first and foremost pancreatic malignancy must be excluded.

2. The fact that the mass contains some fluid; neither the biliary system nor the pancreatic duct is obstructed.

3. Inflammatory masses, pseudocysts, perampullary lesions, peripancreatic lymphatic mass.

4. The mass would be markedly reduced in size.

Cross-Reference

Gastrointestinal Imaging: THE REQUISITES, ed 3, p 154.

Comments

On rare instances pancreatic carcinoma may present as acute pancreatitis. When there is no etiologic basis for acute pancreatitis in a middle-aged or older adult, it is a consideration. Acute pancreatitis has a variety of imaging presentations, including disease seemingly limited to the pancreatic head, as seen in this case. In most cases more of the gland is involved with edema and even hemorrhage and necrosis in a small number of patients. Necrosis and sepsis constitute the leading causes of death in acute pancreatitis.

Most acute pancreatitis involving the pancreatic head can have a very adverse effect on the biliary system, compressing the common bile duct just as a pancreatic malignant mass might. However, that is not always the case, as in this case. These lesions always present a dilemma and are often biopsied to rule out carcinoma. About 25% to 30% of all cases of pancreatitis will present with findings limited to the pancreatic head. Gallstones passing through the shared ampulla of Vater can also give rise to inflammatory changes in the pancreatic head as well as throughout the entire gland. The stone does always have to be present. Some stones will lodge, cause havoc with pancreatic drainage, and then pass. Over 80% of patients with gallstone pancreatitis will have stones detected in stool. However, most of these will have accompanying bile duct obstruction and some degree of distal pancreatic duct obstruction. In this case the lack of biliary involvement, the fluid in and around the tumor, and the normal distal pancreas suggest an inflammatory origin. A calcification in the ampulla of Vater would seal the diagnosis.

Notes

CASE 117

Amebiasis of the Colon

1. Tuberculosis and Crohn's disease and amebiasis.

2. Amebiasis.

3. Dilated terminal ileum (backwash ileitis).

4. Blastomycosis.

Cross-Reference

Gastrointestinal Radiology: THE REQUISITES, ed 3, p 299.

Comments

The coned appearance of the cecum is produced by several diseases, most of which are inflammatory in nature. In determining the exact cause, the radiologist must make a proper evaluation of the region. The most common causative condition encountered in industrialized societies is Crohn's disease. Tuberculosis can present with an appearance virtually identical to that of Crohn's disease, with a coned cecum and inflammation of the terminal ileum. Adjacent inflammatory conditions, such as appendicitis and diverticulitis, are considerations. Neoplasms, such as adenocarcinoma and lymphoma, are also in the differential diagnosis. Long-standing ulcerative colitis may produce a coned cecum but often with a dilated terminal ileum, the so-called backwash ileitis. Other rare conditions that can produce this appearance include anisakiasis, blastomycosis, and *Yersinia* species infection.

Amebiasis is an infection of the bowel produced by the protozoan *Entamoeba histolytica*. It is acquired by ingestion of infected water or soil that contains the cysts. When infection occurs, it can range from very mild or indolent to severe, acute colitis. When cysts spread to the liver or lungs, they can produce abscesses. Changes in the colon include ulceration, which can be either diffuse granularity, collar-button ulcers, or aphthous ulcers. The colon may have skip lesions, with intervening areas of normal bowel, and thus may resemble Crohn's disease. Focal severe inflammation may mimic annular carcinomas. There also may be pronounced granulation tissue formation, leading to protuberant lesions called *amebomas,* which can also mimic neoplasia.

The cecum is invariably infected in amebiasis, and the classic appearance is that of the coned cecum. This abnormality is often seen in the chronic stages of colitis. One strong differential consideration is that amebiasis does not affect the terminal ileum, as do Crohn's disease and tuberculosis. However, amebiasis is seen predominantly in underdeveloped countries and should be considered only if the history is appropriate.

Notes

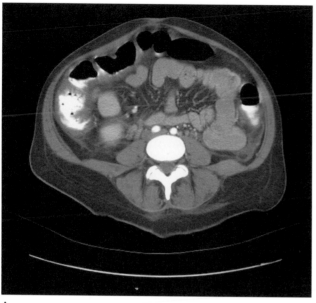

A

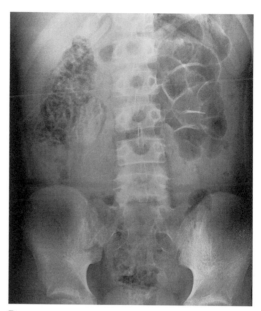

B

1. What are some possible causes of pneumatosis of the colon seen on the conventional image of the bowel?

2. In the pediatric age group, what are the most likely causes?

3. What possible underlying medical conditions may this patient have?

4. Is the course of treatment for this condition surgical or medical?

Typhlitis of the Cecum

1. Ischemia, colitis (inflammatory bowel disease), enterocolitis (infectious), steroid use, endoscopic procedures, and obstructive pulmonary disease.

2. Neutropenic colitis, endoscopic procedures, obstructive pulmonary disease (asthma), and steroid use.

3. Neutropenic colitis is seen in patients with leukemia, lymphoma, and sometimes acquired immunodeficiency syndrome.

4. Medical management is the primary treatment.

Cross-Reference

Gastrointestinal Imaging: THE REQUISITES, ed 3, p 313.

Comments

Neutropenic colitis, or typhlitis, is an inflammatory condition of the right side of the colon that occurs in patients undergoing treatment for leukemia, lymphoma, and sometimes other malignancies. Typically this condition affects the pediatric population, but in some instances it is encountered in the adult population. The clinical findings include fever, abdominal pain, and sometimes diarrhea. CT is the diagnostic modality of choice, demonstrating thickened bowel wall (sometimes with pneumatosis) and pericolic inflammatory changes in the mesenteric fat. These changes in the bowel are the result of a combination of edema, hemorrhage, and inflammatory exudate. Neoplastic involvement is not really a feature of the disease.

Pneumatosis (seen on the conventional image of the abdomen) can be a result of conditions such as asthma or as a sequela of a surgical or endoscopic procedure. If the patient has been taking steroids to treat any medical condition, the medication could be the cause of the pneumatosis. The usual finding when inflammation is the etiology is irregular thickening and inflammatory changes seen involving the cecum (as seen on the CT image). The history of a compromised immune system immediately makes neutropenic colitis the primary diagnostic consideration, however. Interestingly, the treatment of neutropenic colitis is primarily aggressive antibiotic treatment. Surgery is necessary only for those patients with obvious perforation and abscess development. Despite the pneumatosis and pericolonic inflammatory changes, most patients respond well to antibiotics and supportive treatment and do not require surgery.

Notes

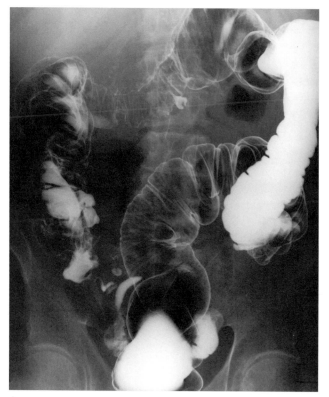

A

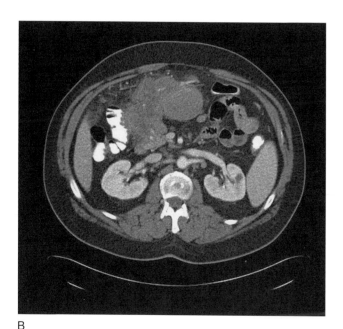

B

1. What is the primary pathologic process demonstrated in these images?

2. What important secondary finding is shown?

3. What are the peritoneal ligamentous connections involving the transverse colon?

4. What comprises the greater omentum?

Spread of Gastric Carcinoma to Colon via Gastrocolic Ligament

1. Large gastric mass with malignant appearance, spreading into the perigastric fat on CT image.

2. Changes along the superior margin of the transverse colon suggest serosal invasion (Fig. 119A).

3. The transverse colon is invested on its anterosuperior surface by the gastrocolic ligament and on its inferoposterior surface by the transverse mesocolon.

4. The greater omentum is made up primarily of the gastrocolic ligament, but also includes the gastrosplenic ligament, the gastrophrenic ligament, and the gastrorenal ligament.

Cross-Reference
Gastrointestinal Imaging: THE REQUISITES, ed 3, p 290.

Comments
The "policeman" of the abdomen, the greater omentum (mostly made up of the gastrocolic ligament) encloses the lesser sac anteriorly while the posterior margin is the transverse mesocolon. A small connection between the lesser sac and the peritoneal cavity is located in the region of the duodenum, the epiploic foramen or foramen of Winslow. Processes affecting the lesser curvature of the stomach are therefore able to reach the transverse colon via the gastrocolic ligament and it would manifest as serosal involvement along the course of the transverse colon, giving the characteristic "crenulated margin," as seen in the barium image.

Peritoneal spread via lymphatics and "drop" metastases are more common than spread down the gastrocolic ligament. However, there are reports of metastatic disease to the stomach (i.e., melanoma) as well as primary gallbladder carcinoma spreading to the colon via the gastrocolic ligament. However, these are rare and the first consideration should be the stomach. Worldwide, gastric carcinoma is said to be the second most common malignancy after lung cancer, but there has been significant drop in the incidence in the Western world over the last 25 years. In general the long accepted "pathway" theory—chronic gastritis, diminished acidity, gastric atrophy, metaplasia, dysplasia, and cancer—is still considered valid. But the pathway may be influenced by several other factors such as *H. pylori,* dietary habits (smoked foods), and of course, long-term cigarette smoking.

Notes

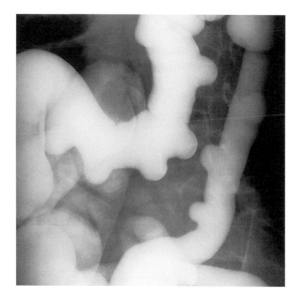

1. Name some disorders that may produce this appearance.

2. What is the difference between true diverticula and pseudodiverticula?

3. What disorders produce wide-mouth sacculations?

4. What may develop within these sacculations?

Scleroderma of the Colon

1. Scleroderma, chronic Crohn's disease, laxative abuse, previous ischemia, and radiation.

2. True diverticula have all three layers of bowel wall. The diverticula of the colon have only the mucosa and submucosa pouching outward through weaknesses in the colonic wall where penetrating vessels occur.

3. Scleroderma, Crohn's disease less commonly.

4. Fecaliths, resembling tumors.

Cross-Reference

Gastrointestinal Imaging: THE REQUISITES, ed 3, p 312.

Comments

The presence of large wide-mouth sacculations in the colon can be an indication of several diseases. Many term these wide-mouth diverticula *pseudodiverticula* because they are not related to the typical diverticula seen in everyday practice. However, they contain all three layers of bowel and thus represent true diverticula. The small diverticula seen in everyday practice are not "true" diverticula. These large-mouth diverticula or sacculations occur when there is eccentric involvement of the bowel wall by some process, producing fibrosis on one side, with eccentric bulging of the opposite wall. A variety of processes can result in the loss of the haustral folds, but only some produce the eccentric diverticula. These processes include scleroderma, Crohn's disease, and laxative abuse. Scleroderma does not involve the colon as frequently as it does other portions of the gastrointestinal tract. Just as it does in other portions of the gastrointestinal tract, however, scleroderma of the colon produces patchy smooth muscle atrophy along with fibrotic replacement of the muscle. This effect leads to the formation of wide-mouth sacculations at weakened areas. There are also abnormalities of transit time, and patients often complain of constipation. The haustral fold pattern is often diminished. Fecal impaction is a complication, and patients may develop benign pneumatosis, which could be the result of a combination of steroid therapy and stasis in the colon. An interesting feature of these wide-mouth sacculations is their ability to retain material. They fail to contract and empty and are found outside the fecal stream in the colon. Thus, these sacculations sometimes develop impacted fecal material or fecaliths within them. These fecaliths can become adherent and resemble polyps or tumors on barium enema studies. Although scleroderma may result in colonic sacculations, the classic "hidebound" appearance of scleroderma is limited to small bowel involvement.

Fibrosis in the wall and folds of the small bowel give rise to this unusual appearance of atrophic folds, seemingly pulled tightly together by the disease. This should not be confused with the "stack of coins" appearance of small bowel intramural hemorrhage in which the folds show no effacement.

Notes

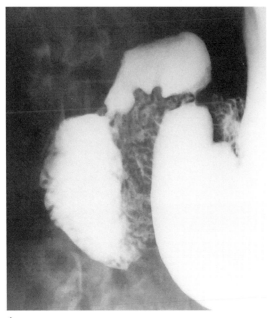

A

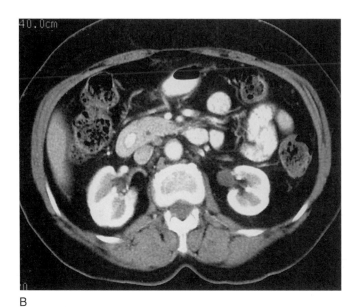

B

1. What anomaly is evident in this patient?

2. What portion of the embryologic pancreas becomes the head and uncinate process?

3. What complication is associated with this condition?

4. In what age group does this condition present?

Annular Pancreas

1. Annular pancreas.

2. Ventral pancreas.

3. Pancreatitis.

4. Half present in neonatal period, half in adulthood.

Cross-Reference

Gastrointestinal Imaging: THE REQUISITES, ed 3, p 152.

Comments

The embryologic development of the pancreas is complex and can lead to a variety of anomalies. Some are of no clinical significance, whereas others may present difficulties early or later in life. The pancreas forms as two distinct buds off the biliary or hepatic bud, which comes from the midgut. These buds are termed the ventral and dorsal pancreatic buds. The dorsal pancreatic bud is to the left of the midline and eventually forms the body and tail of the pancreas. The ventral bud develops to the right of the duodenum. It must rotate, along with the duodenum, to the left. After the ventral and dorsal buds fuse, this ventral bud becomes the head and uncinate process of the pancreas. Failure of fusion will result in pancreatic divisum.

Annular pancreas occurs when there is abnormal rotation of the ventral pancreas or the duodenum, both of which must rotate for proper pancreatic positioning. Some believe that the ventral bud adheres to the duodenum, so that as the structures rotate, the ventral pancreas develops and grows around the duodenum rather than in its normal position. The ventral duct continues to drain into the major papilla and joins with the biliary system, which is its normal embryologic anatomy.

The major pancreatic complication of annular pancreas is the development of acute or chronic pancreatitis. This condition may affect as many as one quarter of patients with annular pancreas. Also, the annular pancreas produces duodenal narrowing or obstruction to varying degrees. About half of the cases of annular pancreas present in the neonatal period with duodenal symptoms. There may be other associated anomalies in the neonate as well. If the condition persists until adulthood, the annular pancreas may be discovered incidentally or when symptoms of pancreatitis or duodenal obstruction occur. These patients may become jaundiced as well. Surgery is necessary to correct the condition.

Notes

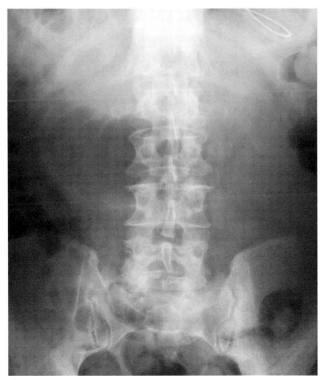

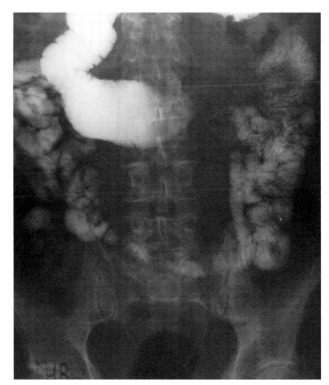

A   B

1. Describe the findings on these AP views of the abdomen.

2. What hollow viscus structures cross the spine transversely?

3. Which structure is this?

4. What is the most common cause of small bowel obstruction?

Primary Carcinoma of Duodenal Sweep

1. Marked dilated loop of bowel crossing the upper abdomen.

2. The stomach, duodenum, and transverse colon can all be said to cross the abdomen transversely.

3. Duodenum.

4. Postsurgical fibrous adhesions. However, this is extremely rare in the duodenum, and the level of suspicion for a malignancy is always higher here.

Cross-Reference
Gastrointestinal Imaging: THE REQUISITES, ed 3, p 91.

Comments

Primary adenocarcinoma, such as demonstrated in this case, is uncommon. It is thought to represent 0.3% of all malignancies of the gastrointestinal tract. Most patients are slow to seek medical aid as the lesion is insidious and the symptoms are nonspecific, and thus it is often fatal by the time of diagnosis. In one study the diagnosis was made post mortem in 25% of cases. At least 50% of patients will have metastatic disease at the time of diagnosis. With the increased use of widespread endoscopy and abdominal CT examinations, these figures should have improved in the last 15 years. However, whether this has affected long-term survival rates is still not clear. The incidence of primary adenocarcinoma of the duodenum, as is the incidence of adenoma, is increased in patients with Gardiner's familial polyposis. The more proximal the lesion, the earlier diagnosis and the better the survival. These patients may also present with biliary symptoms.

Notes

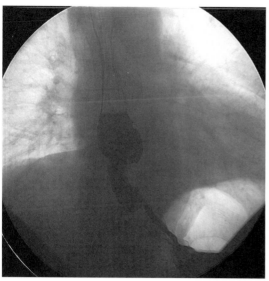

A

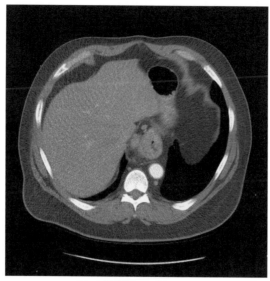

B

1. What type of primary esophageal neoplasm may have this appearance?

2. What metastatic neoplasms can involve the esophagus?

3. What inflammatory process could have this appearance?

4. What common benign condition should also be considered?

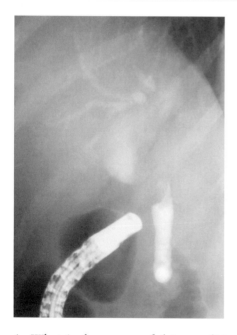

1. What is the name of this condition?

2. What underlying mechanism is producing it?

3. What condition does it mimic?

4. What major complication is associated with this condition?

C A S E   1 2 3

Metastatic Disease of the Esophagus

1. Adenocarcinoma of the lower esophagus and GE junction.

2. Rare, but lymphoma and leukemia, melanoma, and renal cell metastatic lesions of the esophagus have been encountered.

3. GERD and stricture might be a consideration.

4. GIST.

Cross-Reference

Gastrointestinal Imaging: THE REQUISITES, ed 3, p 11.

Comments

Metastatic disease of the esophagus is rare. In many cases it will look like a primary esophageal lesion until histologic examination is obtained. In this case a patient with a large renal cell carcinoma also complained of worsening dysphagia.

Other neoplasms can also affect the esophagus as metastatic lesions. Melanoma has been occasionally seen. Both lymphoma and leukemia can occur in the esophagus when the disease is diffuse and extensive but rarely occur when it is a primary process. Both lymphoma and leukemia of the esophagus typically produce multifocal lesions. These lesions may appear as diffuse fold thickening and irregularity or as multiple nodules, usually submucosal in location. Thus, their radiologic appearance may mimic that of other diffuse esophageal malignancies or hematogenous metastatic processes to the esophagus. These lesions usually regress readily with treatment of the primary tumor but have been known to produce symptoms of dysphagia.

Other causes of multiple filling defects in the esophagus include unusual appearances of squamous esophageal carcinoma, such as varicoid carcinoma or verrucous squamous carcinoma. Squamous papillomas of the esophagus, which is a benign condition, could present as multiple filling defects as well. Probably the most common infectious condition that could have this appearance is candidiasis of the esophagus. Other infectious diseases are less likely. Varices of the esophagus present as multiple submucosal filling defects and have an appearance similar to that shown in this case. Glycogen acanthoses, which produce mucosal nodules in the older population, never become this large.

Notes

C A S E   1 2 4

Mirizzi Syndrome

1. Mirizzi syndrome.

2. A gallstone impacted in the cystic duct with severe local inflammation.

3. Neoplasm of the gallbladder or bile ducts.

4. Surgical ligation of the wrong ducts.

Cross-Reference

Gastrointestinal Imaging: THE REQUISITES, ed 3, p 231.

Comments

This study demonstrates what is termed Mirizzi syndrome. This uncommon condition occurs when a stone becomes impacted in the cystic duct or neck of the gallbladder. This type of impaction is very common, but in the Mirizzi syndrome a severe local inflammatory response occurs. Of course, the affected area is critical because there are several ducts and crossing vessels in the region. The inflammatory response produces a mass or tumor effect in the area. The inflammatory mass impinges on the common hepatic and bile ducts, producing varying degrees of narrowing or even obstruction. The intrahepatic bile ducts may become dilated proximal to the obstruction. There can even be secondary involvement of the major vessels in the area. There is also associated cholecystitis because the gallbladder is now obstructed.

The major concern for physicians dealing with this condition is not the inflammation itself but the difficulty in making an appropriate diagnosis and performing corrective surgery. With the inflammatory mass effect and the bile duct dilation, the condition may mimic a neoplasm of either the gallbladder or bile ducts. Adenopathy also may have a similar appearance. These changes are most confusing on endoscopic retrograde cholangiopancreatography (ERCP). Even if the correct diagnosis is made, prompt surgical intervention is typically warranted. For the surgeon the difficulty arises in identifying and isolating the correct ducts. Often the common hepatic duct is mistaken for the cystic duct, and ligation of the common hepatic duct ensues, producing disastrous complications. When possible, a stent can be placed in the extrahepatic ducts at ERCP to help identify them for the surgeon.

Notes

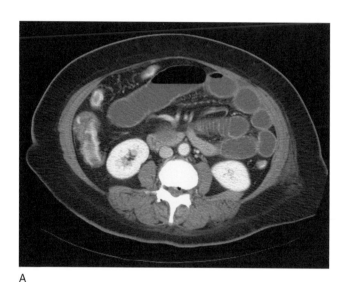

A

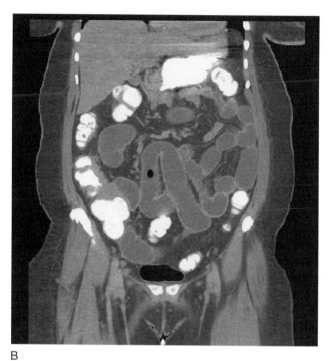

B

1. This is a 65-year-old woman with an advanced breast tumor. Describe the findings on these CT images.

2. What would be your first diagnostic consideration?

3. What the most likely GI organ for spread of breast carcinoma?

4. How often is the colon a site of direct metastatic disease?

Metastatic Disease to the Colon

1. Infiltrating process involving cecum and ileocecal valve causing small bowel obstruction.

2. Colon carcinoma.

3. Stomach.

4. Very rare, but this case is an example of spread of breast carcinoma to left colon presenting as a small bowel obstruction.

Cross-Reference

Gastrointestinal Imaging: THE REQUISITES, ed 3, p 290.

Comments

Breast cancer is the most common malignant lesion in women. Metastatic disease is not uncommon. Most secondary spread involves the bone, liver, lungs, brain, and adrenals, and even the pleural or peritoneal cavities. This can result in serosal invasion of the colon, which is well known. However, a very small number will spread to the gut directly. The most common site for the direct spread of breast carcinoma is the stomach. It can appear as metastatic masses, sometimes with ulceration giving the "bull's eye" lesion of the stomach. In other cases spread can be infiltrative in the stomach and this is one of the causes of linitis plastica. Direct spread to the colon, however, is rare. When it does occur it will have the same presentation as seen in the stomach. It can be one mass or several masses, or it can present as an infiltrative mural process such as in this case. Note the thickened wall of the cecum. The infiltrative involvement of the ileocecal valve has resulted in an unusual presentation in this case. The CT images also clearly show the small bowel obstruction that gave rise to this patient's abdominal complaints. Most malignant lesions of the breast are of the ductal infiltrative type. A smaller number, 10% to 12%, are lobular carcinomas. Some authors think that the lobular types are more likely to metastasize, and that it is the lobular type that almost always results in the uncommon direct metastatic spread to sites in the gastrointestinal tract such as the stomach and colon. Spread to colon is said to occur in 3% to 4% of breast carcinomas. However, this number may include serosal spread as well as direct spread. There are several cases in the literature of direct spread to the colon masquerading as primary colon carcinoma.

Notes

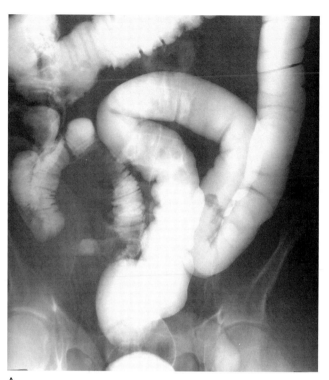

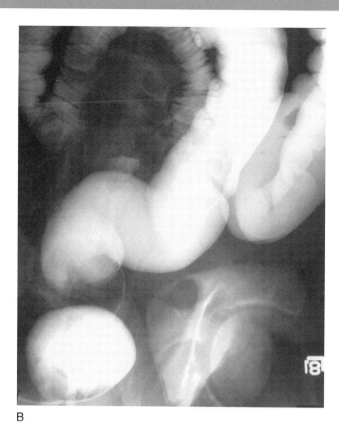

A   B

1. What is the collection of barium seen in the distal ileum low in this patient's pelvis?

2. In patients with gallstone ileus, where do the calculi almost invariably obstruct the bowel lumen?

3. What is the partially patent remnant of the omphalomesentery duct called?

4. What types of mucosa may be found in these remnants?

Meckel's Diverticulum

1. Meckel's diverticulum.

2. Gallstones large enough will be unable to pass the terminal ileum, the narrowest diameter in the gut. Smaller stones will pass. Not all gallstones that erode into the gut cause obstruction.

3. Meckel's diverticulum.

4. All layers of regular small bowel wall. Less than half will have varying degrees of gastric mucosa as well.

Cross-Reference
Gastrointestinal Imaging: THE REQUISITES, ed 3, p 142.

Comments
Meckel's diverticulum is the most common congenital anomaly of the intestines, occurring in up to 3% of the population. It represents incomplete obliteration of the omphalomesenteric duct (also called vitelline duct), which is an embryologic structure. Most Meckel's diverticula do not cause symptoms. However, almost half of these diverticula contain ectopic gastric mucosa that may be functional and may produce pain, ulceration, and bleeding. The Meckel's diverticulum scan, in which technetium-99m pertechnetate is used, is taken up by the gastric mucosa and can detect areas of ectopic gastric mucosa. However, this test is not always reliable. Other complications of Meckel's diverticula include obstruction caused by either invagination and intussusception or formation of a large enterolith. Malignancy is rarely encountered.

Enteroliths are rare, forming in less than 10% of symptomatic Meckel's diverticula, and do not always calcify. When they do calcify, enteroliths may produce bleeding or obstruction. Major differential considerations include a gallstone that has eroded into the gastrointestinal tract, the so-called "gallstone ileus syndrome," or a calcified appendicolith.

Notes

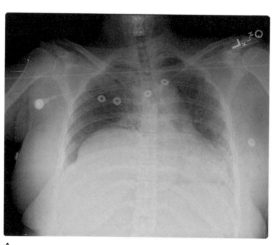

A

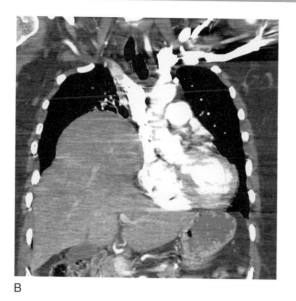

B

1. On which side is diaphragmatic rupture more common?

2. What is the common perception error in right-sided rupture?

3. What is the incidence of post-traumatic diaphragmatic rupture?

4. What are the clinical symptoms of right-sided diaphragmatic tear with liver in the thorax?

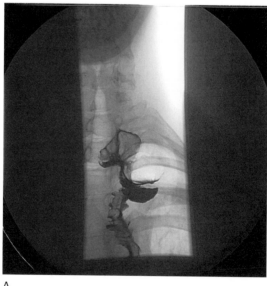

A

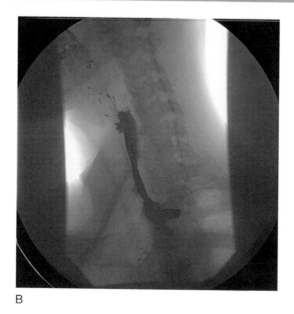

B

1. What congenital malformation was this patent born with?

2. What is the incidence of the malformation? What is the treatment?

3. What is the simplest way to make the diagnosis?

4. How would you perform the procedure?

CASE 127

Diaphragmatic Rupture with Liver in Chest

1. The left side.

2. Commonly mistaken for elevated hemidiaphragm or eventration.

3. Autopsy reports place it between 5% and 6%.

4. May have no symptoms or only vague abdominal pain.

Cross-Reference

Gastrointestinal Imaging: THE REQUISITES, ed 3, p 326.

Comments

Most diaphragmatic ruptures are not as dramatic as the one demonstrated in the case. This patient was involved in a high-speed motor collision. The supine portable image of the chest ought to arouse suspicion immediately because of what appears to be a high, rounded right-sided diaphragm. CT is the examination of choice but even here small diaphragmatic tears can be missed. It is a help for the radiologist to know that the likelihood of a diaphragmatic tear is eight times greater on the left. The thinking here is that the liver absorbs some of the traumatic shock that would have been otherwise transmitted in its entirety to the diaphragm. Although autopsy results put the incidence at between 5% and 6%, it is much lower clinically and radiologically. The reasons are that we probably do not see many of the patients who die before reaching the hospital and that the diagnosis is often difficult, even with CT. When discovered, a diaphragmatic tear should be surgically repaired. Most tears will result in bowel in the lower chest, and the risk of future bowel obstruction, ischemia, or even gastric volvulus is increased. This is generally applicable to right-sided tears as well. Having said that, almost every practicing radiologist has examined patients with bowel and in some cases liver in their chest who have no complaints relative to that finding. It is more than an "incidental" finding and should be handled as a significant finding. Other CT findings would include discontinuation of the diaphragmatic stripe. This should be evaluated in cases of blunt severe abdominal trauma but especially so if a liver laceration is identified.

Notes

CASE 128

Esophageal Atresia with Small Bowel Transposition

1. Esophageal atresia.

2. It is seen in about 1 in 4000 live births. Treatment is gastric or jejunal pull-through, as seen in this case.

3. Try to pass an NG tube.

4. Sit the baby upright and inject a small amount of thin barium through the NG tube. Avoid water-soluble contrast agent, as many of the variations of this malformation will have a tracheoesophageal communication.

Cross-Reference

Gastrointestinal Imaging: THE REQUISITES, ed 3, p 19.

Comments

The surgical repair of esophageal atresia can present the unsuspecting radiologist with some perplexing esophageal findings later in life when the patient undergoes an UGI examination. Again one must emphasize the importance to radiologists in training that we practice the specialty of radiologic imaging in the profession of medicine. Therefore, it is necessary when possible to talk to the patient prior to any examination, to answer all questions or concerns, and to take a concise past and current medical history. Such an approach would greatly reduce the likelihood of the resident being startled by the findings. In this case, this young individual had esophageal atresia at birth which was treated with jejunation interposition between the proximal esophagus and the stomach. Today, in an attempt to maintain the continuity of the bowel most of these surgeries are done using colonic interposition. Such procedures may also be seen in patients who have fibrosis and marked generalized stricturing of the esophagus, as well as in patients with adenocarcinomas of the distal esophagus or GE junction. The haustral fold pattern of the interposed colon is to some extent retained and is usually easily recognizable. In the case of jejunal interposition the normal jejunal pattern alters and is somewhat more difficult to recognize. The major long-term problem is gastric acid reflux, which is severe in almost 25% of these patients. A small number of cases (< 5%) will redevelop a tracheoesophageal fistula. If there is an increased risk of malignancy in these patients, it is with those adults whose interpositions were performed for malignancy. Although there has been some discussion in the literature about the risk of malignancy in interposition done for esophageal atresia, it seems to be minimal.

Notes

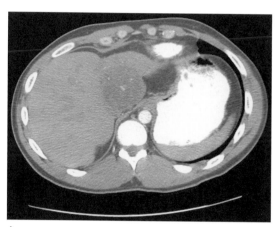

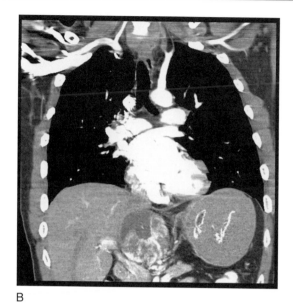

A

B

1. In this young patient with a solitary lesion in the left hepatic lobes, what are the diagnostic possibilities?

2. What is striking about this lesion?

3. What type of hepatoma occurs in young patients?

4. What conditions predispose an individual to develop this lesion?

C A S E   1 2 9

Fibrolamellar Hepatoma in 26-Year-Old Man

1. Focal nodular hyperplasia, hepatic adenoma, and fibrolamellar hepatoma.

2. The lesion is solitary, in a young adult (26-year-old man), and has tiny punctate calcifications on the noncontrasted image, and part of the lesion is very hypervascular on the enhanced image.

3. Fibrolamellar hepatoma.

4. None known.

Cross-Reference

Gastrointestinal Imaging: THE REQUISITES, ed 3, p 196.

Comments

Neoplasms of the liver in young patients can be caused by several different cell types. The most commonly encountered are focal nodular hyperplasia (FNH) and hepatic adenoma. Hemangiomas and metastases also must be considered. The appearance of this tumor in conjunction with a central scar or low-density areas is suggestive of FNH but also can occur in other conditions.

Fibrolamellar carcinoma is an unusual variant of conventional hepatocellular carcinoma (HCC) seen almost exclusively in younger patients. Also, the usual predisposing factors associated with HCC, such as cirrhosis or long-standing hepatitis, are not associated with fibrolamellar carcinoma. There is not believed to be any associated etiologic risk factors for the development of fibrolamellar hepatoma, but this possibility must be a strong consideration when liver masses are encountered in a young adult. The radiologic diagnosis can be difficult to make because the lesion may resemble other liver tumors. It typically has a central "scar" or area of fibrous or necrotic tissue that can resemble FNH in its appearance. Fibrolamellar hepatoma does calcify, as in this case, and has been described in up to 50% of patients. On CT scans the tumor is often hypodense, particularly its central scar. However, delayed images show increasing homogeneity or enhancement of the lesion with the surrounding liver, simulating a hemangioma. A poorly performed CT scan may underestimate the size of the lesion. Nuclear scanning may help differentiate the mass from FNH because fibrolamellar hepatoma does not have Kupffer cells.

The prognosis for patients with fibrolamellar hepatoma is much better than that for patients with HCC, and the lesion is potentially curable with surgery. Vascular invasion and other abnormalities of HCC are much less common in fibrolamellar hepatoma. This lesion also responds well to chemotherapy.

Notes

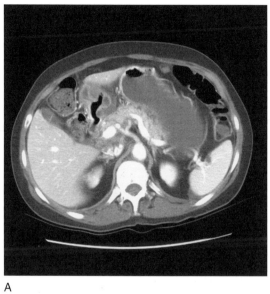

A

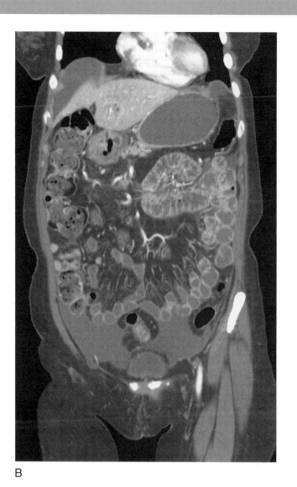

B

1. Describe the findings in this 68-year-old man who is losing weight.

2. Did disease originate in the stomach or duodenum?

3. Which disease is more likely to cross the pyloric channel into the duodenum: adenocarcinoma or gastric lymphoma?

4. What percentage of gastric malignancies are adenocarcinomas?

C A S E   1 3 0

Gastric Carcinoma Crossing Pylorus

1. There is a nodular mural lesion involving the distal antrum, crossing the pylorus, and invading and narrowing the duodenum. There is also evidence of intrapertitoneal spread of disease (fluid and small nodes) and possible liver involvement.

2. The stomach. Malignant disease involving the duodenal bulb with retrograde extension is virtually unheard of.

3. Gastric lymphoma.

4. About 95%.

Cross-Reference
Gastrointestinal Imaging: THE REQUISITES, ed 3, p 68.

Comments
About 95% of gastric malignancies are adenocarcinomas; 2% to 3% are lymphoma, and the rest are a rare assortment of other lesions, mostly malignant GISTs. It has long been taught that adenocarcinomas crossing the pylorus are very rare. Residents are taught that lymphoma has a greater disposition to cross the pylorus and affect the duodenum, adenocarcinomas much less so. This is true, however, when the question is posed: which lesions are found to have crossed the pylorus in more cases? This is simple logic. Although lymphomas have a greater tendency to cross the pylorus, they constitute only a tiny fraction of gastric malignancies compared to lymphomas. Thus the specific answer to a question phrased in such a manner is "adenocarcinoma."

The idea that adenocarcinomas only rarely cross into the duodenum comes from early radiologic literature. Residents were taught that the pylorus was a "barrier" to the extension of the gastric lesion in that direction. However, recent observations with microscopic support have suggested rather a different picture—that transpyloric extension of gastric carcinomas may be more common than we believed. Recent studies have found that transpyloric extension may be as high as 20%. This case demonstrates the point. Thus, lesions in the prepyloric gastric antrum can result in two significant complications. More common is gastric outlet obstruction (often in a patient with no past history of PUD), and now we must consider the possibility of transpyloric extension, even when not macroscopically visible.

Notes

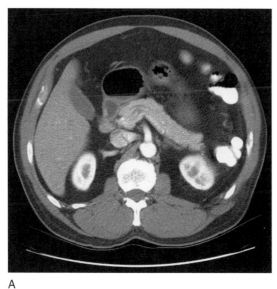

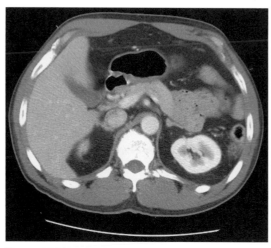

A   B

1. Considering Figure 131A, what might be the clinical history of this patient?

2. Figure 131B was obtained almost a year later. What does this tell you?

3. Approximately how often is this diagnosis missed or not seen on CT scanning?

4. Assuming that most of the time the lesion spontaneously regresses, what are some of the uncommon but serious complications that the patient is at risk for?

Subtle Pancreatic Trauma

1. Blunt trauma to the abdomen such as a motor vehicle collision.

2. It shows complete resolution of the pancreatic contusion and the tiny amount of fluid associated with it on the earlier image.

3. It varies. Some authors contend that subtle pancreatic contusions are missed in excess of 50% of cases.

4. Pancreatitis, bleeding, infection.

Cross-Reference
Gastrointestinal Imaging: THE REQUISITES, ed 3, p 174.

Comments
Pancreatic blunt trauma is not common, coming in at ninth or tenth on the list of organs most commonly injured in blunt trauma. It seems to be more common in penetrating trauma. MDCT (and in some cases clinical suspicions of subtle injury may require thin sections through the pancreas) is the examination of choice at the moment. The pancreas lying across the bony spine would seem to be a most obvious candidate for contusion or fracture in blunt trauma. The fact that it is not injured more often is puzzling. It may be that we are missing the subtle cases or that subtle cases are not seen on current CT technique. Most subtle injuries are located in the body of the pancreas. The intimate relationship of vascular structures to the pancreatic head makes diagnosis and the morbidity and mortality rates of pancreatic injury higher than at other sites in the pancreas. The aorta, subhepatic IVC, the SMA and SMC, and the confluence of the portal vein are all found around and contiguous with the substance of the pancreatic head. In this case the only evidence for pancreatic injury is a small amount of fluid seen paralleling the pancreatic duct in the body of the pancreas. In cases such as this specific treatment is not required and the outcome, as in this patient, is excellent. However, follow-up is recommended to ensure complete healing without complication.

Notes

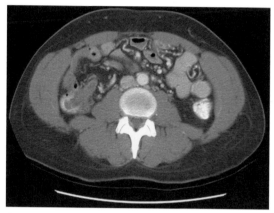

A

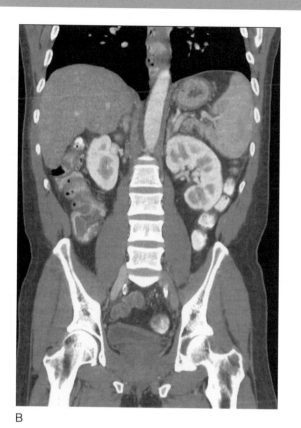

B

1. This patient is referred to you because of an outside diagnosis of cecal mass. What do you think?

2. What might be the cause of this mass?

3. What would you recommend for further workup?

4. What are the physiologic circumstances that might explain these findings?

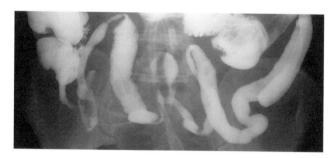

1. What chronic malabsorptive state may produce these changes?

2. What may occur during the acute phase of bone marrow transplantation?

3. When does graft-versus-host disease occur?

4. What organs are involved by graft-versus-host disease?

C A S E   1 3 2

Prolapsed Terminal Ileum in Cecum

1. This is a normal CT study of the abdomen.

2. Prolapse of the terminal ileum into the cecum.

3. None.

4. In some patients when the cecum is empty, parts of the terminal ileum may prolapse into the cecum.

Cross-Reference
Gastrointestinal Imaging: THE REQUISITES, ed 3, p 277.

Comments
With the advent of CT we have had the opportunity of seeing ileocecal function, even with our static imaging. It has long been suspected by fluoroscopists that prolapse through the ileocecal valve occurs when the right colon, and in particular the ileocecal valve, is empty. This must be distinguished from an ileocoloic interception, which is truly pathologic and almost always has an underlying cause and is invariably symptomatic. Conversely when the cecum becomes distended the prolapsed ileum returns to its normal position, and indeed in some patients with incompetent ileocecal valves there may be reflux of colonic material into the terminal ileum. These are things to look for on routine CT studies of the abdomen. The two other possibilities that might warrant consideration are (1) the aforementioned ileocecal intussusception and (2) ileocecal valve masses and true cecal masses. Evaluate the surrounding pericolic fat looking for stranding of small nodes. Evaluate the serosal wall of the bowel to ensure it is crisp. Take care to identify the possibility of ileocecal valve lipomatosis, which is a benign condition. Make sure there is node suggestion of obstruction. If there is any concern, ask for a barium enema for confirmation. In this case the BE was normal with no trace of a cecal mass.

Notes

C A S E   1 3 3

Graft-versus-Host Disease in a Bone Marrow Transplant

1. Sprue (the moulage pattern).

2. Enteritis with diarrhea and pain secondary to radiation or chemotherapy.

3. Typically within 100 days of the bone marrow transplant.

4. Gastrointestinal tract, skin, liver, and lungs.

Cross-Reference
Gastrointestinal Imaging: THE REQUISITES, ed 3, p 125.

Comments
Transplant recipients face a variety of gastrointestinal complications, which are typically related to the immunosuppressive drugs taken to prevent rejection. Peptic ulcer disease, bowel perforation, and opportunistic infections are common. Pancreatitis and hepatitis also occur more frequently in these patients.

In patients who undergo bone marrow transplants for various diseases, another set of complications can occur in addition to those already mentioned. In the initial induction phase of therapy, during which the native bone marrow is destroyed, the patient receives high-dose radiation or chemotherapy. During this phase, acute enteritis with diarrhea, pain, and bleeding may develop because of the loss of mucosal cells lining the bowel. In the latter stages the transplanted marrow (graft) may mount an immune response against the body (host), producing the so-called graft-versus-host (GVH) disease. This rejection typically occurs within the first few months of bone marrow transplant, although later development is possible.

The major organs involved in GVH disease include the skin, gastrointestinal tract, lungs, and liver. Patients develop a diffuse rash, protein-losing diarrhea, and jaundice. Abnormalities encountered in the small bowel include fold thickening, which may progress to complete effacement of the folds; luminal narrowing; and separation of the bowel loops. Similar changes also may occur in the colon, resembling chronic ulcerative colitis. Pneumatosis of the bowel also has been reported. Gastric abnormalities include dilation and delayed gastric emptying. An unusual radiologic abnormality is prolonged barium coating of the mucosa. CT findings include bowel wall thickening, the "halo" sign caused by bowel wall edema, pericolic inflammation, and mesenteric thickening.

Notes

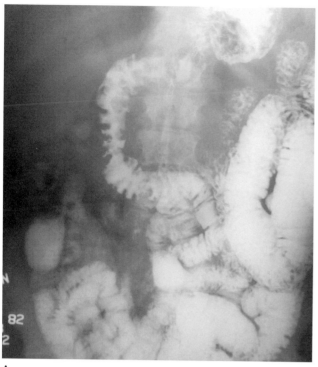

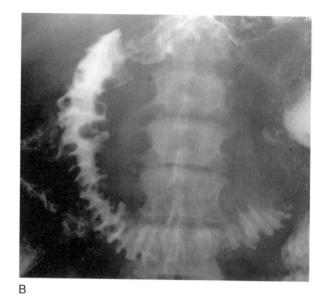

A

B

1. What conditions may produce elevated serum gastrin levels?

2. What are the major symptoms of elevated gastrin levels?

3. What structures in the body contain histamine?

4. What organs are involved in systemic mastocytosis?

Mastocytosis of Small Bowel

1. Gastrinoma, histamine release, achlorhydria, pernicious anemia, and G-cell hyperplasia.

2. Abdominal pain secondary to peptic ulcer disease and diarrhea caused by malabsorption.

3. Mast cells.

4. Skin, gastrointestinal tract, bone, liver, and spleen.

Cross-Reference
Gastrointestinal Imaging: THE REQUISITES, ed 3, p 127.

Comments
A number of clinical conditions produce elevated serum gastrin levels. The best known cause is Zollinger-Ellison (Z-E) syndrome, resulting from a gastrin-producing tumor. Another condition associated with elevated gastrin is mastocytosis. Mastocytosis is an accumulation of mast cells in the skin and various other organs. Mast cells are responsible for storage and release of histamine. Histamine increases gastrin levels, although not to the extent seen in patients with Z-E syndrome (often in excess of 1000 pg/mL).

Mastocytosis typically involves the skin. When the mast cells are disturbed and release histamine, they produce raised elevations, accounting for the disease description urticaria pigmentosa. It is less commonly known that other organs may be involved with a mast cell infiltrate; this occurrence is termed systemic mastocytosis. The gastrointestinal tract (small bowel) is the second most commonly involved organ after the skin; the bone, liver, and spleen also can be involved. There can be both local and systemic release of histamine. Clinically, patients complain of bouts of diarrhea, flushing, and tachycardia. Alcohol consumption may precipitate the symptoms, and the condition is treated with histamine receptor antagonists.

Radiologically, small bowel examination shows thickened folds and sometimes bowel wall thickening. Because of the increased gastrin levels, there is a higher incidence of peptic ulcer disease, as well as increased secretions in the small bowel. All these abnormalities may be present in the individual with Z-E syndrome. However, mastocytosis can involve the bone marrow, producing diffuse sclerotic changes. In this case the vertebral bodies are quite dense. Whenever the diagnostic considerations for thickened small bowel with some nodularity are being pondered, one should always look at the bones. Sclerotic bones, along with the fold abnormalities, suggests the diagnosis of mastocytosis.

Notes

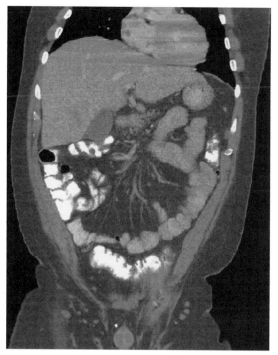

A

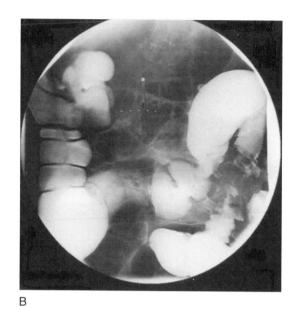

B

1. Both these patients have the same disease. List the findings.

2. What would be your first diagnostic consideration?

3. What inflammatory processs might also have this appearance?

4. Would you consider Crohn's disease?

Actinomycosis of Sigmoid Colon

1. The coronal CT image shows soft tissue density involving the sigmoid colon with pericolonic extension, also invading and breaching the lower muscular abdominal wall. The barium shows segmental involvement with severe spasm and mucosal destruction.

2. Regardless of the lack of classical findings, the first diagnostic consideration must be carcinoma of the colon.

3. Inflammatory processes such as diverticulitis, appendagitis, fungal infections, and actinomycosis would all be possibilities. Tuberculosis might be considered, especially if the focal area was in the right colon.

4. No. The focal involvement may mimic Crohn's disease, but with the remainder of the colon having a normal appearance, it would be an unlikely diagnostic consideration.

Cross-Reference

Gastrointestinal Imaging: THE REQUISITES, ed 3, p 317.

Comments

Actinomycosis is a relatively uncommon inflammatory entity caused by the commonly found anaerobic bacterium, *Actinomyces israeli,* a gram-positive bacillus, which is a component of the normal human flora and can be found in the mouths of most people. When the cellular environment is conducive for anaerobic proliferation, it is possible for *Actinomyces* to proliferate, migrate, and infect tissue. It can occur almost anywhere in the body. Bowel involvement is uncommon, although it has increased in frequency over the last few decades. The most common sites of the disease seems to be the sigmoid colon, although involvement of the right colon has been described in the literature. Actinomycosis, like syphilis, can mimic other diseases, such as colonic diverticulitis, abscesses, appendagitis, and malignant tumors, presenting a diagnostic challenge, and unfortunately often identified postoperatively in many of the cases.

Diagnosis can be determined with endoscopy and imaging techniques, such as CT and MRI, where the striking characteristic of actinomycosis is best displayed; it is the tendency of the disease to routinely breach normal barriers to disease such as muscle and fascial planes. Other common findings in CT scan and barium study include mural invasion with stricture formation, mass effect with tapered narrowing of the lumen, and thickened mucosal folds. In many cases the radiologic findings are similar to those of intestinal tuberculosis and destructive malignant tumors.

Notes

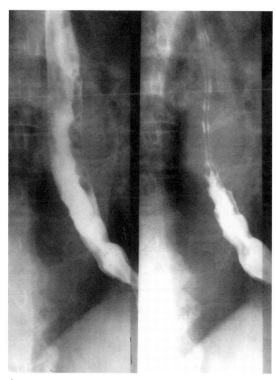

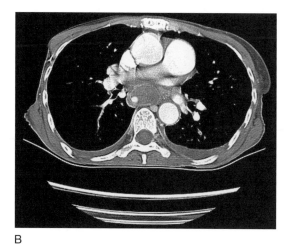

A

B

1. From the barium esophagogram, what are the radiologic findings and most likely diagnosis?

2. The cross-sectional CT image of the lower thorax suggests what serious complication?

3. What underlying condition might this patient suffer from?

4. What forms of treatment are currently available for this condition?

Bleeding Esophageal Varices

1. Uphill esophageal varices.

2. Massive UGI bleeding.

3. Liver cirrhosis and portal venous hypertension would be the primary consideration.

4. Balloon tamponade, IV fluid push, packed red blood cells, vasopressors.

Cross-Reference
Gastrointestinal Imaging: THE REQUISITES, ed 3, p 9.

Comments
The barium esophagogram shows marginal smooth serpiginous lesions of the distal esophagus which seem to change with patient position and Valsalva breathing. These important distinguishing features differentiate it from the so-called "varicoid carcinoma," which spreads linearly along the submucosa and can give a static image similar to varices. The CT image was obtained on a 56-year-old man presenting with hematemesis, which fortuitously shows old blood filling the distal esophagus along with a tiny collection of active bleeding (seen in the lumen as a bright spot). The goal of treatment is to stop the acute bleeding as soon as possible, and treat persistent varices with medicines and medical procedures. Bleeding must be controlled quickly to prevent shock and death. In endoscopic therapy the varices may be injected directly with a clotting medication or a rubber band placed around the bleeding veins. This procedure is used in acute bleeding episodes and as prophylactic (buying time) therapy.

Acute bleeding may also be treated by a balloon tamponade, a special tube that is inserted through the nose into the stomach and inflated with air to produce pressure against the bleeding veins.

In the transjugular intrahepatic portosystemic shunt (TIPS) procedure, a catheter is extended through a vein across the liver where it connects the portal blood vessels to the regular veins in the body, and decreases pressure in the portal vein system. In addition, medications may be used to decrease portal blood flow and to slow bleeding.

In addition to TIPS, intra-abdominal emergency surgery may be used (rarely) to treat patients if other therapy fails. Portacaval shunts or even surgical removal of the esophagus are two surgical treatment options, but these procedures have a high death rate.

Patients presenting with moderate to severe bleeding from esophageal varices can cause a dramatic and messy ER situation. Some patients can exsanguinate before treatment can stanch the loss of blood. It is estimated that of people in the United States with portal hypertension 5% to 15% will have esophageal varices. CT images of the active variceal bleeding in the esophagus are unusual, but may be seen if the bleed is small and continuous, such as in this case. Each episode of variceal hemorrhage carries a 20% to 30% risk of death, and up to 70% of patients who do not receive treatment die within 1 year of the initial bleeding episode.

Notes

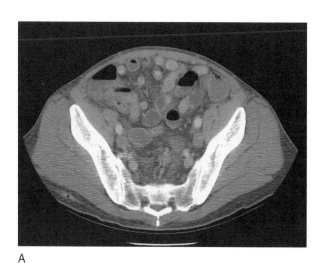

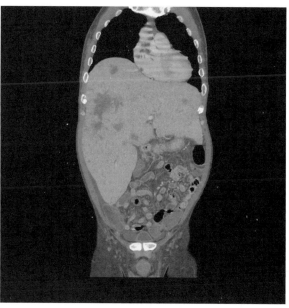

A   B

1. This person was seen in the ER with RLQ pain. How would you describe the appearance of the appendix in the transaxial image?

2. Could this be simple appendicitis?

3. What is the most common neoplasm of the appendix?

4. What percentage of GI malignancies are appendiceal in origin?

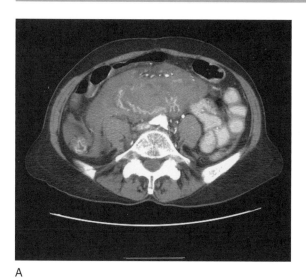

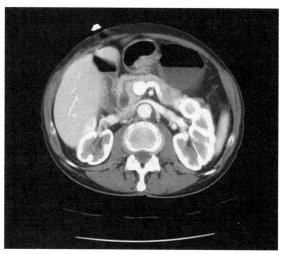

A   B

1. What is the radiopaque material seen in the huge upper abdominal mass in Figure 138A?

2. What might be the clinical history of this patient?

3. What other secondary diagnoses should be considered with an upper abdominal mass of this size?

4. Figure 138B was obtained 6 weeks later. How does this affect your diagnosis?

CASE 137

Appendiceal Carcinoma Presenting Clinically Like Acute Appendicitis

1. Swollen with some air-fluid levels in the area.

2. On the transaxial image it might be tempting to say it was simple appendicitis, but the mesentery is not clean, raising some suspicion. On the other hand, the coronal image shows widespread disease.

3. Benign carcinoid.

4. Slightly less than 1%.

Cross-Reference

Gastrointestinal Imaging: THE REQUISITES, ed 3, p 280.

Comments

Primary neoplasm of the appendix is uncommon, representing fewer than 1% of all GI tumors. The most common are benign carcinoids. The most common of the primary malignant lesions of the appendix is adenocarcinoma, most frequently a mucinous adenocarcinoma. Because of this and other mucoid lesions of the appendix, the presence of pseudomyoma peritonei is always a possibility. Most patients, as in this case, present with acute appendicitis-like symptoms. The lesions are often found on routine appendectomy. Most of the carcinoids are found incidentally during postmortem examination. The primary lesions are often small, but upon inspection of the appendix and abdomen during surgery the appendix is found to be thickened and hard and the leaves of the mesentery are studded with innumerable tiny yellow metastatic deposits. There will often be ascitic fluid. CT is the examination of choice. Although the disease is rare, if the thickened wall appendix does not look like edema, or there are adjacent nodes, hazy density of the mesentery, or evidence of distal disease, the diagnosis should be considered. An inflamed appendix may weep small amounts of fluid into the peritoneal cavity which collect in the pelvic recesses, and unless the ascites is significant, it is a lesser sign.

Notes

CASE 138

Huge Duodenal Hematoma Resolved after 6 Weeks

1. Gastrografin within the lumen of the duodenum.

2. A large lymphomatous mass might be a consideration; however, this patient was in a motor vehicle collision and the possibility of a huge upper adominal hematoma of duodenal origin must be considered.

3. Gastric outlet obstruction and biliary obstruction, both of which this patient had.

4. The mass is almost completely resolved except for some residual duodenal wall thickening confirming the diagnosis of a huge hematoma.

Cross-Reference

Gastrointestinal Imaging: THE REQUISITES, ed 3, p 97.

Comments

Numerous references in the literature discuss large duodenal hematomas being mistakenly diagnosed as upper abdominal masses. These hematomas are present without a history of trauma, but from this case we can see why such a diagnostic mistake is possible, even with the history of motor vehicle collision. Huge lymphomatous masses (root of mesentry and retroperitoneal adenopathy) through which the duodenum passes unobstructed, the so-called "sandwich sign," is a good example. This patient experienced both gastric outlet obstruction and a degree of obstruction of the biliary duct, was decompressed with an NG tube, and was treated conservatively and continuously improved. No bile duct intervention was required and a CT obtained 6 weeks later shows almost complete resolution of the hematoma. However, not all large upper abdominal hematomas present with a history of trauma. Sometimes the history is suppressed. Sometimes the patient has a coagulability problem. Sometimes it is entirely idiopathic. Some of these patients, unfortunately, are diagnosed at surgery.

Notes

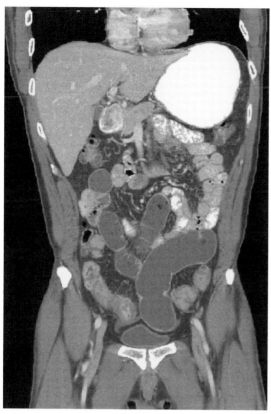

A

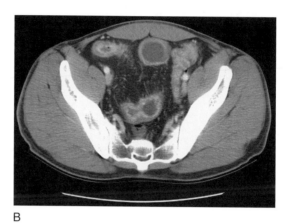

B

1. What is the most striking feature shown on these images?

2. What is the most common cause of small bowel obstruction in young adults?

3. What inflammatory processes can result in SBO?

4. From these images what might you postulate the cause of the SBO to be?

Crohn's Disease Presenting as a Small Bowel Obstruction

1. High-grade small bowel obstruction, with normal caliber small bowel distally.

2. The same as in older adults, postoperative adhesions.

3. Crohn's disease, acute appendicitis, and even some cases of acute diverticulitis have been reported as presenting with SBO.

4. The distal ileum shows thickened walls and some stranding in the surrounding fat, all very suggestive of Crohn's disease, which this patient had.

Cross-Reference
Gastrointestinal Imaging: THE REQUISITES, ed 3, p 114.

Comments
It is unusual for Crohn's disease to present as a small bowel obstruction. However, a small percentage of patients will present in just such a fashion, often creating some diagnostic confusion. Why this occurs is not absolutely clear. It is probably a true inflammatory stricture further complicated by additional inflammation and edema, possibly around the site of a developing sinus or fistulous tract. CT imaging, and especially MDCT multiplanar imaging, has greatly increased the diagnostic capability of the physician. Although uncommon, a young patient presenting with small bowel obstruction and no history of prior abdominal surgery should raise the possibility of Crohn's disease or acute appendicitis. Crohn's patients presenting with acute small bowel obstruction represent about 2% of all newly seen disease. It is one of the few reasons that the treatment of these patients may be surgical. In some patients NG suction and high-dose steroids may relieve obstructive symptoms.

Notes

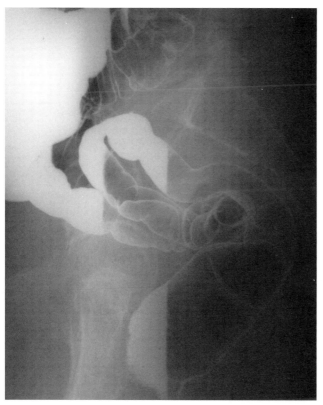

A

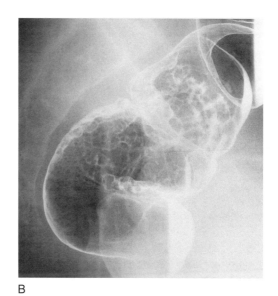

B

1. What do these radiographs of the rectum have in common?

2. What is the most frequent histologic diagnosis?

3. What is the incidence of carcinoma in these lesions?

4. What condition may have similar appearance in the ascending colon and cecum?

C A S E 1 4 0

Carpet Lesions of the Rectum

1. Superficial carpet lesions of the rectum. One is more obvious, the other more subtle. Can you find it?

2. Villous adenoma.

3. 20% to 40%.

4. So-called urticaria of the colon.

Cross-Reference
Gastrointestinal Imaging: THE REQUISITES, ed 3, p 268.

Comments
Neoplastic lesions of the colon usually present as polypoid protuberances into the lumen of the bowel. On occasion they grow superficially or even infiltrate through the wall of the bowel. The "carpet" lesion of the colon results when a neoplastic growth develops superficially along the mucosa rather than growing in a polypoid fashion. This growth produces a subtle irregularity of the mucosal surface, and the barium that becomes entrapped within the interstices of the lesion has the appearance of shag carpet, hence the terminology. The more subtle lesion is on the anterior rectal wall, which is slightly flat (instead of the usual concavity) and slightly irregular. Tumors that develop in this fashion typically occur in areas of the colon where the diameter is quite large. Most are found in the rectum and cecum and to a lesser extent in the ascending colon. These areas are where peristaltic activity is least likely to push an intraluminal lesion distally, which may promote intraluminal growth as seen in other areas.

Pathologically these tumors tend to be predominantly villous adenomas and are potentially dangerous, as many will contain foci of malignancy. Some authors consider villous adenoma as a premalignant lesion. It would be extremely rare for these lesions to be simple adenomas. The lesions typically are larger than 3 cm because they are often difficult to diagnose when they are small. Lacking the intraluminal component, only with good double-contrast technique can the subtle mucosal irregularity be appreciated. It is a well-known fact that the incidence of carcinoma in colonic adenomas increases with increasing size as well as with villous histologic findings. Some large carpet lesion may have villous histologic features but turn out not to be malignant. Carcinoma in these lesions should be considered potential carcinomas until proved otherwise. These lesions are usually too large to be removed endoscopically and because of their lack of intraluminal components are not amenable to endoscopic removal.

Notes

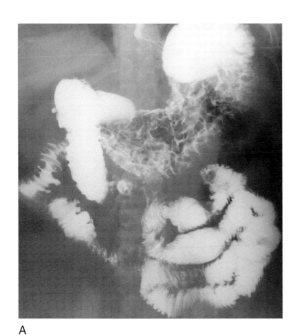

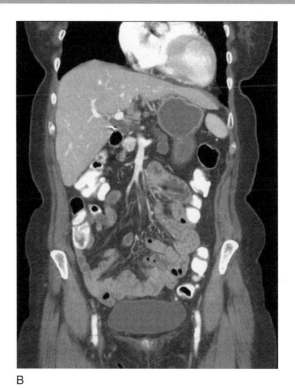

A   B

1. In multiple endocrine neoplasia (MEN) syndrome I, what organs are involved by tumors?

2. What are the locations and incidence of extrapancreatic gastrinomas?

3. Approximately what percentage of gastrinomas are malignant?

4. Besides multiple ulcers, what is another common symptom of gastrinomas?

Zollinger-Ellison Syndrome

1. Pancreas (gastrinoma), parathyroid, pituitary, and adrenal gland.

2. Duodenum (about 15%) and other organs (about 10%), such as para-aortic region, bladder, and ovaries.

3. Approximately 60%.

4. Diarrhea.

Cross-Reference
Gastrointestinal Imaging: THE REQUISITES, ed 3, p 98.

Comments
Zollinger-Ellison (Z-E) syndrome is caused by gastrin secretion from non–islet cell tumors of the pancreas, so-called gastrinomas. The large majority (> 75%) occur in the pancreas, but this tumor is also known to occur in ectopic locations. Approximately 15% of gastrinomas are found in the duodenum, and the remainder are in the para-aortic region, bladder, ovaries, and even liver. About one quarter are associated with multiple endocrine neoplasia syndrome I (MEN-I), which also causes tumors of the parathyroid, pituitary, and adrenal glands. The majority of gastrinomas are malignant and have a propensity for early metastases. Those tumors associated with the MEN-I syndrome have a lesser incidence of malignancy, however. On CT the gastrinomas are usually hypervascular and are best seen on the arterial phase of scanning. The small enhancing mass is seen in the pancreatic head just to the right of the origin of the SMA on the coronal CT image in this case.

Clinically, patients develop peptic ulcer disease because of the acid hypersecretion related to the elevated gastrin levels. Most ulcers in patients with Z-E syndrome occur in the gastric antrum and duodenal bulb. Occasionally, ulcers occur in the distal duodenum. Although they are uncommon even in patients with Z-E syndrome, distal duodenal ulcers are so rare in healthy patients that they are considered a feature of the disease. Serum gastrin levels can be variable in patients with Z-E syndrome, although any level above 1000 units is indicative of the condition. Often a gastrin-provocative test using secretin is necessary to determine the presence of a gastrinoma. (This test produces a dramatic rise in serum gastrin levels in affected patients.)

The gastric acid hypersecretion may present as increased fluid in the stomach, along with thickened rugal folds. Many gastrinoma patients also complain of diarrhea. The increased acidity in the small bowel interferes with the function of the small bowel enzymes, resulting in diminished intestinal absorption. In severe cases a spruelike condition may ensue, with villous atrophy, malabsorption, and steatorrhea.

Notes

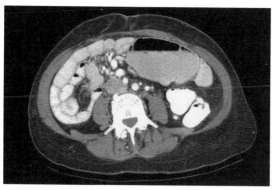
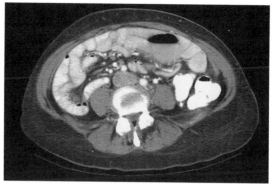

A   B

1. What strikes you as "unusual" in these images?

2. On Figure 142B, what are the relative positions of the SMA and the SMV?

3. How does this condition manifest itself clinically?

4. What other anatomic anomalies might be associated with this condition?

CASE 143

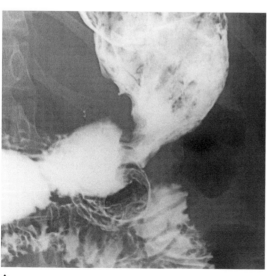
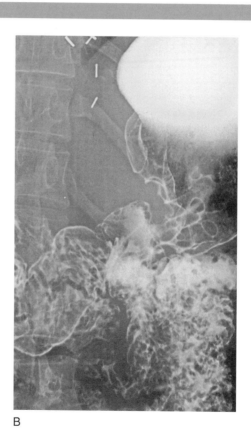

A   B

1. Describe the findings in these images.

2. What do they imply about the patient's past medical history?

3. What is a pseudolymphoma of the stomach?

4. What activity is responsible for these findings?

Midgut Malrotation

1. The position of the small bowel and cecum are abnormal. The cecum is seen on the left side of the abdomen and the small bowel is almost entirely on the right in this case of midgut malrotation.

2. They are reversed. The SMA should normally be to the left of the SMV.

3. In adults it is almost always an incidental finding. In children it is associated with midgut volvulus (life-threatening condition) and duodenal obstruction secondary to Ladd bands.

4. Congenital anomalies such as congenital heart disease, abdominal wall defects, imperforate anus, annular pancreas, and biliary atresia.

Cross-Reference

Gastrointestinal Imaging: THE REQUISITES, ed 3, p 146.

Comments

It is important to remember that the human gut herniates into the umbilicus at about 6 weeks of intrauterine life. This herniation results in 270 degrees of counterclockwise rotation around the superior mesenteric artery before re-entering the coelomic cavity at 12 weeks. The process can be faulty in about 1 in 500 live births with failure of achieving the full 270 degrees, resulting in degrees of malrotation abnormality.

In adults the finding of midgut malrotation often is an incidental finding. The colon is usually found on the left. The small bowel is on the right and the positions of the SMA and SMV are reversed. In addition, the position of the ligament of Treitz can be located in the midline or even the right upper abdomen. About 60% of all symptomatic midgut malrotations are diagnosed by one year. A barium upper GI study is still the fastest and most inexpensive method of diagnosis. In some adults there may be vague symptoms present that bring the patient to a diagnostic workup, such as low-grade chronic recurrent abdominal pain and symptoms suggestive of malabsorption.

Notes

Pseudotumor of the Stomach

1. Nodular marginal mass on the distal lesser curvature of the stomach.

2. The "nodular mass" is a prominent plication defect secondary to a prior Billroth I surgery for PUD.

3. Pseudolymphoma is a confusing benign lesion of the stomach that mimics malignant disease in its appearance. It is also known as lymphoreticular hyperplasia.

4. Surgery.

Cross-Reference

Gastrointestinal Imaging: THE REQUISITES, ed 3, p 86.

Comments

The most important aspect of this case is the importance of having a correct and relevant patient history prior to doing a procedure. In this particular case the history was not given with the imaging request and the radiologist failed to get the history of prior gastric surgery from the patient. Thus, the "heaped up" nodular appearance of the lesser curvature of the distal stomach was misdiagnosed as a possible malignancy. In fact, it is a pseudotumor of the stomach caused by the large plication defect that results from anastomosing a large lumen to a smaller lumen. This case is a reminder to residents in training that they are physicians and that no procedure should ever be undertaken without first talking to the patient (if possible) and obtaining a short, concise, and relevant history. Pseudotumor of the stomach should not be confused with pseudolymphoma of the stomach, the appearance of which mimics an aggressive lymphoma or even adenocarcinoma. Pseudolymphomas of the stomach are fortunately rare, but should be included (near the bottom of the list) in the differential diagnosis of any large aggressive appearing, seemingly destructive lesion of the stomach.

Notes

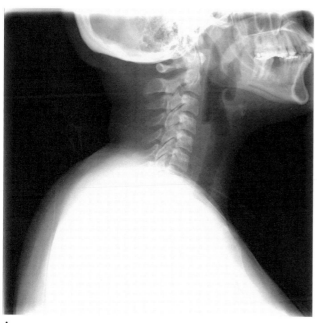

A

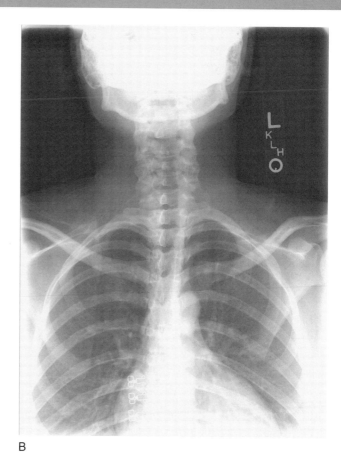

B

1. What might this patient's story be?

2. Describe the finding.

3. Is this the best way of imaging the finding?

4. What complications can result from this finding?

Fishbone Stuck in Upper Esophagus

1. Patient was at a picnic and got something caught in the throat.

2. A slender linear radiopacity is seen in the soft tissues (esophagus) anterior to the C6-C7 disk space, and behind the tracheal airway is a chicken bone.

3. CT.

4. Esophageal perforation, mediastinitis, mediastinal abscesses, and even vascular penetration or injury if the point of the chicken bone lodges at the level of the aortic arch and penetrates both the esophagus and the arch.

Cross-Reference

Gastrointestinal Imaging: THE REQUISITES, ed 3, p 37.

Comments

Fish or chicken bones caught in the cervical esophagus are a problem, first, because they are the most common foreign body seen in the upper esophagus, and second, because they are among the hardest to see on routine imaging. They may not be radiopaque enough to see. There may be laryngeal calcifications that obscure them. Plain images of the neck have a low yield (approximately 20%). The contrast agent–soaked cotton pledgets used prior to the advent of high-quality CT were virtually useless and a waste of time and radiation. For as many times as I have been asked to do this examination for the suspicion of a fish or chicken bone lodged in the upper esophagus, I have never seen a positive result. The idea was that the contrast agent–soaked pledget would hang up on the bone. Plain images may still be used as a screening tool, but ultimately the examination of choice is CT of the neck and upper esophagus. CT not only will identify the foreign body in almost every case but also will assess the area around the bone for penetration and complication. When a fish or chicken bone passes and is in the distal GI tract, the problem is usually solved. However, it should be remembered that the lodging and then passing of sharp objects may cause an abrasion of the upper esophageal mucosa. In these cases the patient's symptoms will not abate with the passing of the bone, but may continue until the healing of the abrasion.

Notes

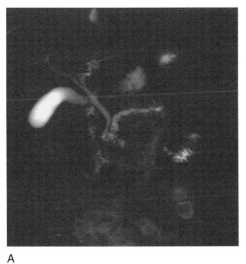

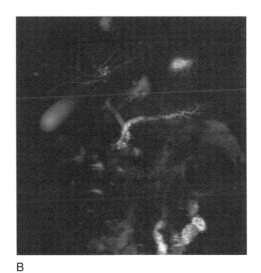

A   B

1. What does MRCP stand for?

2. How can you know with some degree of confidence if you are dealing with a pancreatic head mass or chronic pancreatitis?

3. What might a lesion in the pancreatic head look like on MRCP?

4. Currently, what is the best imaging modality for evaluating the pancreas for potential malignancy masses?

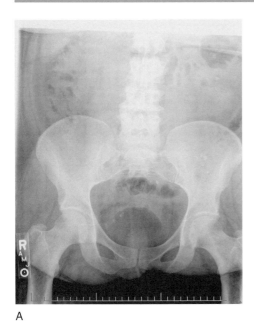

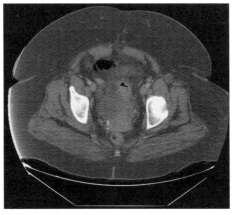

A   B

1. What is the significant finding on the plain image of the abdomen?

2. What symptoms might this patient report?

3. What conditions might result in such symptoms and radiologic findings?

4. What is the most common cause?

MRCP Chronic Pancreatitis

1. Magnetic resonance cholangiopancreatography.

2. One can never know with absolute certainty, but the lack of intra- and extrahepatic bile duct dilatation and the presence of a dilated tortuous pancreatic duct with the secondary ducts visible are very suggestive of chronic pancreatic inflammation.

3. Pancreatic ductal dilatation is usually uniform distal to the lesion, the lesion is often visible, and bile duct obstruction is common.

4. At the moment MDCT with multiplanar capacity is the best way to image a possible lesion of the pancreas.

Cross-Reference

Gastrointestinal Imaging: THE REQUISITES, ed 3, p 158.

Comments

Although there is still considerable controversy as to the role of MRCP in the workup of biliary and pancreatic lesions, it can be summed up with this straightforward question: Will MRCP replace ERCP (endoscopic retrograde cholangiopancreatography)? The question begs an answer, in that any noninvasive diagnostic procedure that has the potential to replace an invasive procedure and achieve the same results is a straightforward patient care issue. ERCP is currently considered the "gold standard" for diagnosis of biliary obstruction and some pancreatic processes. However, it carries with it the same risks of perforation of the bowel as routine endoscopy. Today MRCP is often used for failed ERCP or patients who might not tolerate the procedure. However, this may change. No patient preparation is required for MRCP, usually no sedation is necessary, and contraindications of MRCP are fewer than ERCP. Because of all this, studies to compare the sensitivity and specificity of the two techniques are ongoing. The initial results suggest that MRCP is a comparable examination for diagnostic purposes to ERCP without many of the associated risks. However, ERCP can also be an interventional procedure (used to place a stent, remove a stone, etc.) and will remain an important part of biliary-pancreatic medicine.

Notes

Enterocystic Fistula

1. Air in the urinary bladder. Ovoid air-filled structure in the base of the midpelvis.

2. Pneumaturia, abdominal pain, fever which broke about the time the patient experienced pneumaturia.

3. Tuberculosis, Crohn's disease, actinomycosis, diverticulitis, neoplastic disease, and postradiation treatment of the pelvis.

4. Sigmoid diverticulitis.

Cross-Reference

Gastrointestinal Imaging: THE REQUISITES, ed 3, p 141.

Comments

Of the many things to consider in the radiologic evaluation of the plain image of the abdomen is the question, "Is there air in unexpected places?" In this case, allowing for exclusion of other innocuous causes such as bladder catheterization, air is seen in the urinary bladder and must be considered abnormal, and a pathologic fistuluous connection to an air-containing adjacent hollow organ viscus is a prime diagnostic consideration. When considering the diagnostic considerations, age and medical history become important. In a young patient, one might consider Crohn's disease and possibly tuberculosis. If the patient has had a pelvic neoplasm treated with pelvic radiation, it raises the possibility of a radiation-induced fistulous connection to bowel. Older patients would be more likely to have colonic diverticulitis as the underlying process. From the plain film it is not difficult to ascertain that we are dealing with an older patient (73-year-old woman). The transaxial image confirms pelvic inflammation with an air-containing tract. Sigmoid diverticulosis was the underlying cause. The paracolic abscess pointed to and connected with the bladder. With the naturally occurring abscess drainage, the patient reported feeling better, but experiencing pneumaturia.

Notes

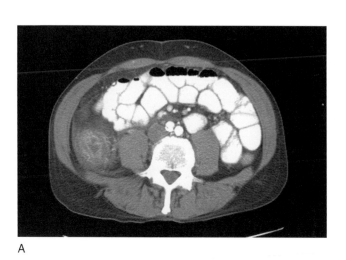

A

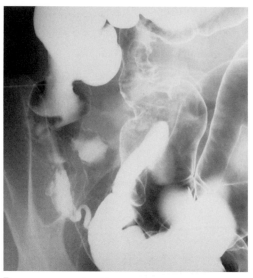

B

1. What neoplastic processes may produce multifocal involvement of the colon?

2. Name some infectious processes that may have this type of appearance.

3. What type of inflammatory bowel disease should be considered?

4. If the patient has pulmonary disease, what is a likely diagnosis?

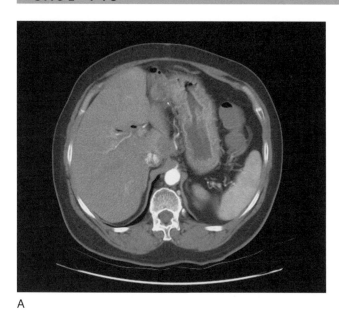

A

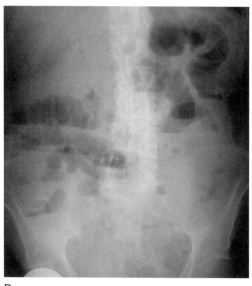

B

1. What is this condition called?

2. What are the three radiographic features associated with this condition?

3. Where does the stone most often impact itself?

4. What is necessary for the condition to develop?

Tuberculosis of Cecum

1. Lymphoma and serosal metastases.

2. Tuberculosis and amebiasis.

3. Crohn's disease.

4. Tuberculosis.

Cross-Reference

Gastrointestinal Imaging: THE REQUISITES, ed 3, p 300.

Comments

The barium enema illustration in this case shows some deformity of the cecum. If you look carefully you will see there is also an irregular area of narrowing in the transverse colon. The CT image shows thickening and deformity of the cecum with a narrowed lumen. These findings indicate that the process is multifocal in nature. A variety of conditions must be considered in this instance. One of the most common inflammatory processes of the ileocecal region is Crohn's disease. It also can affect any portion of the gastrointestinal tract, and the colon is a likely area for further involvement. Possible infectious processes include amebiasis and tuberculosis. Both of these conditions can affect the ileocecal area, as well as the rest of the colon. Of the possible neoplastic processes, the most likely is serosal metastasis, which has an affinity for the cecal region. Lymphoma must always be considered in the differential diagnosis of multifocal gastrointestinal lesions.

The final, correct diagnosis for this patient was tuberculosis. When a chest radiograph was finally obtained, the patient had upper lobe pulmonary findings consistent with tuberculosis. However, a normal chest x-ray film should not preclude this diagnosis because intestinal tuberculosis can occur without an abnormal chest film, especially in HIV patients. Most intestinal tuberculosis occurs as a result of the patient with pulmonary tuberculosis swallowing infected sputum; the intestinal tuberculosis is usually secondary. Adenopathy may occur in patients with intestinal tuberculosis but also occurs in those with Crohn's disease or lymphoma and therefore does not help differentiate the conditions. Patients with these findings in the right lower quadrant are often misdiagnosed as having Crohn's disease.

Notes

Gallstone Ileus

1. Gallstone ileus.

2. Gallstone in the bowel, small bowel dilation, and air in the biliary system.

3. Terminal ileum.

4. Cholecystenteric fistula must develop and the stone must be large enough to become impacted in the terminal ileum.

Cross-Reference

Gastrointestinal Imaging: THE REQUISITES, ed 3, p 136.

Comments

The term "gallstone ileus" refers to an unusual set of circumstances that develop in conjunction with chronic gallbladder disease and stone formation. In this condition a large gallstone or gallstones develop. There must also be associated chronic cholecystitis. During this inflammation, a portion of the bowel becomes adherent to the gallbladder, which is actually a common occurrence in patients with chronic gallbladder inflammation. With time, the gallstone erodes through the gallbladder wall and into the lumen of the bowel, resulting in a cholecystenteric fistula. The fistula most commonly extends into the duodenum, but extension into the colon and even the stomach also has been reported. As the large gallstone travels through the bowel lumen, it becomes impacted at a site where the lumen narrows, resulting in bowel dilation or obstruction.

The classic triad in this condition consists of air in the biliary system, bowel obstruction, and a radiopaque stone evident in the abdomen. The biliary air is seen in about 50% of cases and is secondary to the fistula that is open between the gallbladder and bowel. Often, the amount of air is quite small. The stone is the most difficult finding to establish because of the bowel dilation. If it is not obscured by the contrast material, the stone often can be demonstrated on CT. Finally, the bowel obstruction usually occurs in the terminal ileum at the ileocecal valve. Rarely, the stone obstructs the third portion of the duodenum, or the sigmoid colon. Infrequently (probably less than a third of the time) the entire triad of radiologic findings is present. Any time two of the entities are visible, the diagnosis of gallstone ileus should be considered.

Notes

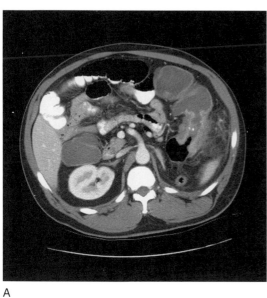

A

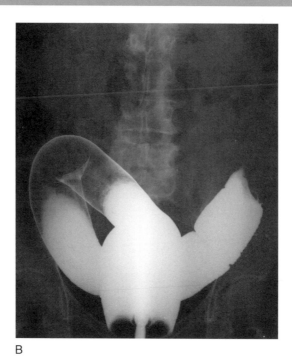

B

1. What do these two patients have in common?

2. What is the outstanding difference in how they might clinically present?

3. How do left-sided colonic carcinomas usually present?

4. What is the significance of this difference in the radiologic findings between the patient with the CT image and the one with the barium enema image?

251

Left-sided Colonic Obstruction without Antegrade Obstruction

1. They both have left-sided colonic adenocarcinoma.

2. The patient with the CT image clearly shows obstruction above the lesion. The patient having the barium enema shows no evidence of obstruction above the lesion.

3. Most common presentation of left-sided lesions is antegrade obstruction.

4. The difference will address the question of whether the proximal colon will be examined during barium enema examination.

Cross-Reference

Gastrointestinal Imaging: THE REQUISITES, ed 3, p 302.

Comments

The general thinking regarding the clinical differences in right versus left colonic carcinomas relates to the following factors:

The wider right-sided lumen and relatively thinner wall of the left colon.

The fact that the bowel content being delivered to the right colon from the terminal ileum is mostly fluid in nature.

The fact that one of the main physiologic functions of the colon is water reabsorption.

Thus, most right-sided lesions can grow quite large and still not be obstructive. Most left-sided lesions present with rectal bleeding. On the other hand, the lumen of the left side is smaller and water absorption has resulted in stool formation, and as a result the left-sided lesion often presents as an obstructive process such as seen on the CT image in this case.

However, a slowly growing indolent lesion of the left colon may present as an exception to the rule. Because of slow growth the luminal contours of the lesions are affected by the fecal stream and develop a "flap valve" configuration. As a result such patients may be shown to have complete retrograde obstruction to the flow of barium, while there is *no* evidence of antegrade obstruction (i.e., dilated fluid-filled loops of bowel, air-fluid levels, etc.) as seen in the barium enema included in this case. Study the image and you see no evidence of antegrade obstruction. This addresses the age-old issue of "should I stop the barium flow when I encounter an incomplete colonic obstruction?" The answer is clear. If there is evidence of antegrade obstruction, one should cease the barium flow immediately. Putting barium on the proximal side of an obstructing lesion can complicate the situation. However, if there is no evidence of antegrade obstruction on plain images of the abdomen, one can feel quite free to continue to examine the proximal colon without fear of causing harm.

Notes

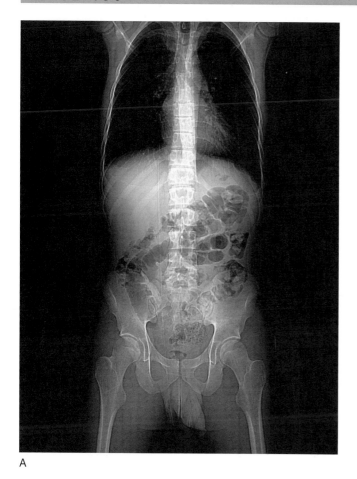

A

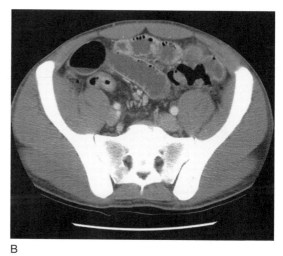

B

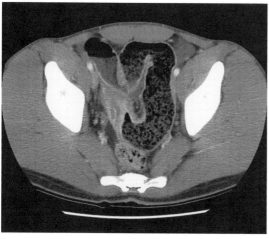

C

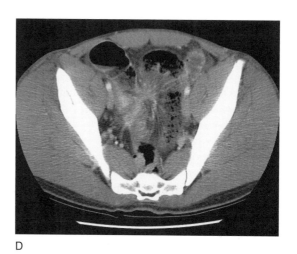

D

1. What does the mottled mixed density and lucency seen in this patient's pelvis on the topogram most likely represent?

2. What pathology might have this appearance?

3. What if you were told that this patient was not septic, had Crohn's disease and SBO, and showed a sigmoid colon largely empty of stool?

4. How often does this finding occur in patients with SBO?

Small Bowel Feces Sign in Crohn's Disease

1. Stool in the sigmoid colon.

2. Abcess.

3. The finding might be the small bowel feces sign (SBFS) seen in chronic SBO.

4. This finding has been reported in up to 55% of CT examinations of small bowel obstruction, although other authors consider it a much less frequent finding (5–8%).

Cross-Reference

Gastrointestinal Imaging: THE REQUISITES, ed 3, p 137.

Comment

Despite its appearance, what looks like stool in the patient's pelvis (Fig. 150A) is actually fecal-like material backed up behind a stricture in the distal ileum of a young male with Crohn's disease. Note the thickened inflamed bowel in Figure 150B. You will also see a severe stricture with proximal dilatation and feces-like material distending the loop of obstructed small bowel (Figs. 150C, 150D). This finding, the small bowel feces sign (SBFS), although not rare, is relatively uncommon. It is most likely to occur in patients with long-standing moderate to severe narrowing of the small bowel. Since Crohn's disease often includes fistulous communications that can partially decompress the SBO (as in this patient), SBFS is often seen in patients with Crohn's disease. However, it has also been described in small bowel obstruction secondary to adhesions, ischemia, hernias, and cystic fibrosis. Any chronically slow-developing obstruction may result in this finding. The SBFS is helpful in that it occurs at the level of the obstruction, with the distal tip of the feces-like material tapering down to the exact obstructive site. In general, CT is a fast and effective way of evaluating for potential small bowel or even colonic obstruction. It can be done quickly without luminal contrast, as dilated bowel proximal to the obstructing site is usually distended with air or, more likely, fluid. The identification of normal caliber bowel and its relation to fluid-filled distended bowel can often identify the obstructing site and, in some cases, the offending agent. Adhesions are difficult to see with CT, and the absence of any other cause of a sudden transition is suggestive of adhesions. As adhesions are the most common cause of SBO and approximately 20% of hospital admissions are the results of some form of SBO, CT evaluation is becoming an increasingly important diagnostic tool in these cases.

Notes

Challenge

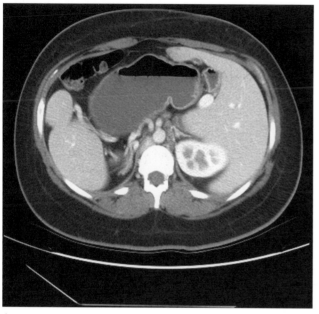
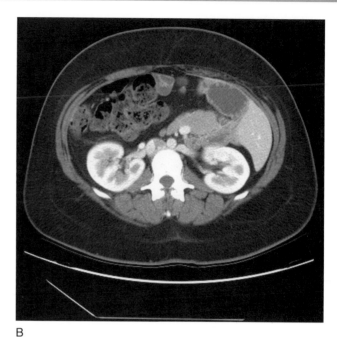

A

B

1. What is the risk of congenital heart disease in this patient?

2. On what side of the chest would you expect to find the cardiac apex located?

3. How would you describe the origins of the celiac axis and SMA in this patient?

4. Describe the anatomy of the pancreas shown in these images.

Situs Ambiguous

1. Increased.

2. On the right, dextrocradia.

3. They have a common trunk arising from the anterior aorta.

4. The pancreatic head is located in the left upper quadrant while the pancreatic body is severely truncated.

Cross-Reference

Gastrointestinal Imaging: THE REQUISITES, ed 3, p 146.

Comments

The reverse of the normal arrangement of organs in the chest and abdomen (situs solitus) is called situs inversus and sometimes situs ambiguous, although situs ambiguous (heterotaxia) is usually reserved for conditions that fall outside the mere orderly mirror arrangement of situs inversus, such as seen in this patient. This would include such an array of anomalies that may or may not be present in any predictable frequency. These anomalies would include such features as discontinuous IVC, azygos continuation, and common or shared trunk for the celiac and superior mesenteric arteries, as seen in this patient. Situs ambiguous can also occur with asplenia, and these patients have an extremely high incidence of congenital heart disease (85–95%); situs ambiguous is more commonly seen in the pediatric population. The other main division of situs ambiguous is situs ambiguous with polysplenia, such as in this adult patient. The incidence of heart disease is much lower. This patient is somewhat unusual as he does not have dextrocardia. Most of these patients will have levocardia. The condition of situs ambiguous is somewhat vague, in that not all the characteristics of the conditions may be present. Multiple spleens and a left-sided liver as well as bowel situs inversus are usually seen. However, IVC interruption with azygos continuation, truncated pancreas, as well as dextrocardia may not always be present,

Situs ambiguous with asplenia is almost universally associated with some form of congenital heart disease and is uncommon in the adult population. This probably relates to the high mortality rate in infancy of situs ambiguous and asplenia.

Situs ambiguous with polysplenia may be an asymptomatic condition if not associated with a congenital cardiac defect. The organ arrangement may be an incidental discovery. Occasionally these patients are referred for vague abdominal pain.

Notes

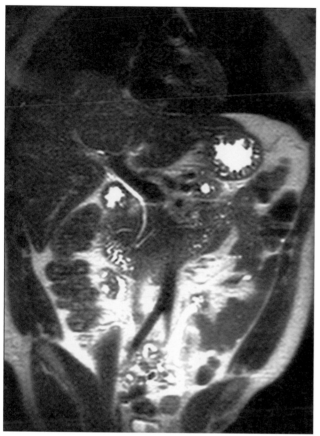

A

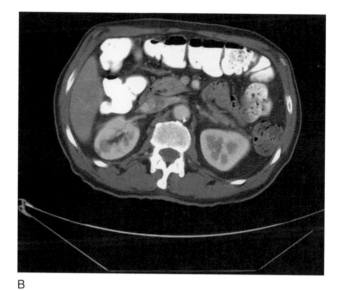

B

1. What is the most common congenital abnormality of the pancreatic ducts?

2. What complication is most often associated with pancreatic anomalies?

3. Which embryologic duct becomes the major duct of the pancreas?

4. Which duct drains the dorsal pancreas?

Pancreatic Divisum

1. Pancreas divisum.

2. Pancreatitis.

3. Duct of Wirsung.

4. Duct of Santorini.

Cross-Reference
Gastrointestinal Imaging: THE REQUISITES, ed 3, p 152.

Comments
The pancreas develops as two separate buds from the mid-gut that appear at about the fifth week of gestation and fuse together shortly thereafter to form a single pancreas. Not only do the two buds fuse their tissue, but the associated ductal structures must also join. Because of the complex nature of the ductal structures, anomalies affecting the drainage of the pancreatic ducts occur in a large percentage of individuals. Embryologically the major, or ventral, pancreatic bud develops into the ventral pancreas. In situations in which the ventral and dorsal buds do not fuse, as the ventral pancreas rotates, its duct becomes the major duct in the head of the pancreas with a foreshortened somewhat arborizing appearance. It also is joined to the biliary system, and these ducts drain through the major papilla. The minor ventral bud of the pancreas develops separately, and drains via the minor papilla. Under normal circumstances, the duct of Santorini fuses to the duct of Wirsung, and the Santorini duct goes on to drain through the Wirsung duct and into the major papilla. The portion of the Santorini duct that did drain into the duodenum usually involutes, and there is no separate papilla.

Pancreas divisum (seen in 4–7% of autopsy cases) may have several variations, the most common of which is when the less prominent ventral duct maintains its separate drainage, along with the bile duct, into the duodenum via the major papilla. The minor papilla is usually proximal to the major papilla and drains the greater dorsal duct. The dorsal duct drains the body and tail, and the ventral duct drains the head and uncinate. In some instances, as in this case, there may be a tiny communicating branch between the two systems.

Most cases of pancreas divisum are discovered incidentally during endoscopic retrograde cholangiopancreatography or, as in this case, MRCP (magnetic resonance cholangiopancreatography). However, there is a higher than normal incidence of pancreatitis in these patients. The exact etiology of pancreatitis in pancreatic divisum, absent all other factors (stones, alcohol, etc.), is unclear. Some researchers think it relates to the major duct attempting to empty its exocrine content into the duodenum via a tiny minor papilla. Acute pancreatitis in a young person should arouse some suspicion for this condition. Although ERCP or MRCP would be the examination of choice, the demonstration of what appears to be three ducts in the pancreatic head is suggestive, as in the CT image of this case.

Notes

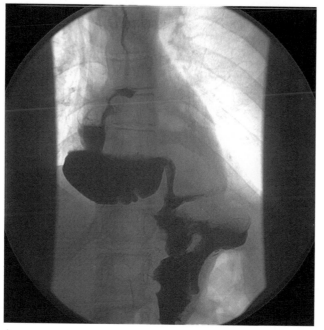
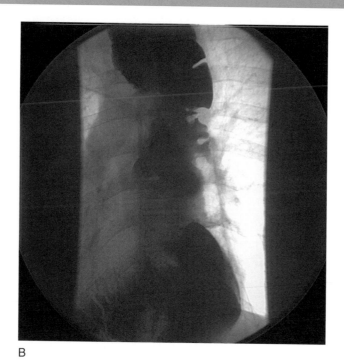

A   B

1. What are the indications for colonic interposition to treat esophageal disease?

2. Name a few of the complications associated with this condition.

3. Does malignancy ever develop within the colonic interposition?

4. When is a mucocele of the bypassed esophagus seen?

Colonic Interposition

1. Typically, benign disease, such as severe strictures, perforation, and failed surgical procedures, and rarely malignancy.

2. Leakage at an anastomosis is the most common; fistulas, strictures, ischemia, aspiration, food retention, and mucocele of the bypassed esophagus also can occur.

3. Rarely, but colonic malignancy has been reported in the colonic interposition.

4. A mucocele may develop within several months of the surgery.

Cross-Reference

Gastrointestinal Imaging: THE REQUISITES, ed 3, p 39.

Comments

The patient with severe esophageal disease may require surgical bypass when the native esophagus is obstructed or no longer functional. Some surgeons use a length of colon and anastomose it from the upper thoracic or cervical esophagus to the stomach. Or they may use jejunum, thus bypassing the diseased esophagus. The remaining esophagus may be surgically isolated but usually is not removed because of potential damage to nerves, lymphatics, and collateral blood flow. This procedure is most commonly performed in patients with benign diseases, such as caustic or peptic strictures, or severe motor disorders. Occasionally it is performed in patients with malignant disease, particularly if there is a good chance of survival, or if a complication, such as perforation, has occurred.

Complications are common because of the complexity of the surgery. Early complications include anastomotic leakage and possible fistula formation. Stenoses also may develop at the anastomotic sites, typically the proximal site. Aspiration of ingested contents is another problem. Later problems include stasis of swallowed material within the interposed segment and reflux of gastric contents into the colonic interposition. Malignancy has been described in these colonic interpositions, but it is rare.

If in the course of the surgery, the surgeon isolates the esophagus by surgically closing its ends, a mucocele of the esophagus may develop. This mucocele consists of mucous or proteinaceous secretions that fill the lumen of the isolated esophagus and have nowhere to drain. Usually the phenomenon is self-limited because increasing pressure within the lumen causes cessation of the mucous secretion. Rarely the mass continues to increase in size, leading to symptoms. However, the presence of a transposed colon or jejunum in the chest may occasionally present the resident or radiologist with a surprise when an adequate history was omitted. Talking to the patient prior to the examination is very good. Being surprised during the performance of the examination is not.

Notes

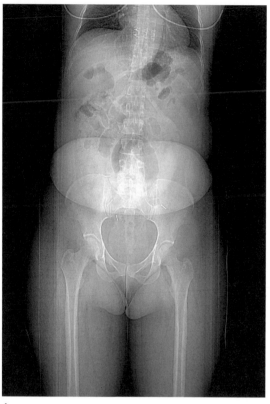

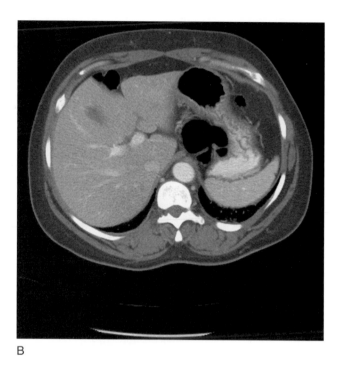

A   B

1. What is the bowel derangement seen in these images?

2. What is the peritoneal space posterior to the stomach and anterior to the pancreas called?

3. Where is the foramen of Winslow located?

4. What is the incidence of internal bowel herniation?

Foramen of Winslow Internal Bowel Hernia

1. Colonic gas is seen behind the stomach.

2. The lesser sac.

3. Posterior to the edge of the lesser omentum, just to the right of the spine.

4. 1% to 2%. They are relatively uncommon.

Cross-Reference

Gastrointestinal Imaging: THE REQUISITES, ed 3, p 331.

Comments

The foramen of Winslow (also known as the epiploic foramen) lies at the right free edge of the hepatogastric and hepatoduodenal ligaments in the region of the underside of the liver. It is normally a little larger than the width of a finger, but can be much larger in some people. It is highly unusual to see bowel herniation via the foramen into the lesser sac. One must take time to evaluate carefully, as a right paraduodenal hernia can have a similar appearance. If the herniated bowel crosses the midline to the right, it is evidence of a foramen of Winslow hernia. In most cases, such as this case, it is redundant transverse colon or right colon with little or no retroperitonization that herniates through the foramen. If the bowel becomes strangulated, it becomes a surgical emergency. A BE would be very helpful, but as seen in this case, plain film and CT suggest the diagnosis. On plain film, the gastric air bubble is seen as well as a collection of air overlying but not in the stomach. Likewise, on the CT image, air is seen behind the stomach in the region of the gastrohepatic ligament and the foramen itself. Internal bowel hernias are not common and foramen of Winslow hernias even less so. Most internal hernias are paraduodenal or transmesenteric. Many are asymptomatic and are discovered incidentally. The hernia can also be transient and be the cause of endless workups for the patient with vague abdominal complaints and transient obstructive symptoms. It is also possible for the herniated bowel to compress the common bile duct, and a few cases of jaundice relating to foramen of Winslow hernias have been reported.

Notes

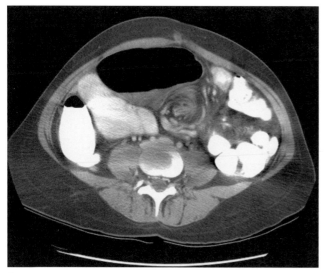

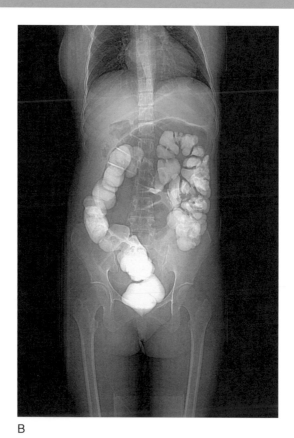

A

B

1. What is the unusual configuration seen at the root of the mesentery on the CT image?

2. Is the patient obstructed? If so, what type of obstruction might you suggest here?

3. In what age group is this condition most commonly seen?

4. What imaging examination might you suggest next?

Mesenteric Volvulus

1. The "swirl" sign at the root of the mesentery indicates rotation of the mesentery and the bowel.

2. Yes. A closed loop obstruction. The grossly dilated bowel in the midabdomen is clearly not colon. Contrast agent is seen in a collapsed colon.

3. Children in the first years of life.

4. None. Such findings warrant an immediate surgical consultation.

Cross-Reference

Gastrointestinal Imaging: THE REQUISITES, ed 3, p 110.

Comments

Small bowel, or mesenteric, volvulus is a life-threatening condition that occurs when a loop or loops of small bowel twist around its mesenteric root. When complete occlusion occurs it is, in effect, a "closed loop obstruction" and requires immediate treatment to avoid compromise of the vascular pedicle, bowel necrosis, perforation, peritonitis, and death. The condition may be transitory in some. However, even when the bowel is unobstructed, CT imaging may suggest the possibility of the diagnosis by the somewhat swirling appearance of the root of the mesentery, even if the patient is unobstructed. In this case the swirling configuration of the mesenteric root is quite pronounced and the patient is experiencing a closed loop obstruction with gross dilatation of loops of small bowel in the midabdomen.

The condition is most frequently seen in infants with mid-gut malrotation, Ladd's bands, and the attendant increase in mid-gut volvulus. This is sometimes referred to as secondary mesenteric volvulus. That is to say, there are underlying congenital causes for the volvulus. However, it is occasionally seen in the older population as a primary volvulus in which no congenital abnormalities are present. It is thought that conditions such as an extra long mesentery, high fiber diets, or even anorexia may contribute to the development of the condition. This is all speculation and we do not know why some patients will develop this condition. Mesenteric volvulus is not common and represents about 1% to 2% of small bowel obstructions. However, a full-blown twist of the mesenteric root and the resulting closed loop obstruction can lead to mesenteric infarction in almost half of such patients. There is probably a direct correlation of morbidity to the length of the interval between diagnosis and treatment.

Not all swirling seen at the mesenteric root is a small bowel volvulus. As just indicated, it may be a transient process that results in complicated workups without significant results. Like transient intussusception, seeing the patient between episodes can be problematic.

Notes

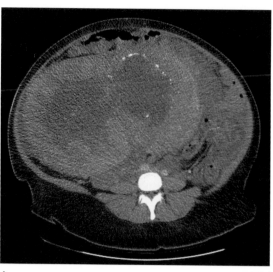

A

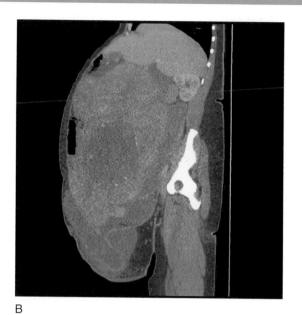

B

1. What is the probable organ of origin of the huge mass in this young woman?

2. What is the most common gynecologic tumor in women over age 30?

3. What are the symptoms that brought this woman to medical attention?

4. What percentage of women with this condition have symptoms?

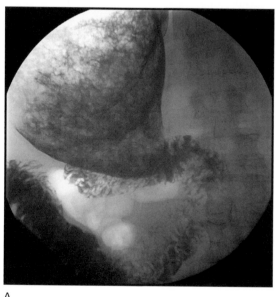

A

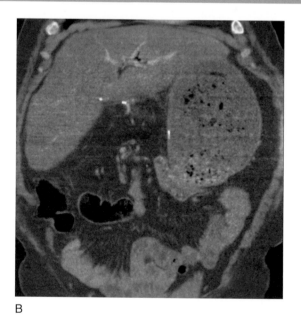

B

1. What is unusual about this patient's stomach?

2. What might you surmise as a past history for this patient?.

3. What are the common symptoms seen with this condition?

4. What do you call a collection of hair in the stomach?

CASE 156

Huge Myometrial Leiomyomas

1. The pelvis, most likely uterine.

2. Uterine fibroids, seen in about 25% of women over 30.

3. Abdominal pain and pressure effect of mass in this patient. Menorrhagia can also be a presenting complaint.

4. Most uterine fibroids cause no symptoms. Only about 15% of patients require treatment.

Cross-Reference

Gastrointestinal Imaging: THE REQUISITES, ed 3, p 308.

Comments

Uterine fibroids do not usually present a problem for either patients or radiologists. They are commonly a secondary finding noted at the time of examination (especially in CT). This patient's huge myometrial leiomyoma is unusual and malignancy was suspected. However, a 30-pound fibroid along with adhesions and fluid were found at surgery and pathologic examination showed no evidence of malignancy. There is a small malignant risk in uterine fibroids usually given as about 1%. Most are asymptomatic. Some are implicated in infertility states. Common treatments include selective resection or total hysterectomy, if deemed necessary. An estimated 600,000 hysterectomies occur annually in the United States and approximately a third are for uterine leiomyomas (fibroid). In recent years treatment by uterine artery embolization has proved helpful in the treatment of symptomatic lesions.

CT and ultrasound are often used in the evaluation of this condition. However, MRI may also be very helpful. Fibroids tend to enhance on the margins when gadolinium enhancement is used. The rim may be seen in unenhanced cases with T_2 imaging. Their tissue signal is usually lower than the surrounding tissue on both T_1 and T_2 imaging. Small linear arrangements of calcification can be seen in this lesion which might suggest benignity but cannot rule out malignancy.

Alternative diagnostic considerations in this patient would be ovarian mass, tumor originating from ovary or uterus, uterine leiomyosarcoma, and adenomyosis of the uterus.

Notes

CASE 157

Gastric Bezoar in Post-Billroth I Stomach

1. The stomach is distended with material with air in the substance of the material.

2. The distal stomach is missing and the patient has had a partial gastrectomy.

3. Fullness, vomiting, and abdominal discomfort.

4. Trichobezoar.

Cross-Reference

Gastrointestinal Imaging: THE REQUISITES, ed 3, p 78.

Comments

Gastric bezoars represent one of the complications of gastric surgery relating to disordered motility. However, bezoars can be seen in stomachs with normal anatomy as well. Bezoars are a ball of foreign or nondigestable material which will not pass the pylorus or the stoma in the postoperative stomach. Most bezoars are seen as a complication of gastric surgery or as the result of the ingestion of nonfood items, such as hair (trichobezoars) or indigestible fiber (phytobezoars). The fruit of the ever-famous persimmon tree is almost always used as an example and is probably the most common cause of bezoars in nonsurgical stomachs in the Unites States. Bezoars have been reported with other accumulations of fiber in the stomach as well, including psyllium fiber powder laxatives ingested with insufficient water.

After gastric surgery the occurrence of bezoars is thought to range between 5% and 12%, although this can seem somewhat high, given day-to-day experience with these patients. Such indigestibles as orange, orange peels, potato peels, and laxative fiber probably account for most bezoars in this setting. The bilateral vagotomy, which usually accompanies the gastric resection, leading to the resultant alteration in gastric emptying, is in large measure the source of the problem.

After gastric surgery patients with a gastric bezoar will often complain of abdominal discomfort, pain, fullness, and vomiting. Rarely, bezoars can occur in other parts of the GI tract. Also found in the literature are reports of unusual types of bezoars such as varnish bezoars in detail painters for fine furniture.

Notes

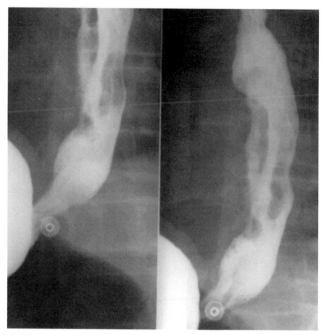

A

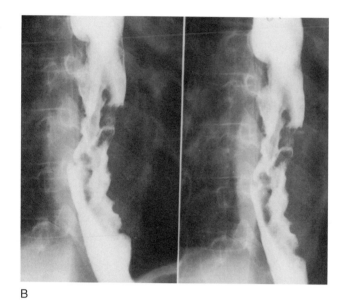

B

1. Based on these findings made on a 58-year-old male alcoholic, what is his condition?

2. What disease is the world's most common cause of portal hypertension and varices?

3. What part of the bowel wall is not found in the esophagus?

4. Why do "jump" metastases occur in esophageal carcinoma?

C A S E   1 5 8

Varicoid Carcinoma of the Esophagus

1. Varicoid appearing filling defects in the margin of the esophagus.

2. Schistosomiasis.

3. Serosal layer.

4. Because the lymphatic plexus of the esophagus extends longitudinally.

Cross-Reference
Gastrointestinal Imaging: THE REQUISITES, ed 3, p 32.

Comments
Esophageal carcinoma can appear in many different forms. The most common is that of a stricture, usually irregular in nature. It also may be an eccentric mass or even a polypoid mass within the lumen. It may ulcerate, with resultant bleeding. The anatomy of the esophagus is somewhat different from that of the remainder of the gastrointestinal tract, which results in the rapid spread of the neoplasm and the resultant poor prognosis.

Unlike the rest of the gastrointestinal tract, there is no serosal layer in the esophagus, and neoplasms are known to directly invade the adjacent structures, resulting in a high rate of morbidity. Also, the lymphatic drainage of the esophagus is complex. There is an extensive network of lymphatic channels in all layers of the esophagus. This characteristic results in metastases spreading circumferentially and to adjacent lymph node groups in the mediastinum. The tumor may "jump" or disseminate throughout the length of the esophagus via these channels. There may be intervening normal mucosa between these areas of tumor. This pattern of spread is believed to result in the varicoid appearance of esophageal carcinoma seen in this patient. Despite the history of alcoholism, varicoid carcinoma of the esophagus can be distinguished by the fact that the pattern does not change whether the patient is upright or recumbent, does not change with Valsalva respiration, is not pliable, and carries no peristaltic waves.

Varicoid carcinoma is an unusual variant of esophageal carcinoma. The tumor spreads submucosally down the length of the esophagus, producing thickened folds. The appearance closely mimics esophageal varices, hence the name. Because of this pattern of spread, dysphagia is usually a late symptom, and the disease has usually spread extensively before being diagnosed. Thus, the patient with this form of esophageal neoplasm has a poor prognosis.

Notes

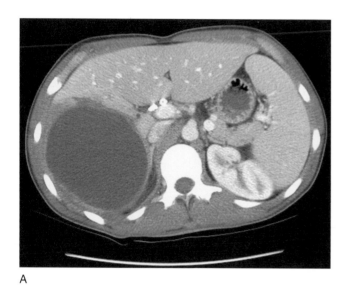

A

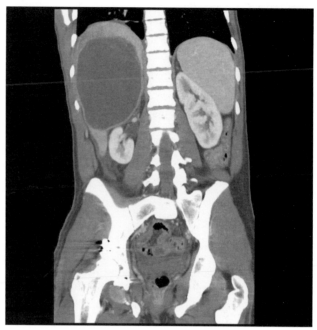

B

1. What is the most common neoplasm of the liver?

2. Apart from bleeding following trauma or in a postprocedure period (i.e., liver biopsy, ERCP), what might give the appearance seen on these images?

3. What are the usual etiologic origins of this condition?

4. What complications may be associated with this condition?

Intrahepatic Biloma

1. Hemagiomas.

2. An intrahepatic biloma.

3. Intraoperative, procedural, or post-traumatic damage to the bile ducts.

4. Infection or biloma formation that bursts into the peritoneal cavity resulting in a bile peritonitis.

Cross-Reference

Gastrointestinal Imaging: THE REQUISITES, ed 3, p 241.

Comments

The CT images demonstrate a large cystic well-defined lesion taking up considerable space in the liver. Major diagnostic considerations include some type of cystic structure communicating with the biliary system. Simple hepatic cysts, although lined by biliary tract epithelium, rarely communicate with the biliary system, despite their common occurrence. Echinococcal cysts may communicate with the biliary system, and one of their major complications is spontaneous rupture into the bile ducts or peritoneal cavity. Necrotic tumors or metastases rarely communicate with the biliary tract.

The most common cause for this intrahepatic cystic lesion, which was later drained, was due to the accumulation of bile as a result of a ruptured bile duct sustained in the initial injury. This injury may be seen following the course of cholecystectomy. During cholecystectomy, the surgeon often inserts probes or catheters into the bile ducts to identify possible retained calculi or debris. Sometimes a small endoscope is inserted into the ducts. Because intrahepatic ducts often taper rapidly, some of these small intrahepatic ducts may rupture during passage of some of these instruments. If a cholangiogram is obtained in the immediate postoperative period, a small area of extravasation may be identified.

Usually these small intrahepatic duct perforations close spontaneously after 2 to 3 weeks. Problems arise if pressure in the biliary system is increased because of obstruction, as in this patient. In that scenario, the size of the bile collection may increase and form a biloma. If the biliary tract also is infected, the bile may become infected and form an abscess. The radiologist must recognize this complication and accurately identify its true nature. This study usually can be followed by drainage of the biloma and injection into the evacuated cavity to see if the leaking bile duct can be identified. If so, repeat injections of the drained biloma over the course of the next few weeks may be undertaken to show healing and integrity of the biliary system. Similar but more expensive mechanisms for following the healing biliary system would be serial CT and MRI studies. The most worrisome complications of a biloma are infection and leakage into the peritoneal cavity.

Notes

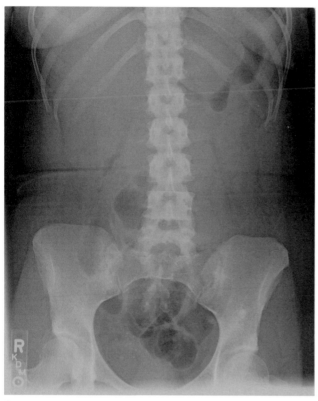

A

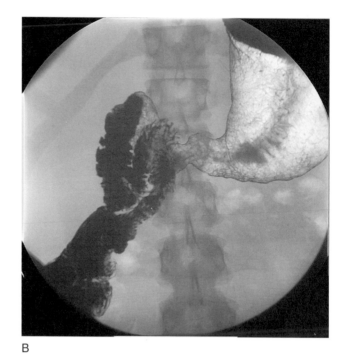

B

1. What is the most common cause of gastric erosions?

2. In patients with Crohn's disease, what area of the stomach is most commonly involved?

3. How often does Crohn's disease of the stomach occur as an isolated finding?

4. What is meant by the "ram's horn" sign?

Crohn's Disease of the Stomach

1. Peptic ulcer disease.

2. Antrum.

3. Almost always occurs in conjunction with ileal or colonic Crohn's disease.

4. Chronic Crohn's disease and deformity of the stomach, resulting in an appearance resembling a ram's horn.

Cross-Reference
Gastrointestinal Imaging: THE REQUISITES, ed 3, p 69.

Comments

Crohn's disease of the stomach is usually found in the distal aspect of the stomach but rarely may involve the entire organ. The antrum is first to become involved, and the disease may spread more proximally. Fundal involvement is unusual. Many patients also have associated involvement of the duodenum. Rarely is the stomach the only part of the gut that is involved by Crohn's disease; most often there is ileal or colonic Crohn's disease as well, and it should be assumed that there will be disease in other portions of the gastrointestinal tract, too. As a corollary, the incidence of Crohn's disease involving the stomach can range between 5% and 40% of cases and a much higher incidence is reported in Japan than in North America.

The most common presentation of Crohn's disease in the stomach is that of gastric erosions. These erosions are identical to other types of erosions in the stomach, and there is no way to radiologically distinguish them. As the disease progresses, the severity of the inflammation may increase, and ulcers may become confluent and linear or stellate in configuration. As with other portions of the gastrointestinal tract, the inflammation is transmural, resulting in fibrosis and scarring. Typically (according to some reports in more than half of the cases of gastric Crohn's disease) there may be involvement of the adjacent duodenum. When Crohn's disease is long-standing, the antrum and duodenum become a featureless rigid tube; this presentation is called the "ram's horn" sign because of the conical antrum and widening funnel of the body and fundus. This configuration may be so severe that it resembles a scirrhous carcinoma or any condition that might give a linitis plastica appearance to the stomach.

Fistulas are a rare complication of gastric Crohn's disease but can develop into the transverse colon. Postinflammatory polyps may develop as a sequela of Crohn's disease of the stomach as they do elsewhere in the gut, especially in the colon.

Notes

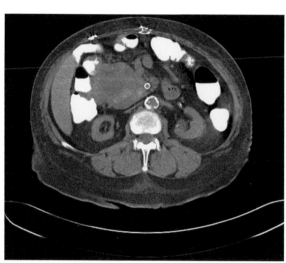

A

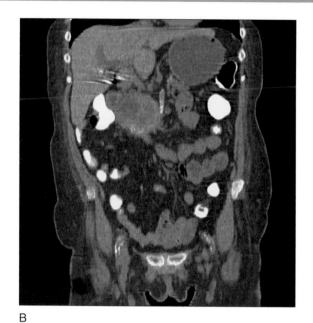

B

1. Describe the findings on the two CT images provided for this case.

2. What might be the complaint that caused this patient to seek medical help?

3. Does the size of the lesion help in the differential diagnosis?

4. What endocrine activity do you expect to find in this lesion?

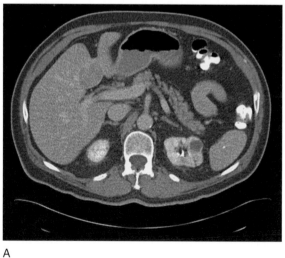

A

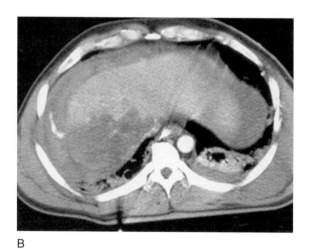

B

1. What do these two patients have in common?

2. What is the predisposing condition most commonly associated with this lesion?

3. What elevated serum factor is commonly seen with this disease?

4. How would a medical student in South Korea answer question 2?

CASE 161

Nonfunctioning Islet Cell Tumor of Pancreas

1. A large mass with central necrosis seen arising from the pancreatic head.

2. Vague abdominal discomfort, no pain or weight loss.

3. Yes.

4. None.

Cross-Reference

Gastrointestinal Imaging: THE REQUISITES, ed 3, p 164.

Comments

About 20% to 25% of all islet cell tumors of the pancreas are nonfunctioning islet cell tumors. Because they are relatively asymptomatic (they do not produce and secrete endocrine products) they can grow to large size, such as in this case. Please note that the biliary system is not invaded and there is no biliary dilation within the liver. Because these tumors grow slowly and quietly over a long period, they are not only quite large when discovered, but also they may be malignant at that time as well. Some studies have shown that almost 50% are malignant at the time of discovery, mostly by contiguous spread or from metastatic disease to the liver. Most of the tumors will be large enough to have necrotic centers at the time of discovery. In addition nonfunctioning islet cell tumors may a have cystic component, which can confuse and delay diagnosis. Nonfunctioning islet cell tumors can occur anywhere in the pancreas, with the most popular sites being the head and tail. They can reach sizes of 8 to 20 cm. And even with the high potential of malignancy, the prognosis remains high, which is not the case for ductal adenocarcinomas of the pancreas. Between 20% and 25% of all islet cell tumors, functioning or nonfunctioning, will have some calcifications within them, whereas only 1% to 2% of ductal carcinomas show any sign of calcification. The treatment is surgical.

Notes

CASE 162

Hepatocellular Carcinoma

1. They both have HCC (hepatocellular carcinoma, hepatoma).

2. Chronic alcoholism and cirrhosis of the liver.

3. Elevated serum alpha-fetoprotein (AFP) is seen in 60% to 80% of patients with hepatoma.

4. Chronic hepatitis B and C and parasitic liver infections are far more common causes in Korea than cirrohisis.

Cross-Reference

Gastrointestinal Imaging: THE REQUISITES, ed 3, p 195.

Comments

Hepatocellular carcinoma (HCC) is a primary malignancy of the heptocyte. In the West the disease is relatively uncommon when compared to Asia. However, it is usually associated with alcoholism and cirrhosis in the West. Hepatic infections, especially hepatitis B, as well as parasitic infections of the liver, are thought to be the major etiologic factors in Asia. The disease has a dismal outlook with survival usually not exceeding 6 to 18 months following diagnosis. At the time of diagnosis, at least 50% of patients will have tumor spread to the portal veins. Of note, there appears to be an increasing incidence in HCC in the West, possibly relating to an increasing incidence of hepatitis B and C.

The disease is more commonly seen in men, especially in Asia. The advent of high-quality MDCT and MRI has not changed the mortality rate. One CT image in this case shows the typical HCC mass lesion of the right lobe of the liver with portal vein invasion and active bleeding. The other CT image is much more subtle and the HCC lesion is seen only on delayed images, in which the lesion is seen as a slight blush in the right lobe of the liver. In general, distortion of the liver architecture by cirrhosis further complicates the process of detecting subtle or early lesions. An elevated AFP level is helpful for its positive predictive value, but if serum AFP is normal, it does not exclude the disease. In practice the higher the AFP levels, the greater the likelihood of HCC. CT-guided liver biopsy, if not contraindicated by the possibility of abnormal bleeding and clotting issues, is the most efficient manner of diagnosis.

Notes

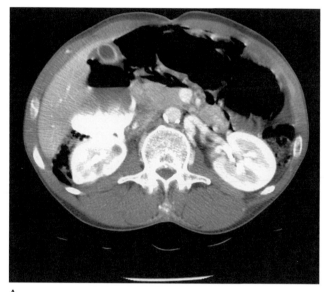

A

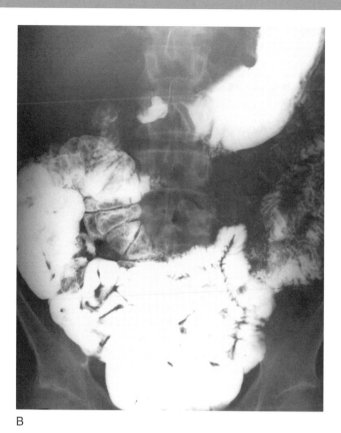

B

1. How would you describe the appearance of the duodenal bulb on the barium image?

2. What is the definition of a giant duodenal ulcer?

3. Where do perforating ulcers most commonly occur?

4. What complication is shown in the CT image?

Giant Duodenal Ulcer and Perforation

1. It retains barium, has something of a duodenal bulb configuration, but shows no fold pattern.

2. A large duodenal ulcer over 2 cm in size, or an ulcer replacing two thirds of the duodenal bulb.

3. Anterior aspect of stomach or duodenal bulb.

4. Perforation and oral contrast material outside the duodenal wall.

Cross-Reference

Gastrointestinal Imaging: THE REQUISITES, ed 3, p 99.

Comments

The barium study on this patient with a giant duodenal ulcer shows retained barium within what appears to be a somewhat duodenal configuration. However, no fold pattern is detected. Postbulbar narrowing can also be frequently seen in giant duodenal ulcer disease. The most important complications are bleeding and perforation. This CT image shown here demonstrates large amounts of free intraperitoneal air and oral contrast agent in a dependent position along the inferior edge of the liver. CT may demonstrate as little as 1 to 2 mL of free intraperitoneal air. Studies have shown that upright or decubitus radiographs also may demonstrate similarly tiny amounts of free intraperitoneal air. However, in practice, CT has proved more sensitive than other modalities in demonstrating small amounts of free intraperitoneal air. Also, patients are often too sick to obtain adequate positional views for abdominal studies, and the CT demonstration of free intraperitoneal air is not dependent on upright positioning. Although, in patients who are too ill to stand, the indirect signs of pneumoperitoneum may be seen on conventional images, CT is very sensitive for the detection of free air regardless of the patient position.

Free intraperitoneal air may be easy to diagnose, but the exact site of perforation may not be so easy. Sometimes the site of perforation is identified at the time of surgery. Plain radiographs of the abdomen reveal only the presence of free intraperitoneal air, which is a nonspecific finding. However, with the increased use of CT in the emergency setting, the detection of contrast material leaking into the peritoneal cavity, as well as the presence of free intraperitoneal air, has become possible. The collection of contrast material along the inferior edge of the liver, as in this case, strongly suggests the diagnosis of perforated duodenum. However, if the contrast agent were in the lesser sac or left side of the abdomen, it would suggest perforation of the stomach. Given the aforementioned findings, and in the right clinical setting, it is not necessary to perform further studies, and surgery should be performed promptly.

Notes

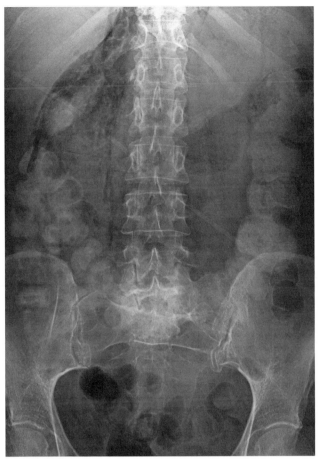

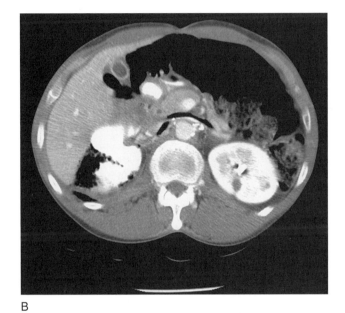

A   B

1. Where does air in the bowel come from?

2. What unexpected places is air seen in these images?

3. What might be some of the clinical causes for these findings?

4. Is there such a thing as benign pneumoretroperitoneum?

Air in Retroperitoneum

1. 99% of air seen in the bowel is ingested.

2. Both the CT and conventional image of the abdomen show air in the retroperitoneum, as well as in the peritoneum.

3. Perforated hollow viscus that is retroperitoneal in location.

4. No.

Cross-Reference

Gastrointestinal Imaging: THE REQUISITES, ed 3, p 98.

Comments

Occasionally one sees a patient with free intraperitoneal air and no symptoms. It is usually the result of a burst serosal bleb in patients with the cystic type of pneumatosis coli. However, air in the retroperitoneum is never benign and is always associated with significant underlying causes. Perhaps the most common cause is perforated holllow viscus that is located behind the posterior peritoneal layer of the peritoneal cavity (the retroperitoneum), in which lie parts of the duodenum, ascending and descending colon, pancreas, kidney, and adrenal glands.

Besides perforation of peptic ulcer disease, other considerations might include perforation secondary to endoscopy or ERCP or trauma. A large pneumomediastinum could also cause some air to percolate through the diaphragmatic hiatus into the retroperitoneum. In cases of significant pneumoretroperitoneum, the air tends to be streaky and linear in nature, following the iliopsoas muscle, perhaps outlining the kidney. There are no Rigler's signs, or air collecting under the diaphragm, or air outlining the falciform ligament, as is seen with a pneumoperitoneum. Blunt trauma to the abdomen affecting the retroperitonized portions of the colon and resulting in leakage of air can produce these findings as well. Streaky linear air collections are seen on the plain image of the abdomen shown with this case. However, CT is much more sensitive in the detection of retroperitoneal air, especially small amounts, and is now the standard study.

Notes

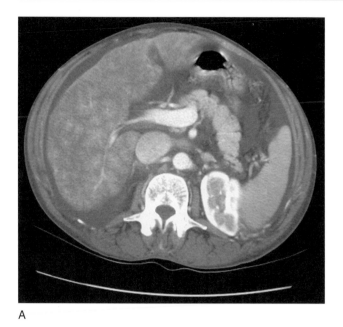

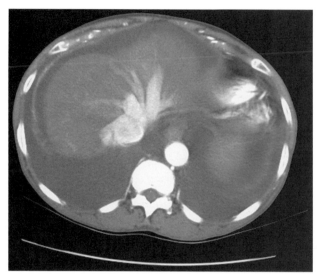

A   B

1. How would you describe the hepatic appearance on these CT images?

2. How does this appearance relate to cardiac function?

3. What processes within the liver give rise to this appearance?

4. What percentage of autopsies demonstrate some degree of this finding?

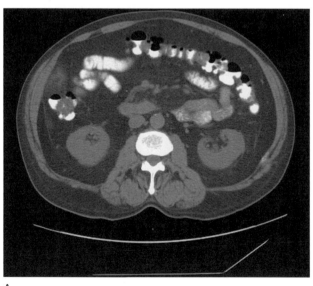

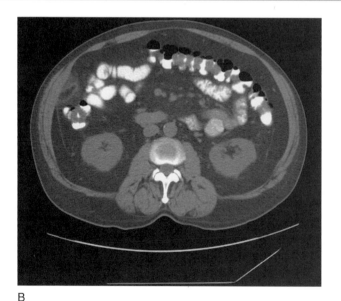

A   B

1. Describe the CT findings in this 68-year-old complaining of lower abdominal pain for 2 to 3 days.

2. What are the etiologic theories for this condition?

3. What conditions can this disease mimic?

4. What is the treatment for this condition?

C A S E   1 6 5

Nutmeg Liver

1. Widespread "mottled" pattern.

2. It is almost always due to right-sided heart failure.

3. Chronic passive congestion of blood in the liver.

4. Almost all.

Cross-Reference

Gastrointestinal Imaging: THE REQUISITES, ed 3, p 383.

Comments

Right-sided heart failure is almost always the basis of a diffuse "mottled appearing," somewhat enlarged liver, with distended hepatic veins. It has been referred to by pathologists as the "nutmeg" liver for over a hundred years and is an extremely common finding at autopsy. Any chronic preterminal event may result in right-sided heart failure, hence the common high incidence seen at autopsy. The nutmeg is a spice, the germ taken from the seed of a tree found in the tropics. The name "nutmeg liver" was used by pathologists to describe sections taken from a chronically passive congested liver, usually due to right-sided heart failure. The congestion and pigmentation about the central veins of the liver lobules gave it a "nutmeg" appearance to the eyes of early pathologists, who were inclined to give food-related names to disease entities in the early days of histopathology (i.e., "bread and butter pericarditis," "anchovy sauce" liver lesions).

This would have continued as an interesting sidelight of histopathology if CT imaging had not come on the scene. When evaluating patients with congestive heart failure, and especially right-sided failure, radiologists began to observe that the liver took on a diffuse "mottled" appearance almost identical to that described by the pathologists. Distention of the hepatic veins and degrees of hepatomegaly are also seen.

The potential problem of the "nutmeg" liver is that it could conceivably mask some other hepatic disease. Notwithstanding, the term "nutmeg" liver has now passed into the lexicon of the radiologists and hepatic imaging.

Notes

C A S E   1 6 6

Appendagitis of Colon

1. CT images show a small projection of fat (epiploic appendage) with surrounding inflammatory changes (epiploic appendigitis).

2. The most favored etiologic possibility is torsion of the appendage. Another is thrombus in the vessels in the appendage. It is quite possible that the former leads to the latter.

3. Appendicitis, diverticulitis.

4. Conservative management.

Cross-Reference

Gastrointestinal Imaging: THE REQUISITES, ed 3, p 319.

Comments

Acute epiploic appendagitis is an unusual self-limiting inflammatory process involving the epiploic appendages of the colon. It is thought to be due to torsion of the appendage pedicle which results in vascular occlusion, thrombus, and inflammation. The epiploic appendages are fatty extensions arising from the two rows of teni coli, which form the well-known haustral pattern of the colon. The teni are peritoneum-covered and are found anywhere along the length of the colon. Prior to laporoscopy and CT imaging the condition went undiagnosed and the patient recovered, or it was mistaken for some other intra-abdominal disease and the patient underwent laporotomy. MDCT imaging is excellent not only for demonstrating the condition but also for the exclusion of other causes of abdominal pain, which might require immediate intervention. As discussed earlier, the treatment is conservative with spontaneous resolution in virtually all patients. CT imaging will show the inflamed appendage, as in this case, apart from the bowel wall and without inflammatory changes of the bowel wall. Follow-up CT studies may show involution with some scar tissue in the pericolonic fat. Tiny calcifications or focal fatty scarring in the fat around the pericolic regions may be indicative of prior epiploic appendagitis.

Notes

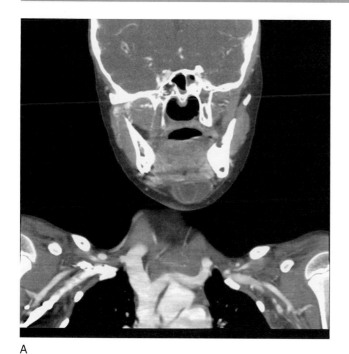

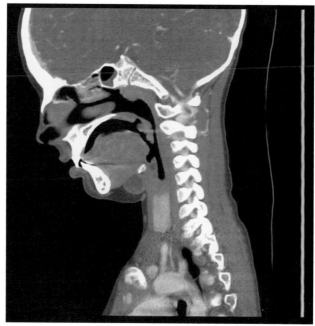

A

B

1. This child with persistent mild dysphasia had a CT study. What are the findings?

2. Is this anomaly more common in males or females?

3. What complications are associated with this condition?

4. What is the definitive treatment?

C A S E   1 6 7

Thyroglossal Cyst

1. A cystic structure at the base of the tongue in the midline adjacent to the hyoid bone: thyroglossal cyst.

2. Females.

3. Infection, and rarely malignancy.

4. Surgery.

Cross-Reference
Gastrointestinal Imaging: THE REQUISITES, ed 3, p 10.

Comments

A thyroglossal cyst is a cystic structure formed in a persistent thyroglossal duct. This duct usually involutes early in embryonic life (8–9 weeks) but may retain some patency in a small percentage of the population, leading to cyst formation at the base of the tongue, often in the midline and occasionally touching the hyoid bone. Most patients are female and asymptomatic. Occasionally it may cause a globus sensation or "dysphagia." Barium swallow is usually normal. CT imaging will demonstrate the mass at the base of the tongue, usually midline, but not always. It rarely exceeds 3 cm in size. Complications include infection, in which case the patient will present with painful swallowing (the cyst moves with the tongue) and a painful lump in the neck in a sublingual location. Rarely, an association of thyroglossal cyst with medullary carcinoma of the thyroid gland has been reported.

Other cystic structures in the neck or upper mediastinum to be considered are foregut cysts such as bronchogenic cysts, duplication cysts, neurogenic cysts, and thymic cysts. Many of these conditions produce no symptoms and are often incidental findings. However, as the individual ages, some of these cystic structures may become symptomatic.

Notes

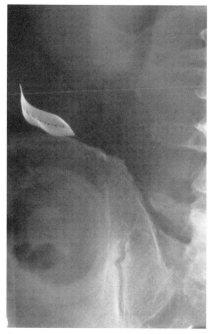

A

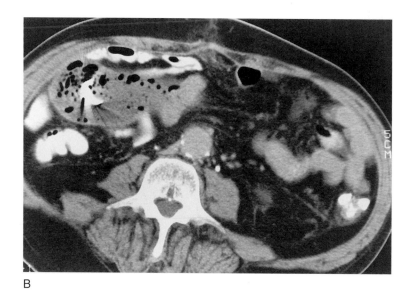

B

1. What abnormality is developing in the anterior abdomen?

2. What is the cause for the high-density focus within this abnormality?

3. Why is it radiopaque?

4. What treatment may be performed by the radiologist?

Gossypiboma (Retained Surgical Sponge and Abscess)

1. Abscess.

2. Retained surgical device (sponge).

3. Radiopaque material is embedded in a portion of it.

4. Drainage and percutaneous removal.

Cross-Reference

Gastrointestinal Imaging: THE REQUISITES, ed 3, p 123.

Comments

This CT scan demonstrates an abnormal collection of fluid and air within the anterior abdomen consistent with an abscess. Of greater importance, however, is the presence of a ribbon-like density within the abscess, which is indicative of some type of foreign object within the abdominal cavity. It can be seen distinctly on the plain image of the abdomen. This constellation of findings along with the prior abdominal surgery (see ostomy on plain image) raises the likelihood of an iatrogenic cause (i.e., the introduction of some object into the peritoneal cavity during a surgical procedure). This object could be a surgical sponge or towel or perhaps a surgical needle that was dropped into the peritoneal cavity. This complication is rare, considering the number of procedures performed daily.

A retained surgical sponge (also known as a gossypiboma) can sometimes be difficult to diagnose. On plain film motion artifact can make the radiopaque ribbon all but disappear. Thus, an intraoperative image obtained for possibility of retained sponge must be obtained during complete suspended respiration. Motion artifact has been known to make the radiopaque ribbon virtually disappear. The radiopaque ribbon is placed in surgical sponges so that they can be identified on radiographs of the abdomen. The intraoperative radiographs are obtained if the sponge count taken during surgery is incorrect. This study usually detects most sponges that are lost within the abdominal cavity. However, often, because of incorrect counting, the surgeon may be unaware that a sponge has been lost within the abdominal cavity. Some of these objects produce no symptoms and are retained within the abdominal cavity until they are later discovered incidentally during a radiologic examination. Others may serve as a nidus for infection, leading to the development of an abscess, as in this patient. Surgery is the primary treatment when complications, such as abscess formation, occur as a result of a retained foreign object. However, in some instances, the retained sponge can be removed percutaneously during drainage of the abscess.

Notes

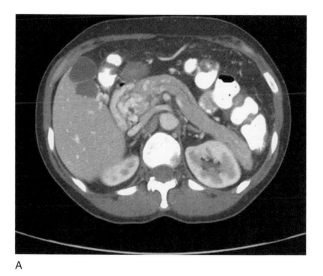
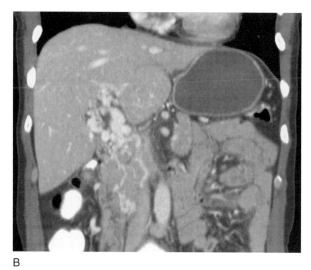

A   B

1. What is the underlying cause of the findings shown on these CT images?

2. What are some of the causes of this condition?

3. What does this appearance say about the acuteness or chronicity of the process?

4. What radiologic intervention has been associated with this condition?

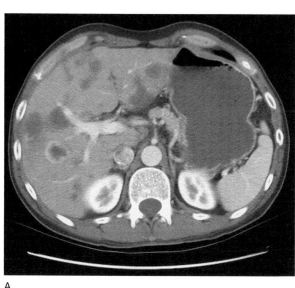
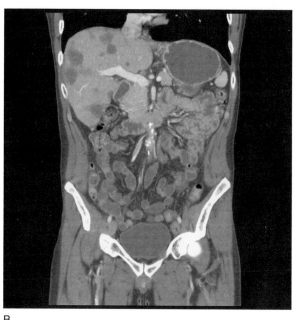

A   B

1. What would be your first diagnostic choice in these two CT images?

2. What is the most common tumor of the liver of vascular origin?

3. What would a tumor of mixed angiomatous and epithelioid elements and of mild local malignant character be called?

4. What would be the most common site of such a neoplasm?

Cavernous Transformation of the Portal Vein

1. Portal vein thrombosis and occlusion and cavernous transformation of the portal system as in this patient.

2. Any condition which might reduce portal vein flow or affect coagulability of the portal system.

3. Slowly progressive chronic nature of the process.

4. The condition has been reported following transjugular intrahepatic portosystem shunting (TIPS).

Cross-Reference

Gastrointestinal Imaging: THE REQUISITES, ed 3, p 205.

Comments

Cavernous transformation of the portal venous system is defined as the formation of numerous serpiginous "worm-like" venous channels between the liver and spleen as a result of chronic portal vein occlusion. This is usually due to portal vein thrombosis. The occlusive process is usually not acute and some time is required to allow formation of prominent venous collateralization. Not all cases of portal vein thrombosis will result in cavernous transformation. It has been reported in cases of chronic portal hypertension due to fibrosing liver disease, chronic pancreatitis, pancreatic carcinoma, HCC, perinatal omphalitis in newborns, pregnancy, hemolytic anemias such as thalassemia, and hypercoagulable diseases as well as systemic sepsis. It can also progress to such conditions as esophageal varices and gastric varices and gastrointestinal bleeding. The diagnosis of both portal vein thrombosis and cavernous transformation can usually be made using Doppler ultrasound. CT can also demonstrate these changes, as well as demonstrate the underlying cause in some instances.

Notes

Epithelioid Hemangioepithelioma

1. The first consideration would be malignant metastatic disease.

2. Hemangioma.

3. Epithelioid hemangioendothelioma.

4. Mostly in bone and soft tissue; very rarely in the liver or lungs.

Cross-Reference

Gastrointestinal Imaging: THE REQUISITES, ed 3, p 205.

Comments

You will note that the hepatic lesions are of soft tissue density and that some have a well-defined "halo" around them. This ought not to dissuade the radiologist from considering metastatic disease as the first thing to be excluded. However, no primary disease was present in this patient, and biopsy of the liver lesions revealed the multinodular lesions of the liver to be epithelioid hemangioendotheliomas (EHE). This is a rare condition mostly seen in bone and soft tissues. Its involvement of the liver will look like metastatic disease. Although metastatic lesions can have an enhancing halo, EHE seems to have a more prominent halo sign. Unfortunately, this does not necessarily apply in all the hepatic lesions as seen on the transaxial image of the liver. In a setting in which a primary lesion is not evident, and well-defined peripheral enhancement that is brighter than usual is present (and is not the "puddling" effect seen with benign hemangiomas), EHE is a consideration. The tumor is an unusual vascular lesion characterized by epithelioid endothelial cells. It has been described in adults, both young and older. The tumor histologically has the features of a low-grade malignancy. The World Health Organization (WHO) in 2002 defined "hemangioendothelioma" as a definitive locally aggressive malignant tumor that rarely metastasizes.

In the liver EHE is seen as multiple indolent slow-growing progressive lesions, which on CT may demonstrate a bright, well-defined halo effect. It is extremely rare to see spread of the tumor beyond the liver.

Notes

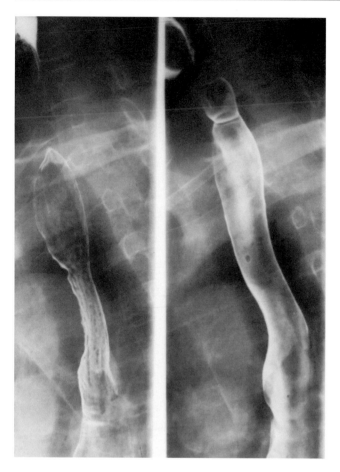

1. What is the striking finding in this barium swallow of young women complaining of dysphagia?

2. Where in the esophagus are strictures most commonly seen?

3. What syndrome can this be associated with?

4. What is the treatment for this particular problem?

Esophageal Web

1. A well-defined circumferential web or ring is seen in the cervical esophagus.

2. Mostly in the distal esophagus.

3. Plummer-Vinson syndrome.

4. Usually endoscopic passage through the web will be curative.

Cross-Reference

Gastrointestinal Imaging: THE REQUISITES, ed 3, p 32.

Comments

These images from a barium esophagogram show a well-defined web or ring structure in the proximal esophagus. These proximal webs are not common. If the web is small or noncircumferential, the patient may be asymptomatic. However, if the lumen is sufficiently compromised, such that a 13-mm barium tablet will be held up by the web, the patient will complain of dysphagia. In Plummer-Vinson syndrome (also known as Paterson-Kelly syndrome in the United Kingdom), these webs are seen, accompanied by iron deficiency anemia. The condition is sometimes referred to as sideropenic dysphagia. The exact cause of this condition is unclear. Indeed, some doubt the validity of the association or the syndrome altogether. Plummer-Vinson syndrome has been speculated to be an autoimmune phenomenon, but no conclusive evidence has been offered to prove this hypothesis. The condition was first described and named in the early 20th century, when the incidence was thought to be relatively common. It is now seen rarely, possibly because fewer barium esophagograms are being done and endoscopy may not see the web or may push by it (and thus effect a cure), or alternatively, Plummer-Vinson syndrome may indeed be a nonentity. For those who have described the condition it has mostly been as a result of an esophageal web seen in the cervical esophagus during a barium esophagogram. It has been said to be found in a predominantly white female population with a predisposition for an increased risk of squamous cell carcinoma of the esophagus. However, this risk factor is also in dispute. For the radiologist, it is important to rule out strictures related to other conditions, such as skin lesions, epidermolysis bullosa, and pemphigus as well as strictures related to gastroesophageal reflux.

Notes

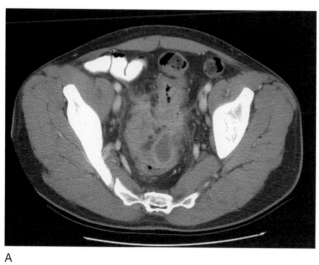

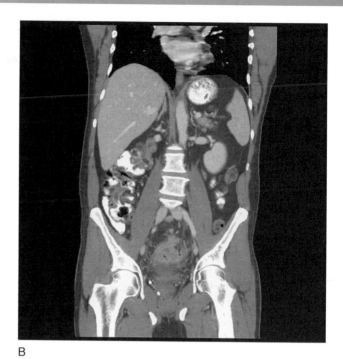

A

B

1. This 68-year-old man presents with peritoneal signs, pain, and fever. What is your diagnosis?

2. What does the fluid collection seen in the paracolic area represent?

3. What differential diagnosis might you consider?

4. Could this be carcinoma of the colon?

Carcinoma of Sigmoid Mimicking Diverticulitis

1. The first consideration would have to be diverticulitis.

2. An abscess.

3. Iatrogenic or trauma perforation of the sigmoid, actinomycosis, an inflammatory process from above collecting in the pelvis.

4. Yes.

Cross-Reference

Gastrointestinal Imaging: THE REQUISITES, ed 3, p 302.

Comments

This patient's CT images show inflammatory changes in and around the sigmoid colon as well as a pericolic abscess. The radiologic diagnosis of diverticulitis was offered. However, the radiologist should keep in mind that, although the usual presenting symptoms of obstruction and bleeding (occult or frank bleeding) account for the vast majority of colonic malignant lesions, perforation is the presentation in a small but significant number of cases (< 1%). In most cases, such as in the case presented here, the perforation site will be at the site of the tumor. However, perforation proximal to the tumor can be seen in about 30% of these patients. Perforation distal to the tumor is extremely rare. Secondary perforation following radiation treatment has been reported but is also rare. Perforation linked to colonic carcinoma occurs slightly more frequently on the right side. In such a scenario the question of a perforated carcinoma is always an issue and must be excluded before considering right-sided diverticulitis. However, when the perforation is left-sided and especially in the sigmoid colon, it can mimic diverticulitis almost perfectly.

Notes

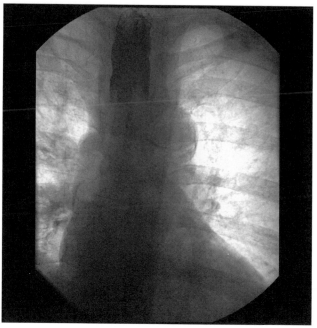

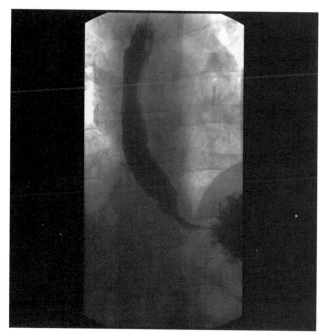

A

B

1. From this sequence of images, formulate a plausible history.

2. What does the presence of the filling defect in the esophagus say about the esophagus itself?

3. What factors contribute to this situation?

4. What is the treatment?

Food Impaction in Esophagus Secondary to Stricture

1. The patient was eating solid food (i.e., steak) and experienced chest pain, gagging, and inability to swallow.

2. Food impaction in the esophagus is almost always indicative of an area of narrowing in the esophagus.

3. Swallowing too large a solid food bolus, sometimes while intoxicated.

4. If not passed after an adequate waiting period, endoscopic removal or push through the GE junction may be necessary.

Cross-Reference
Gastrointestinal Imaging: THE REQUISITES, ed 3, p 37.

Comments

Esophageal food impaction is not uncommon. In virtually in every case, there is some underlying disease. Usually this is in the form of a mild area of narrowing or stricture that is usually located in the distal esophagus, associated with chronic reflux disease. It can often turn out to be the symptomatic form of the esophageal "B" ring, referred to as Schatzki's ring. This condition is sometimes referred to the "steakhouse syndrome," suggesting that the patient has swallowed a large, inadequately chewed solid bolus of food. The reasons for this can vary from the patient perspective. Mild intoxication has often been implicated such as in the "café coronary" in which the bolus becomes stuck in the cervical esophagus or the esophagopharyngeal junction, occluding or compressing the airway. In such cases the more dramatic Heimlich maneuver is called for to prevent asphyxiation.

The capacity for the human gastroesophageal junction to stretch to accommodate a large bolus of food is surprisingly high. The esophagus may be anatomically divided into the tubular and vestibular esophagus. The vestibule is a short segment of natural widening of the esophagus just above the GE junction and should not be confused with a small hiatal hernia. No gastric folds are present in this natural widening and it is more prominent in some patients than in others. Because of this, even a large bolus can usually safely pass the GE junction. When a solid bolus becomes impacted near the GE junction, the radiologist should appreciate the extremely high probability that some underlying narrowing is present. If the narrowing is mild, it can easily be missed at endoscopy. In follow-up studies, a barium tablet (12.5 mm) should be utilized and will often hang up in the narrowed area and subsequently, washed down with warm water. The radiologist should explain to the patient that it is not a medication.

Notes

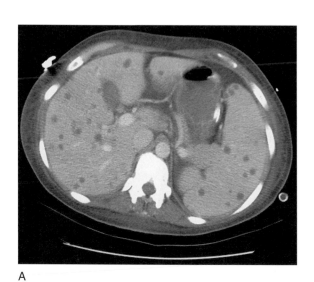

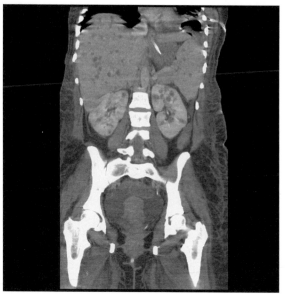

A   B

1. What underlying clinical state in this young man with leukemia may result in these findings?

2. What common disease may mimic this condition?

3. What is the most common causative organism?

4. What other organisms also produce this appearance?

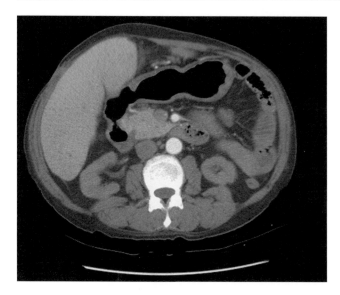

1. Describe the appearance of the stomach in this CT image.

2. How would you describe the gastric fold pattern?

3. If the stomach does not change shape, what might you call this condition on a barium examination?

4. What are some of the conditions that might cause this appearance?

CASE 174

Microabscesses of the Liver and Spleen

1. Immunosuppression.

2. Metastases.

3. Candidiasis.

4. *Aspergillus* and *Cryptococcus*.

Cross-Reference

Gastrointestinal Imaging: THE REQUISITES, ed 3, p 216.

Comments

Multiple low-density areas throughout the liver or spleen may be the result of metastasis, which is the most common cause. However, when there are numerous tiny low-density areas occurring diffusely, the possibility of microabscesses must be seriously considered. The lesions almost always occur in the setting of some type of immunosuppression (i.e., patients with acquired immunodeficiency syndrome, transplant recipients, those with leukemia, and cancer patients undergoing chemotherapy). Patients on steroid therapy compose another subgroup to be considered. The microabscesses develop as the result of a systemic sepsis with a micro-organism, usually fungal. However, many patients may have no irregular findings on blood cultures.

Candida albicans is the organism that most commonly produces this type of appearance. It is believed that the organism often resides in the immunosuppressed patient, and when the immune status of the patient decreases to a certain threshold, a systemic infection occurs. Other organisms that also have been implicated include *Cryptococcus* and *Aspergillus* species. Rarely can this radiologic appearance be attributed to some type of bacterial infection. On ultrasound these abscesses have a bright central echogenic focus with a surrounding hypo-echoic band and "bull's eye" lesion. Hepatic or splenic enlargement may be present. CT often reveals multiple low-density areas in the liver or spleen that often do not exceed 1 cm in diameter. Sometimes there is a central area of high density. The major differential considerations include metastases, and lymphoma may have a similar appearance.

Notes

CASE 175

Severe Uremic Gastritis

1. Air-filled with uniformly mild thickening of the wall.

2. Atrophic

3. Linitis plastica.

4. Severe uremic gastritis (as in this case), gastric sarcoidosis, eosinophilic gastritis, Crohn's disease, radiation, syphilis, severe corrosive gastritis.

Cross-Reference

Gastrointestinal Imaging: THE REQUISITES, ed 3, p 70.

Comments

The usual cause of an atrophic, rigid nonpliant stomach is generally primary or metastatic malignancy. It cannot be totally excluded here, but the lack of mass makes it much less likely. Other conditions that diffusely involve the stomach and result in a ridged "linitis–like" picture must be considered. In this case the patient was a sickle cell patient with chronic renal failure. In such patients chronic severe gastritis is common. Many will also have chronic duodenitis, such as this patient. Uremic gastritis is mostly seen in patients on long-term dialysis. There is also thought to be a higher incidence of peptic ulcer disease in such patients. There would appear to be a correlation between elevated serum creatinine levels and serum gastrin levels, although its is not clear that this is an instigating factor involved with uremic gastritis. Increased urea in the blood may affect the gastric mucosa directly. Endoscopically, uremic gastris has been described as atrophy and hemorrhagic erosive gastritis. *Helicobacter* involvement as a causative effect in uremic gastritis has also been looked at and found to occur with about the same frequency as in other patients with peptic ulcer disease. However, whatever the cause, there seems to be little doubt that patients undergoing chronic dialysis have a higher level of chronic gastritis, duodenitis, and peptic ulceration and erosions and are more predisposed to GI bleeding than the normal population.

Notes

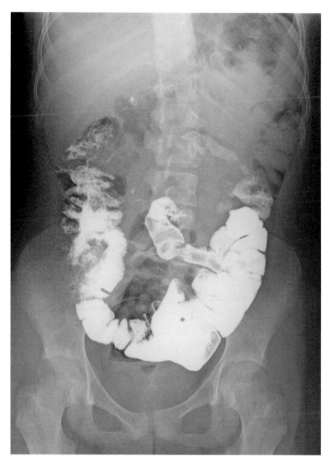

A

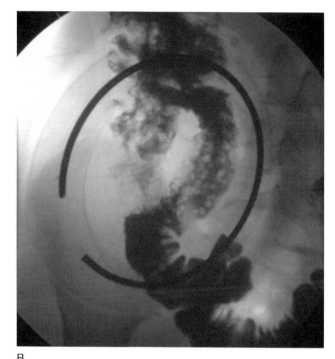

B

1. Describe the appearance of the terminal ileum in this 22-year-old man.

2. What idiopathic complication might this condition be associated with in the pediatric age group?

3. What are normal lymphoid aggregates in the ileum called?

4. Is there any relationship between this finding and IBD (inflammatory bowel disease)?

Lymphoid Hyperplasia of Terminal Ileum

1. Abnormal terminal ileum with numerous 2- to 3-mm nodules scattered through the terminal ileum without evidence of ulceration or inflammation, lymphoid nodular hyperplasia (LNH) best seen with compression view.

2. Ileocolic intussusception.

3. Peyer's patches.

4. Not directly.

Cross-Reference

Gastrointestinal Imaging: THE REQUISITES, ed 3, p 127.

Comments

The condition of lymphoid hyperplasia is often a normal finding in children. It is thought by some that it might act as a nidus for childhood idopathic ileocolic interception. The pattern has also been described in patients with immunodeficiency or giardiasis infestation as well as in *Yersinia* infections of the small bowel (usually the TI), Whipple's disease, and Waldenström's macroglobulinemia. Some investigators feel there is an association of lymphoid hyperplasia of the terminal ileum with the development of Crohn's disease in the distal small bowel. These nodules can range in size from 2 to 5 mm and usually involve the distal small bowel. Cross over into the colon is unusual, although colonic lymphoid hyperplasia is a known entity. In most cases they are regarded as a reactive hyperplasia secondary to bowel response to some viral infectious or inflammatory process which is generally self-limiting, and eventually disappears. There is a significant school of thought that in some cases nodular lymphoid hyperplasia is a presenting sign of small bowel multifocal lymphoma. Another unusual association that has been reported is lactose intolerance. In some instances in adults the condition has been pronounced and symptomatic with weight loss, diarrhea, and abdominal pain to the point at which resection of the terminal ileum was undertaken with varying results. Recently a controversial linkage of childhood autism, LNH, and childhood immunization in Europe was made and has sparked considerable debate.

Notes

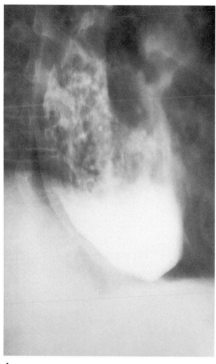

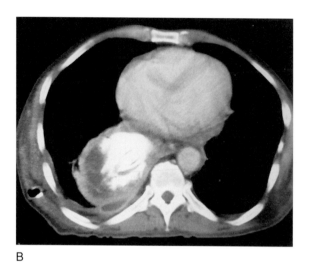

A   B

1. What is the underlying pathophysiologic defect in this patient?

2. What other disorders may mimic this condition?

3. What is an important complication of this disease?

4. Name other conditions that are associated with an increased risk of esophageal carcinoma.

Esophageal Carcinoma Developing in Achalasia

1. Absent or decreased number of ganglion cells in the esophagus.

2. Scleroderma, Chagas' disease, carcinoma of the gastroesophageal junction, and peptic stricture.

3. Esophageal carcinoma.

4. Lye strictures, celiac disease, radiation, head and neck tumors, Plummer-Vinson syndrome, and palmar and plantar hyperkeratosis.

Cross-Reference

Gastrointestinal Imaging: THE REQUISITES, ed 3, p 2.

Comments

Achalasia is a fairly common but poorly understood disorder of esophageal motility, producing life-long dysfunction. It is a neurogenic disorder marked by a decrease or absence of ganglion cells in the esophagus. Abnormalities also have been found in the vagal trunks and nuclei. The underlying etiology for this loss of innervation is uncertain. The result is decreasing esophageal peristalsis and failure of the lower esophageal sphincter to relax. Achalasia occurs almost equally among men and women. Onset is typically in early adulthood, and later onset should raise suspicions of carcinoma, which may mimic the condition (secondary achalasia). With long-standing achalasia, the esophagus becomes markedly dilated and food is retained in it. Scleroderma, peptic strictures, and intramural spread of carcinoma at the gastroesophageal junction may produce a similar appearance.

One of the unusual complications of this condition is the development of esophageal carcinoma secondary to chronic stasis. This complication is said to affect approximately 5% of achalasia patients, although there are many who feel the incidence to be much less. Some authors do not classify cancer as a complication of this condition and consider its prevalence in those with achalasia no higher than in the general population. The duration of the achalasia is usually 20 or more years before carcinoma is found. Typically, squamous cell carcinoma is present, but adenocarcinoma also has been reported. Other conditions that have a proven association with an increased incidence of esophageal squamous carcinoma include lye strictures, head and neck tumors, celiac disease, Plummer-Vinson syndrome (Paterson-Kelly syndrome), radiation exposure, palmar and plantar hyperkeratosis, as well as skin conditions such as epidermolysis bullosa.

Notes

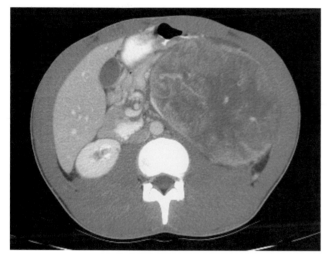

A

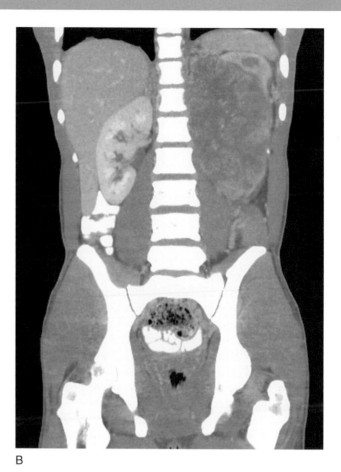

B

1. This 19-year-old man presents with weight loss and abdominal mass. Describe the findings and effects on the GI tract.

2. Is this a gastrointestinal lesion?

3. Are you able to identify the left kidney?

4. Given the patient's age, what prior history would you want to know?

Recurrent Wilms' Tumor Affecting Stomach and Bowel

1. Large inhomogeneous mass is seen in the LUQ compressing stomach and displacing bowel. Recurrent Wilms' tumor

2. No.

3. No. The compressed stomach is the structure seen above the lesion.

4. Any history of childhood tumors?

Cross-Reference

Gastrointestinal Imaging: THE REQUISITES, ed 3, p 59.

Comments

Wilms' tumor is a solid tumor arising from kidney seen in children and infants. It is the fifth most common cancer in children. It is diagnosed and treated in childhood. Today it is a treatable and curable condition. Almost 90% of these patients survive 5 years following diagnosis as opposed to the poor prognosis of even 25 years ago. In this case the patient had a Wilms' tumor of early childhood that was successfully treated. Almost 15 years later the tumor has recurred, as these tumors are known to do (2–3% after nephrectomy) with a much reduced survival rate (20–40%). This tumor falls into the category of large extrinsic masses affecting the bowel. In the left upper quadrant such things as splenomegaly, pancreatic pseudocysts, pancreatic masses, subphrenic processes or process relating to the proximal jejunum, or splenic flexure of the colon would be considerations. In a young patient with a large abdominal mass, the questions of recurrent childhood tumors would be raised. This is unusual but obviously does occur. Most of the extrinsic processes mentioned will compress or displace the adjacent bowel. Rarely there may be contiguous invasion. In this case the stomach can be seen sandwiched between the diaphragm and the tumorous mass without local invasion.

Notes

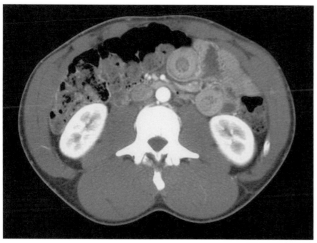 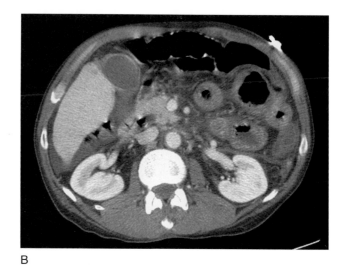

A   B

1. Describe the findings on these two CT images of two different patients.

2. What would be your diagnostic considerations if these patients were immunodeficient?

3. What is the most common organism involved in AIDS-related SB enterolitis?

4. What other types of infectious processes can affect the small bowel of the immunocompromised patient?

AIDS Patient with Small Bowel Infection

1. Bowel wall thickening and edema as well as some ascitic fluid.

2. Small bowel opportunistic infections.

3. *Mycobacterium avium* complex (MAC)

4. Cryptosporidiosis, cytomegalovirus (CMV) infection, microsporidiosis.

Cross-Reference

Gastrointestinal Imaging: THE REQUISITES, ed 3, p 342.

Comments

In patients with acquired immunodeficiency syndrome the small bowel is a common site for infection by opportunistic pathogens. The presenting symptoms are almost always abdominal pain and diarrhea. Although MAC appears to be the most common cause, other considerations would have to include cryptosporidiosis, CMV infection, giardiasis, microsporidiosis, and histoplasmosis. The organism is usually identified by small bowel aspirates or biopsy. Both the images shown in this case were AIDS-related enteric infections. Both barium studies and CT will show abnormal small bowel, as in these cases, that is nonspecific. In cases of enteric involvement of the small bowel with MAC, barium small bowel studies have described the changes in the small bowel as being similar to those seen in Whipple's disease. Cytomegalovirus (CMV) infections are well known in the colon and less frequently the esophagus and small bowel of AIDS patients. Bowel obstructions relating to CMV small bowel infection have been described. When seen on CT images the small bowel will appear thickened and edematous in most of these patients. The possibility of small bowel lymphoma (non-Hodgkin's lymphoma is not uncommon in AIDS patients) must always be considered. Obstruction is uncommon. In older non-AIDS patients, ischemic changes may have a similar appearance. Other neopastic lesions described in the small bowel of AIDS patients include Kaposi sarcoma.

Notes

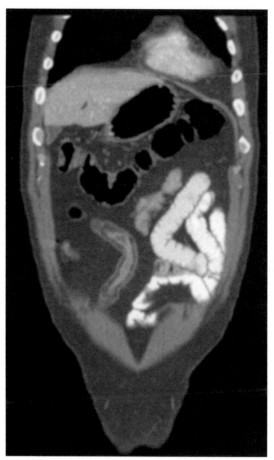

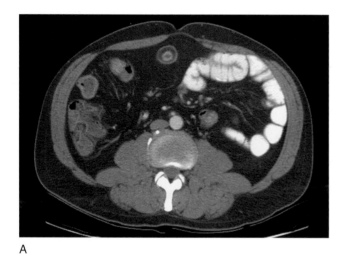

A

B

1. This young patient complains of abdominal pain and diarrhea. What are the CT findings?

2. What is unusual about the thickened ileum wall?

3. What percentage of Crohn's patients present after 50 years of age?

4. Could this be ulcerative colitis?

C A S E   1 8 0

Intramural Fat in Crohn's Disease

1. Thickened ileum with a patternless "pipe–like" appearance of the bowel.

2. Lucency in the submucosa that has the appearance of fat.

3. About 10% to 15%.

4. No.

Cross-Reference

Gastrointestinal Imaging: THE REQUISITES, ed 3, p 294.

Comments

The ring of fat tissue seen in the submucosa of this patient is fast becoming an important CT sign of inflammatory bowel disease. In general, the "halo" sign of submucosal fat is not specific for any particular disease and has been described in several inflammatory entities including Crohn's disease and ulcerative colitis as well as several other inflammatory processes including radiation enteritis. It has been described in normal bowel! This is not the "creeping fat" sign described by pathologists and relating to the gross anatomy of Crohn's disease. Here mesenteric fat around the diseased bowel becomes thickened and rubbery, and appears to extend over the inflamed sersoal surface like "fingers of fat" creeping across the surface of the bowel. The "halo" sign (as seen in this case), on the other hand, is seen in GI inflammatory conditions as a well-defined ring of submucosal lucency, usually of fat density. Its appearance has become more noticeable since the advent of high-resolution CT imaging. It has also been described in intestinal lymphangiectasia. Some authors think of the "halo" sign as nonspecific submucosal edema. It is difficult to actually measure Hounsfield numbers of the lucent ring, but it appears, in this patient, to be of fat density. Subsequent biopsy of this bowel showed this to be Crohn's disease. Edema of the bowel wall usually affects all layers, as shown in Case 179. Moreover, the "halo" sign has been described in patients with no evidence of bowel disease. It may be a finding related to obesity in such cases. If one accepts the fact that the halo sign can represent either fat or a ring of edema, then other possibilities must be considered, such as ischemic bowel or pseudomembranous colitis. Some authors have deemed the rings of lucency as a "double halo" sign when edema is seen between the mucosa and submucosa. In general, a thin single fatty submucosal layer is yet another manifestation of bowel wall inflammation. In a young patient, such as in this case, with the halo sign involving the TI, Crohn's disease must be considered first.

Notes

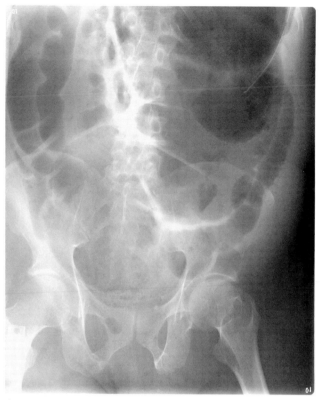

A

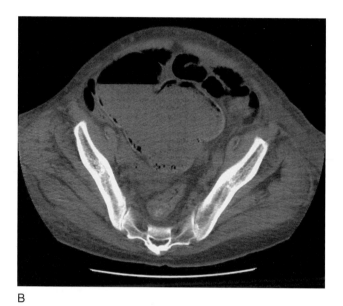

B

1. What is the most common cause of colon obstruction?

2. What percentage of colon obstructions are due to postoperative adhesions?

3. Your next step is a contrast enema to rule out obstruction. True or false?

4. Does the bowel gas pattern suggest a cecal or sigmoid obstruction?

Volvulus of the Transverse Colon

1. Tumor.

2. Rare. Less than 1%.

3. False. It is contraindicated.

4. Neither. The patient has a transverse colon volvulus.

Cross-Reference

Gastrointestinal Imaging: THE REQUISITES, ed 3, p 310.

Comments

The plain conventional AP image of this 74–year-old man, presenting with a distended abdomen and severe pain, shows dilated loops of colon and some small bowel. Because CT imaging of the abdomen is now routinely done on all patients with abdominal complaints or signs, we are able to see air in the cecal wall, indicating probable ischemic changes. We are probably witnessing, via CT imaging, the natural history of colonic obstruction and dilatation of the cecum leading to perforation. The pneumatosis is not apparent on the plain image, obtained about the same time. However, the finding makes a contrast enema contraindicated, in that it will put the patient in immediate risk of perforation. The patient immediately went to surgery where he was found to have a volvulus of the transverse colon. The most common cause of colonic obstruction is cancer, followed by diverticulitis and volvulus. Most commonly volvulus is in the sigmoid (80%) but is also seen in the cecum (15%) and the transverse colon (5%). Predisposing factors are an extra long mesocolon and marked redundancy in the transverse colon. Some authors feel that patients with colonic interposition anterior to the liver (Chiladiti syndrome), reaching the diaphragm, puts patients at increased risk for volvulus. However, this is disputed by other authors, who consider the interposition a variant, with no clinical significance. Splenic flexure volvulus, which may be considered a form of transverse volvulus, is the least common type of colonic volvulus. Surgery is the most acceptable form of definitive treatment. The bowel may be complicated by vascular compromise, as in this patient. In such an event, mortality and morbidity rates are high. Simple reduction of all types of colonic volvulus carries a high recurrence rate.

Notes

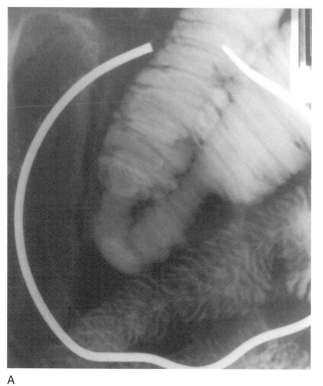

A

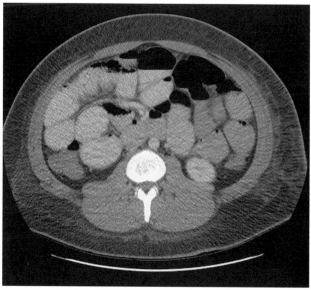

B

1. In general, what might your diagnosis be in this case?

2. What does the spot film from the barium study of the small bowel tell you?

3. How common is this condition?

4. What is the most common predisposing condition associated with this finding?

Ischemic Stricture of Small Bowel

1. Small bowel obstruction.

2. That there is focal narrowing, but no destructive changes.

3. Uncommon.

4. Mesenteric insufficiency, healing, and residual focal scarring and narrowing.

Cross-Reference

Gastrointestinal Imaging: THE REQUISITES, ed 3, p 115.

Comments

This patient presented with an incomplete small bowel obstruction (CT image). A barium small bowel examination showed a focal area of narrowing in the ileum. Please note that the fold pattern is distorted but intact without evidence of mucosal destruction, suggesting this is not a malignant obstruction. The possibility of an inflammatory obstruction was considered. The segment of involved ileum was resected and pathologic examination of the narrowing showed it to be an area of fibrosis and scarring, resulting from prior ischemic disease. These types of small bowel obstructions are uncommon when compared to postoperative adhesions causing small bowel obstruction. It is seen mostly in the elderly population resulting from occlusive or low flow mesenteric arterial disease. However, focal ischemic and resultant fibrotic strictures of the small bowel have been reported in such conditions as collagen vascular disease and any condition resulting in a vasculitis, such as rheumatoid arthritis, post-transplant cases and trauma without perforation, radiation, and even some malabsorption processes. Ischemic disease of the colon is more apt to result in a residual stricture (up to 40%). Small bowel obstruction is also a well-known complication of neoplasms, such as primary adenocarcinoma and carcinoids, as well as inflammatory processes such as Crohn's disease.

Notes

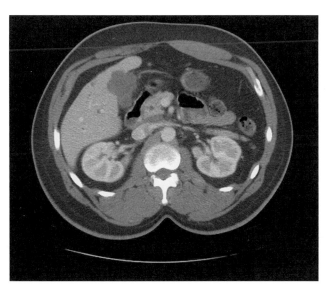

A

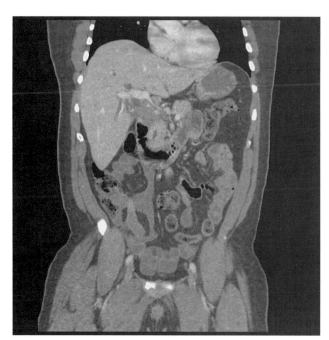

B

1. What is the most common malignancy of the biliary tract?

2. What is the mean survival rate for the condition shown here?

3. What risk factor has been implicated in this disease?

4. Is CT specific for this condition?

Carcinoma of the Gallbladder

1. Gallbladder carcinoma, as in this case.

2. Mean survival time is about 6 months.

3. Porcelain gallbladder.

4. No.

Cross-Reference

Gastrointestinal Imaging: THE REQUISITES, ed 3, p 250.

Comments

Carcinoma of the gallbladder is not common, but it is the most common malignant biliary disease. It is generally an adenocarcinoma. Patients present with symptoms that are very similar to pancreatic head lesions; jaundice, weight loss, and abdominal pain. The condition of chronic cholecystitis that leads to cystic duct occlusion and (if it does not result in a septic catastrophe) can eventually result in a calcified gallbladder wall (porcelain gallbladder). The risk of gallbladder cancer in this setting is high (about 12%). However, other conditions (if not being direct risk factors) are certainly associated with carcinoma of the gallbladder. About 75% of patients with gallbladder cancer will have gallstones, especially a high percentage of cholesterol stones. Owing to the anatomic position of the gallbladder in or around the porta hepatis, the dissemination of the disease to important contiguous structures makes the outlook for survival bleak. CT is not specific but is suggestive. In some cases a soft tissue–filled gallbladder, still maintaining its gallbladder configuration (the "jam packed gallbladder") may be seen, such as in this case. In many instances the finding will be an amorphous mass in the porta hepatis with bile duct obstruction. The origin may be pancreatic or biliary. Depending on the clinical presentation, severe gallbladder inflammation would also be a consideration.

Notes

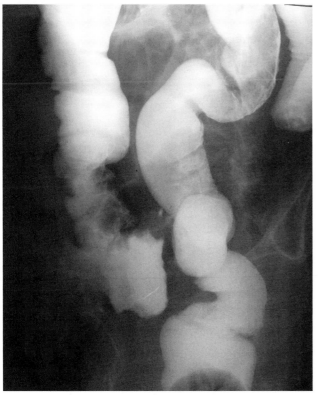

A

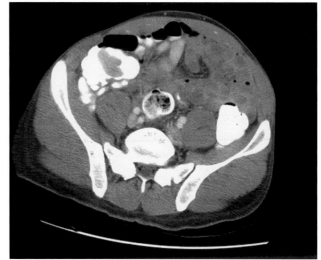

B

1. What is the most common primary malignancy affecting the cecum?

2. How often will lymphoma affect the colon?

3. What structures does Burkitt's lymphoma in Africa most often involve?

4. What virus is associated with Burkitt's lymphoma?

Burkitt's Lymphoma of Cecum

1. Adenocarcinoma.

2. Less than 1% of colonic malignancies.

3. Facial bones, especially mandible, mostly in children.

4. Epstein-Barr virus.

Cross-Reference

Gastrointestinal Imaging: THE REQUISITES, ed 3, p 282.

Comments

This young patient has a destructive colonic mass in the cecum. The obvious possibility would be colonic adeno-carcinoma, which is by far the most common malignant lesion of the colon. Lymphoma is not common. However, among the various types of lymphomas seen in the colon is Burkitt's lymphoma, named after Denis Burkitt, a pathologist who first described the relationship of this highly aggressive tumor, affecting mostly children in equatorial Africa in areas of endemic malaria. The lesion usually involved the mandible in these children. Burkitt's lymphoma is one of the most aggressive tumors known, with a doubling rate much greater than the usual adenocarcinoma of the colon.

The type found in North America usually presents as an intra-abdominal process in the distal ileum or proximal colon and can be seen as a mass in the right lower quadrant. It is extremely typical of Burkitt's lymphoma to involve this area, and the diagnosis should be strongly considered in any child who has a painless palpable mass in the region with heme-positive stool. However, in North America the disease is seen more commonly in young adults. In the type of lymphoma which Burkitt described in Africa, the jaw and retroperitoneal lymph nodes were frequently involved in children, but this is not typical of the type of Burkitt's lymphoma common in North America. The tumor is usually intra-abdominal and often associated with the Epstein-Barr virus, as are some other lymphomas and cancers. As mentioned above, a distinctive feature of this lymphoma is its rapid doubling time. It grows in an extremely aggressive fashion, involving and displacing bowel loops in the region. It also responds fairly dramatically to chemotherapy. HIV patients are particularly susceptible to this tumor.

Notes

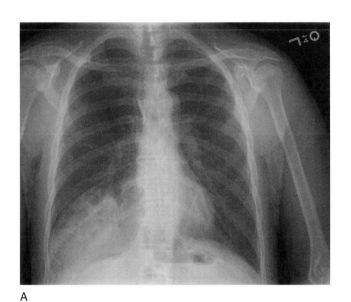

A

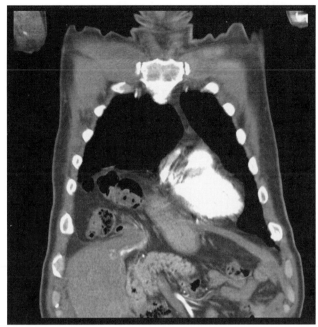

B

1. What is the most common congenital hernial defect in the diaphragm?

2. What is the most common cause of acquired diaphragmatic hernias?

3. Which side is most commonly affected in traumatic defects of the diaphragm?

4. What portion of the diaphragm is most affected with a Bochdalek hernia? What part of the diaphragm is affected in this case?

Morgagni Hernia of the Diaphragm

1. Bochdalek hernia, almost 90%.

2. Trauma, blunt or penetrating.

3. The left side in over 70% of cases.

4. Bochdalek hernias affect the posterior lateral aspect of the diaphragm, mostly on the left lung. In this case the defect is in the anterior right diaphragm, a Morgagni hernia.

Cross-Reference

Gastrointestinal Imaging: THE REQUISITES, ed 3, p 326.

Comments

Congenital diaphragmatic hernias are a major issue in neonates and can be associated with other congenital abnormalities such as pulmonary hypoplasia and gastro-intestinal and cardiac abnormalities. The subsequent migration of the abdominal content into the chest can also compromise breathing. Some of these defects may go undetected into adult life and, indeed, may be discovered as an incidental finding. The same may be true about acquired diaphragmatic hernias, following blunt trauma to the abdomen. With CT, diaphragmatic trauma may be missed at initial imaging, even with multi-planar imaging if there has been no migration of abdominal content through the rent in the diaphragm. These patients will invariably have other life-threatening injuries, which must be addressed first. The right diaphragm is the side most commonly affected with trauma. It is thought that the liver confers some protection to the left. The diagnosis is sometimes made at surgery. In many instances in adult life, abdominal content will migrate through a defect in the diaphragm, congenital or acquired, and cause no symptoms. In other patients there may be vague upper abdominal discomfort. However, some patients will eventually develop an incarceration of bowel in the lower chest with obstructive symptoms and potential vascular compromise. In this lady a defect in her anterior right diaphragm, a Morgagni hernia, was discovered incidentally on routine chest image. Barium studies have always been a definitive way of evaluating the type and amount of bowel entrapped with the hernia. However, in recent times CT, because of its speed and its ability to evaluate for the presence of other organs besides bowel (spleen and liver), is being used with greater frequency with satisfactory results.

Notes

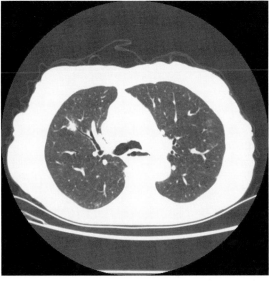
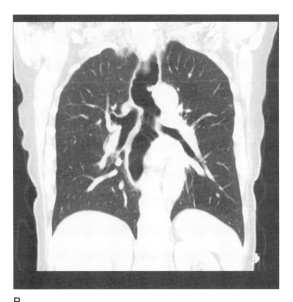

A B

1. This male patient, being treated for lung cancer, now complains of swallowing problems. What do the CT images demonstrate?

2. What are the secondary conditions sometimes associated with a malignancy, and for which there is no well-understood explanation?

3. What is the most common malignancy that gives rise to this relationship?

4. What is the incidence of this unusual relationship?

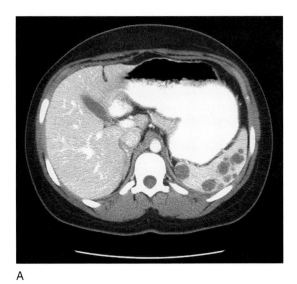
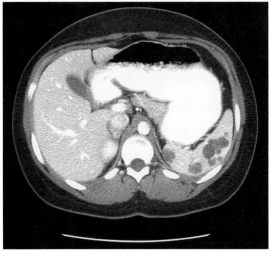

A B

1. What are the chances of these defects in the spleen being simple cysts?

2. What is the most common cause of perfusion defects in the spleen?

3. What percentage of patients with metastatic disease will have splenic involvement?

4. What is the most common tumor seen in the spleen?

CASE 186

Paraneoplastic Syndrome

1. CT images show a lung lesion (carcinoma of lung) and dilated air-filled esophagus.

2. Paraneoplastic syndromes.

3. Small cell carcinoma of the lung.

4. Not well quantified. Some think about 10% of cases.

Cross-Reference
Gastrointestinal Imaging: THE REQUISITES, ed 3, p 27.

Comments
In some malignant conditions, secondary (nonmetastatic) systemic effects can be seen accompanying primary malignant disease. The achalasia-like appearance of the esophagus, as seen in this case, is one such example and is most commonly seen in patients with small cell carcinoma of the lung. However, the paraneoplastic syndromes may encompass much more than the neuromuscular functions of the esophagus. They can affect skin, muscle, joints, kidneys, and even endocrine function. Some cases of scleroderma have been determined to be a paraneoplastic syndrome, secondary to a primary lesion elsewhere in the body. The exact mechanism of paraneoplastic manifestations is not well understood. It may be that the tumors excrete hormones, which affect a specific target organ. There is considerable discussion in the literature of tumor antibodies produced by the body to resist the tumor, but which have a secondary effect in the body. The patient with carcinoma of the lung who has concomitant achalasia-like symptoms and findings, is not common but is not rare. Other gastrointestinal manifestations of paraneoplastic syndrome have been reported, including malabsorption in the small bowel (some say the most common) and unexplained diarrhea. This is an area which is currently of great interest and to which researchers are devoting considerable time. It is possible that the problem is much larger than we currently know. Although lung tumors have been mostly shown to be involved with the paraneoplastic syndromes, recent work has shown that malignancies from almost every body system have that capability. Imaging may be utilized to show either the primary lesions or paraneoplastic manifestations. However, laboratory studies have been where the most of the paraneoplastic effects have been detected.

Notes

CASE 187

Splenic Metastatic Disease

1. Unlikely, as the defects are multiple.

2. Probably splenic infarctions.

3. Rare, around 1% seen in imaging, as in this case; 2% at autopsy.

4. Hemangioma.

Cross-Reference
Gastrointestinal Imaging: THE REQUISITES, ed 3, p 212.

Comments
Marginal perfusion defects in the spleen, often wedge-shaped, are a common finding in the spleen at CT imaging. These defects are almost always old splenic infarcts. Despite the vascularity and the hematogenous "filter" function of the spleen, metastatic disease is extremely uncommon. Several theories as to why this seemingly unusual situation should be the case have been proffered; from the angle of the splenic artery from its takeoff from the celiac axis, to the high concentrations of lymphoid tissue in the spleen. As in this case the most common primary cancer is lung cancer followed by gastrointestinal tumors. To have splenic metastatic disease apparently without liver involvement is especially rare, representing less than 5% of cases of reported splenic metastatic disease.

Other differential considerations would have to include splenic cysts, congenital and acquired (usually secondary to trauma). These cysts are almost entirely solitary. Hydatid cyst may also be seen in the spleen as a solitary lesion. Abscesses, which are encountered with more frequency in immunocompromised patients, may be single but are usually multiple and often tiny. Hemangiomas, the most common benign tumor of the spleen, can be solitary or multiple. Involvement of the spleen with lymphoma or leukemia usually takes the form of splenomegaly. However, if the spleen is of normal size with multiple defects, these possibilities must also be considered. Pancreatic pseudocysts have been reported as intrasplenic lesions.

Notes

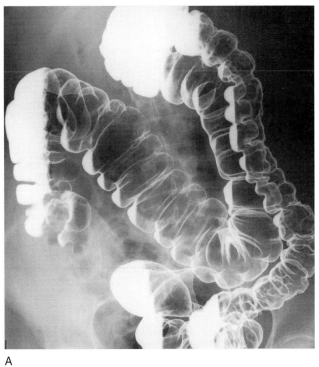

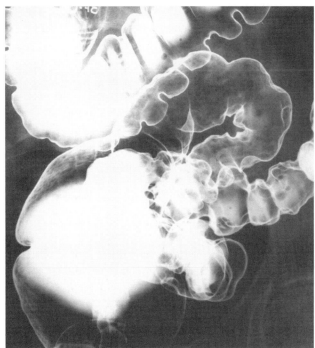

A   B

1. This patient presents with rectal bleeding. What part of the colon is primarily involved with this process?

2. What is the most common colon polyp?

3. What conditions might qualify as diagnostic considerations here?

4. If you knew the patient was in her late 30s and had recently traveled abroad, would it affect your differential considerations?

Schistosomiasis of the Colon

1. The distal colon is involved.

2. Hyperplastic polyps.

3. Hyperplastic polyps, adenomas, polyposis syndromes, and pneumotosis coli.

4. Yes, if she was in North Africa, where she unknowingly contracted schistosomiasis.

Cross-Reference
Gastrointestinal Imaging: THE REQUISITES, ed 3, p 290.

Comments
Polypoid processes limited to the distal colon, as in this case, are usually hyperplastic in nature. However, hyperplastic polyps, although the most common colonic polyp, are mostly small (<5 mm) and difficult to image. The polyps shown in this case are larger with a mostly smooth elevated surface. Some have tiny collections of barium, indicating ulceration. The patient presented with rectal bleeding. Adenomas, which represent about 10% of all colonic polyps, can bleed. However, a cluster of adenomatous polyps limited to the distal colon would be extremely unusual, even in the various polyposis syndromes. The patient's history of foreign travel and "swimming in the Nile" must be considered in the differential possibilities. Schistosomiasis is endemic in several places in the world and, until recently with the return of malaria to the world scene, was the most common infectious (parasitic) disease in the world. Even a single exposure to fresh water in these endemic areas can result in infection, such as in this patient. Humans are the host for this parasitic infection; and with world travel becoming virtually commonplace, physicians and particularly radiologists ought to be aware of the possibility of tropical diseases in our own "backyard," especially the new outbreaks of malaria in travelers coming home to the United States. In schistosomiasis the organisms are *Schistosoma mansoni* and *S. japonicum*. In fresh water the tiny worms penetrate the human skin, seek the vascular system of the host, and migrate to the liver, lungs, and bladder, as well as other organs. Bladder involvement is associated with an increased risk of bladder cancer. When in the host organ, in this case the lower colon (usually *S. mansoni*), they infest the venules of the colon wall, and eventually mature eggs will be deposited in the wall (hence the polyps) and will then rupture into the lumen (hence the ulceration on the polyps and bleeding).

Notes

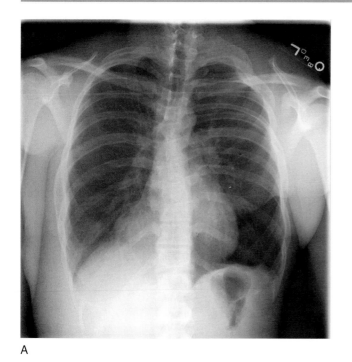

A

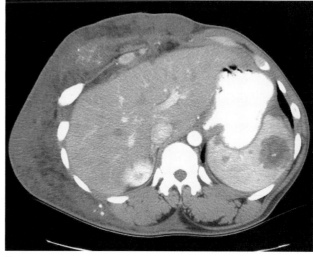

B

1. What is the most common neoplasm found in the spleen?

2. Why is it likely that this is not the lesion shown here?

3. This 20-year-old man also has dysphasia. How can that be accounted for?

4. What congenital conditions can this lesion be associated with?

Lymphangioma of Spleen

1. Hemangiomas.

2. The lesions are multiple and unlike hemangiomas in their appearance. Also, there is soft tissue thickening over the lower chest wall.

3. Cystic hygromas are seen in this condition.

4. Lymphangiomas involving spleen, soft tissue, and bone are seen with greater frequency in Down syndrome, fetal alcohol syndrome, Turner syndrome, and several other congenital conditions.

Cross-Reference

Gastrointestinal Imaging: THE REQUISITES, ed 3, p 214.

Comments

Lymphangioma of the spleen is an unusual condition that rarely involves the spleen. The splenic lesions can be solitary or multiple as in this case. Lymphangioma is a congenital malformation of the lymphatic vessels and system. It can be focal or widespread lymphangiomatosis, as in this example. Even so, the lesion is entirely benign with no malignant potential known. Perhaps the most common manifestation of this in infants is a cystic hygroma, which is thought to represent a form of focal lymphangioma in the neck. Histologically, lymphangiomas are thought to be harmatomas rather than neoplasms. The involvement of the spleen can be a solitary organ involvement or part of lymphangiomatosis. Bone can also be involved. Please note the deformities of the ribs in this patient. Lytic expansile lesions of bones in this condition has been called Gorham's disease. However, these bones appear deformed rather than replaced or destroyed. In some cases of splenic lymphangioma, splenectomy has been necessary when the lesion is symptomatic or diagnosis is questionable. The skin thickening seen over this patient's body is a manifestation of lymphangiomatosis, as is the mediastinal and neck involvement. This condition has been classified into three groupings: (1) lymphangioma circumscriptum, (2) cavernous lymphangioma (this patient), and (3) cystic lymphangioma (cystic hygroma, which can also be seen in some cases of cavernous lymphangioma).

Notes

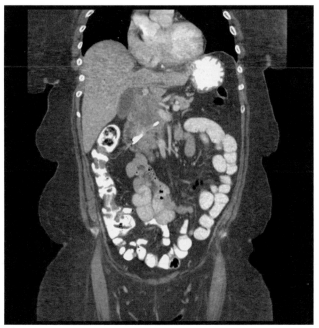

A

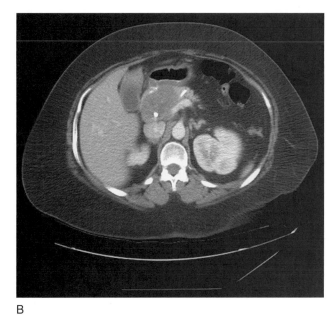

B

1. What is the finding and what would be your first diagnostic consideration?

2. What other condition might give such an appearance?

3. What do the images show that might make you reconsider your initial diagnosis?

4. What might be the clinical presentation in this 32-year-old woman?

T Cell Lymphoma of Pancreatic Head

1. A large soft tissue mass in the pancreatic head, most likely pancreatic carcinoma.

2. An inflammatory mass, an aggregate of peripancreatic lymph nodes, peripancreatic metastatic disease, and infiltrating lymphoma of the pancreatic head, which was the histologic diagnosis in this patient.

3. Ductal adenocarcinoma of the pancreas tends to be a hypovascular lesion, whereas this mass has a more uniform appearance. Also lack of pancreatic duct dilatation.

4. She presented with mild jaundice. Note the biliary stent in place.

Cross-Reference
Gastrointestinal Imaging: THE REQUISITES, ed 3, p 169.

Comments

Primary pancreatic head lymphomas are rare, thought to make up about 0.5% of pancreatic head masses. Secondary involvement of the pancreas by a non-Hodgkin's lymphoma resulting from gross peripancreatic lymphadenopathy is more common. However, in cases such as shown here, in which the mass is entirely within the pancreatic substance and there is no evidence of lymphoma elsewhere, pancreatic lymphoma is a possible differential consideration. In this case the lesion was a T cell lymphoma. Most pancreatic lymphomas are B cell lymphomas. Diagnosis usually results from CT-guided needle aspiration or surgical pathology. MDCT and routine as well as endoscopic ultrasound have also been useful in the diagnosis of pancreatic head masses. However, none of these imaging modalities can be considered specific. Nevertheless, MDCT imaging obtained here shows a more than expected homogeneous appearance than might be expected with a hypovascular ductal adenocarcinoma. In addition, the small portion of the distal pancreas included in the images shows no evidence of pancreatic duct obstruction. Moreover, the biliary duct obstruction that brought the patient to medical attention and resulted in stent placement has completely resolved in a few days. This would be highly unlikely for the usual ductal carcinoma of the pancreas. All these observations, although not specific, might suggest alternative diagnostic possibilities. The incidence of lymphoma is increased in AIDS patients and the incidence of pancreatic lymphoma may also be increased.

Notes

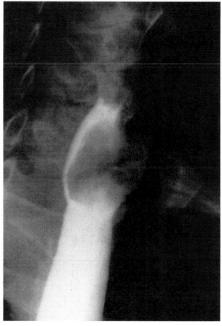

A

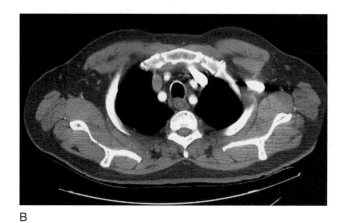

B

1. This patient complains of a globus sensation during swallowing. What are the findings?

2. What is the significance of polyps of the esophagus?

3. What is the most common benign neoplasm of the esophagus?

4. What other types of tumors might have this appearance?

Fibrovascular Esophageal Polyp

1. Filling defect in the esophagogram and intraluminal soft tissue density on the CT image.

2. Polyps of the esophagus must always be viewed with suspicion of malignancy until proved otherwise.

3. Leiomyoma or benign stromal cell tumor.

4. Spindle cell tumors (carcinosarcoma), leiomyosarcoma, adenocarcinoma, and even foreign bodies. Also, stromal cell tumors, fibrovascular polyps, granular cell polyps, and rarely, squamous papillomas.

Cross-Reference
Gastrointestinal Imaging: THE REQUISITES, ed 3, p 10.

Comments

Polyps of the esophagus are unusual, the most common of which is the benign leiomyoma, or stromal cell tumor. They are usually solitary, but multiple leiomyomatosis of the esophagus has been encountered on rare occasion. Fibrovascular polyps, which are composed of fibrovascular tissue, are also rare. Because of the presence of fatty tissue in some of these tumors, fibrovascular polyps may appear to have low density on CT examination. They have a propensity to develop in the upper portion of the esophagus, as seen in this case, in two different patients, particularly in the cervical region of the older population, which is the opposite of most esophageal tumors, typically seen in the middle to distal esophagus. These polyps occur more commonly in men.

Because of their soft nature, these tumors can grow quite large before producing symptoms. The cervical location exposes the polyps to repeated peristalsis and dragging by ingested materials that may cause the tumors to become pedunculated or mobile. Thus the most dramatic clinical finding is when the patient states that he or she has regurgitated a mass into the oropharynx and then swallowed it. These tumors may cause bleeding, but malignant transformation is rare, although if large enough, airway obstruction has been reported in these very mobile tumors. Granular cell tumors are also rare, and are felt to originate in Schwann cells. However, only about 10% occur in the GI tract, usually the esophagus. Squamous cell papillomas in the esophagus have been reported, more frequently in men. Most are asymptomatic. It is not clear whether papillomas are true neoplasms.

Notes

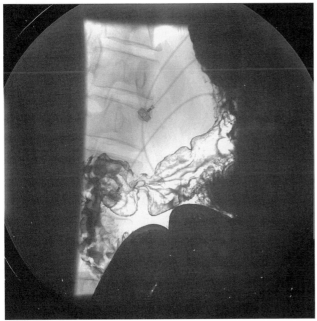

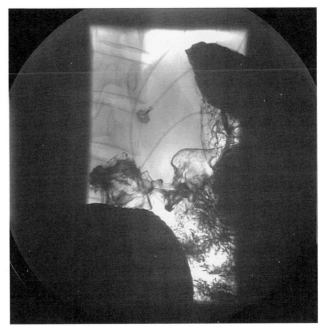

A

B

1. What is the pertinent finding on these compression spot films of the distal stomach?

2. Define a "Dragstead ulcer."

3. What are the possible complications of the ulcer in this case?

4. Define the difference between a "filling defect" and a "barium collection" and give examples of both.

Pyloric Channel Ulcer

1. The pyloric channel is well displayed and a small persistent barium collection is seen in the channel.

2. A penetrating ulcer that extends from the distal gastric antrum to the base of the duodenum, paralleling the pyloric channel, thus giving the so called "double pyloric channel" sign.

3. Bleeding, perforation, and gastric outlet obstruction.

4. A cavity in the GI tract that collects barium is called a barium collection and includes such things as ulcers and diverticula. On the other hand, things that displace barium are called filling defects; these include polyps, masses, and bowel content.

Cross-Reference
Gastrointestinal Imaging: THE REQUISITES, ed 3, p 97.

Comments

This UGI double contrast barium examination clearly shows a persistent collection of barium in the pyloric channel. Ulcers collect barium because they are essentially holes in the mucosa. In the same manner in which a pothole in the road may collect water, so will an ulcer collect barium. Moreover, the granulation tissue that forms the base of the ulceration tends to cause the barium to become adherent to the ulcer crater. Diverticula also collect barium in the same manner. On the other hand, space-occupying lesions such as polyps and masses will displace barium, which is called a filling defect. Although this was basic knowledge a decade ago, it seems less basic to current residents. The widespread use of endoscopy and decreased number of UGI examinations done by radiologists as well as the great interest in newer, more exciting modalities seem to have relegated expertise in barium procedures to a small niche in the radiology department of the 21st century. Nevertheless, the examinations will not go away and we are still required to have some basic knowledge. L. Dragstead, who connected hyperacidity to peptic disease (although to some extent this had been done by Beaumont in 1835), was a surgeon whose name is attached to a penetrating ulcer that connects the gastric antrum to the base of the duodenum; the double pyloric channel sign. Dragstead's work was done before Marshall made the connection between *Helicobacter pylori* and peptic ulcer disease. Ulcers in the pyloric channel often present as gastric outlet obstruction (GOO) after a chronic history of PUD. Beware the patient who presents with GOO with no history of PUD, as this is an ominous sign of possible malignancy.

Notes

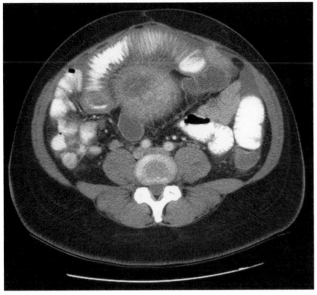 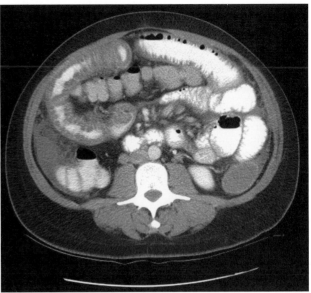

A   B

1. What might be the presenting signs and symptoms of this young patient?

2. What phrase is used to describe the appearance of the affected small loops?

3. What are some causes for this condition?

4. What differential diagnostic considerations would you entertain?

Small Bowel Intramural Hemorrhage

1. Abdominal pain, falling hematocrit.

2. "Stack of coins" appearance, a phrase used primarily in barium studies.

3. Mesenteric ischemia, anticoagulant therapy, trauma.

4. Edema, infiltrative processes such as carcinoma, carcinoid, or lymphoma or metastatic disease.

Cross-Reference

Gastrointestinal Imaging: THE REQUISITES, ed 3, p 144.

Comments

The patients presenting with abdominal pain and CT findings such as in this case must raise many diagnostic possibilities in the mind of the radiologist. The fact that this patient is relatively young lessens, but does not exclude, the possibility of ischemic disease and intramural hemorrhage. Hypoperfusion, such as in hypovolemic shocked bowel would be a consideration. Disease that manifests as an intramural vasculitis such as Schönlein-Henoch purpura affecting the bowel with intramural bleeding may also give such a picture. The CT images in this case show thickened small bowel wall and folds. The folds are "stacked" together such as might be seen in a barium small bowel study, the well-known "stack of coins" sign. In fact, this patient did indeed have a severe intramural hemorrhage of the small bowel. MDCT showed no evidence of arterial occlusion of the major mesenteric vessels. The length of involved bowel would make blunt trauma less likely. The possibility of an infiltrative process, neoplastic or non-neoplastic, is always a consideration. Such things as carcinoid involvement of the bowel might be considered, although the desmoplastic distortion of bowel loops is not present in this case. Metastatic disease would not likely affect such an extended length of bowel. Non-neoplastic diagnostic considerations would be intramural edema, intramural bleeding, and other less likely possibilities such as lymphangectasia and amyloid of the bowel. In this case all findings were the result of mesenteric and intramural small bowel bleeding. A CT examination repeated 3 weeks later showed normal small bowel throughout, an almost sure diagnostic sign of bleeding.

Notes

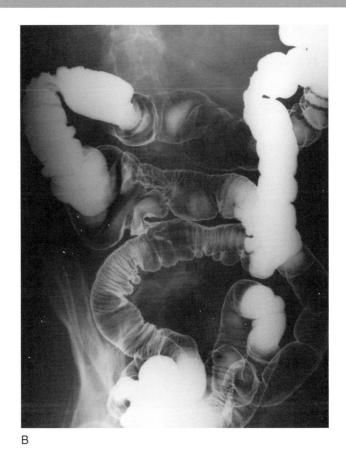

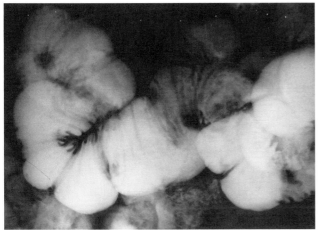

A

B

1. What disorders make up the CREST syndrome?

2. In mixed connective tissue disease, what intestinal organ is most commonly involved?

3. What are the underlying pathologic changes seen in the bowel as a result of scleroderma?

4. What is meant by the term "hidebound" in reference to the appearance of the bowel?

Scleroderma of the Small Bowel and Colon

1. Subcutaneous calcinosis, Raynaud's phenomenon, esophageal dysfunction, sclerodactyly, and telangiectasia.

2. Esophagus.

3. Fibrosis and small vessel vasculitis.

4. Crowding of the valvulae and rigidity of the bowel.

Cross-Reference

Gastrointestinal Imaging: THE REQUISITES, ed 3, pp 89, 113.

Comments

A number of connective tissue diseases can affect the small bowel and colon. Scleroderma is caused by abnormal deposition of collagen in the skin, adjacent to blood vessels, and in various visceral organs. It may be isolated or may occur as part of the CREST syndrome, which includes changes caused by calcinosis, Raynaud's disease, sclerodactyly, esophageal dysmotility, and telangiectasia (CREST). Mixed connective tissue disease (MCTD) is considered a distinct disease that has features of several connective tissue diseases, including systemic lupus erythematosus, scleroderma, polymyositis, and rheumatoid arthritis. In this condition, as in scleroderma, the esophagus is the organ most often involved, with dysmotility being the main feature.

The major abnormality of scleroderma is the abnormal deposition of collagen into various tissues including the bowel. Thus, fibrosis is a major feature of this disease and although the esophagus is most commonly involved, fibrosis can also be seen in both colon and small bowel. However, there is also associated small vessel damage, particularly to the intestines, because much of this deposition produces vasculitis-type changes, with resultant long-term ischemia of the bowel. Malabsorption results because of stasis of the bowel contents, bacterial overgrowth, poor absorption of bile salts, and impaired lymphatic drainage. Diarrhea, weight loss, and bloating are all symptoms of this condition. Radiologically the changes of fibrosis, muscle atrophy, and vasculitis produce dilation of the small bowel, which is often termed "pseudo-obstruction." Pneumatosis is a known finding, especially pneumatosis coli, but its underlying cause not clear. A pathognomonic change seen in the bowel is crowding of the valvulae, or a "hidebound" appearance. The fibrosis of the bowel draws the valvulae closer together, producing more valvulae (> 5) per inch than normal. The margins of the intestines also may be flattened. This flattening gives the bowel an accordion-pleated appearance. In the colon the changes will often be a diminished or disordered haustral pattern with wide mouth diverticula-like deformities.

Notes

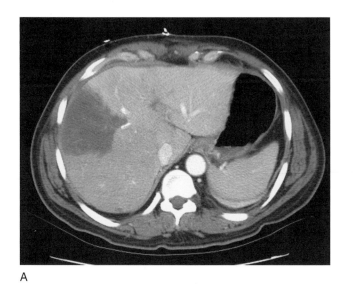

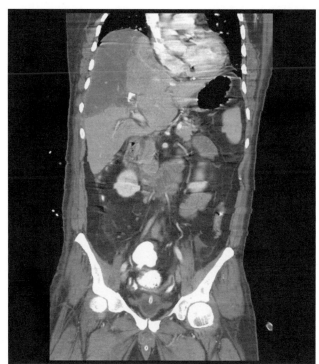

A   B

1. Describe the configuration of the findings in these images.

2. What is this most suggestive of?

3. What conditions might give rise to this finding?

4. What is the primary blood supply of the liver?

Focal Hepatic Artery Occlusion

1. Wedge-shaped perfusion defects in the peripheral right lobe of the liver.

2. Occluded hepatic artery with liver infarction.

3. Thrombosis or occlusion related to surgery, septic emboli, trauma.

4. The portal veins supply as much as 80% of the blood perfusion of the liver.

Cross-Reference

Gastrointestinal Imaging: THE REQUISITES, ed 3, p 177.

Comments

The patient shown in this case developed the wedge-shaped defect following surgery as a result of an hepatic artery vessel being ligated. The wedge-shaped defect is the hepatic infarction resulting from the interruption of arterial blood to the involved segment. One might think that because the liver has two blood supplies, the portal venous and the hepatic arterial, such things might be impossible. However, it has been shown that the portal venous system alone will not protect the liver from possible infarction if there is occlusion of the hepatic artery or its branches. This may relate to function. While the portal veins are transporting absorbed content from the GI tract to the liver for metabolism, the hepatic artery, rich in oxygen, has the primary function of delivering that oxygen to the hepatocyte. Most infarcts occur in the right lobe of the liver and because it is the largest part of the liver that should not be surprising. The best diagnostic tool at the moment is CT with images obtained in the late arterial phase of scanning. However, even in the portal venous phase, tissue damage will still result in the well-described "wedge-shaped" deformity described in imaging literature. In the right clinical setting the diagnosis can be made with confidence. However, it is still not specific, especially in those patients who present with CT findings similar to infarction, but do not have the clinical history. Other etiologic factors must be given some consideration such as hepatic abscess, laceration, or an unusual metastatic lesion and in rare cases, lymphoma of the liver. However, with the continued refinement of CTA (computed tomography arteriography) the ability to trace the hepatic artery as it swings away from the celiac axis, dividing into its right and left branches in the porta hepatis, has vastly improved.

Notes

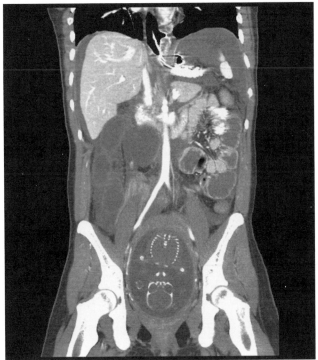

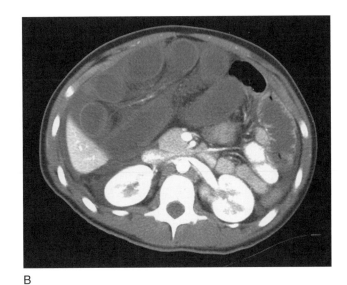

A

B

1. This 17-year-old pregnant patient complained of abdominal pain for several days, collapsed, and was brought to the hospital. What is your assessment of the condition of her small bowel?

2. What risk factors put patients at risk for this condition besides pregnancy?

3. What other CT findings might be expected in such a case?

4. What part of the small bowel is most severely affected by this process?

CASE 196

Mesenteric Venous Occlusion in Pregnancy

1. No perfusion to most of her bowel.

2. Hypercoagulable states.

3. Thrombus seen in superior mesenteric vein, air in bowel wall, thickened edematous bowel wall.

4. The small bowel and ascending colon.

Cross-Reference

Gastrointestinal Imaging: THE REQUISITES, ed 3, p 144.

Comments

Mesenteric venous thrombus is an uncommon form of mesenteric ischemia and infarction. The mortality rate is between 30% and 40%, and it is a deadly condition seen in patients with in hypercoagulable states, such as intraabdominal sepsis, pregnancy, and polycythemia vera, as well as in some women on oral contraceptives. In fact, a few cases of the condition have been reported in pregnant women who have accidentally taken oral contraceptives. Other causes range more widely and include blunt trauma and certain malignancies; rarely it is seen after abdominal surgeries. The striking findings in this case are the complete absence of perfusion of numerous loops of bowel. Note that the descending colon is perfused, suggesting this is a superior mesenteric condition. There is also free fluid in the abdomen, which can be expected in this condition. The high mortality rate associated with this condition is most certainly due to delayed diagnosis and the prolonged time of seeking medical attention.

Notes

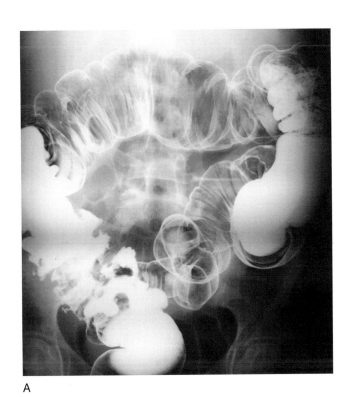

A

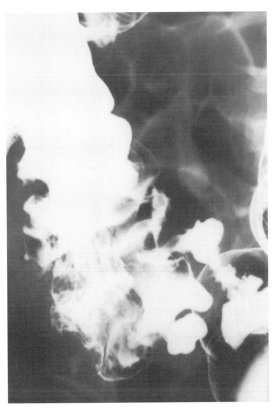

B

1. Describe the findings on this double contrast barium enema.

2. What conditions would you primarily consider?

3. If this patient had oral apthous ulcers, skin lesions, and genital ulcers, would such findings affect your diagnostic considerations?

4. What is "silk route" disease? What is its etiology?

Behçet's Disease of the Colon

1. Severe inflammatory and ulcerative changes that appear to be confined to the cecal region of the colon.

2. Crohn's disease, tuberculosis, possibly amebiasis, or an unusual manifestation of mural infiltrating neoplasm.

3. Yes.

4. Behçet's disease. A vasculitis of unknown cause affecting several organ systems.

Cross-Reference

Gastrointestinal Imaging: THE REQUISITES, ed 3, p 300.

Comments

Behçet's disease is a relatively rare condition in the West, but is seen with more frequency as people move about the world. It is primarily a condition affecting the population living around the Mediterranean Sea, thought to have been brought back in the Middle Ages along the "silk route" pioneered by Marco Polo in his journey to China. A Turkish physician first described it in the literature in the 1930s, and the disease is known by his name. It affects several organ systems, including the eyes, skin, genitals, joints, and gastrointestinal system. Almost always the colon is the GI organ involved, although cases of esophageal involvement have occurred. The most common site of colonic involvement appears to be the ileocecal region. The disease is essentially a vasculitis of unknown origin that leads to inflammation and ulcerative eruptions, many times deep and severe, such as in this case. It may be easily confused with other inflammatory bowel diseases, especially Crohn's disease. The patients usually have other manifestations of Behçet's disease when colonic symptoms manifest. Bowel perforations associated with Behçet's disease have been reported. Occasionally the disease may be seen as an ileocecal inflammatory mass similar to the ileocecal phlegmon seen in Crohn's disease.

Notes

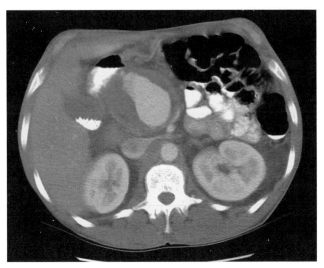

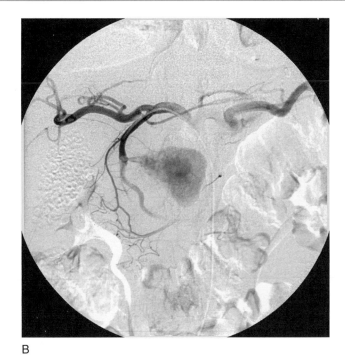

A

B

1. What is the major finding in these images?

2. What might be the accompanying history?

3. What is the incidence of this condition in chronic alcoholism?

4. What is the usual treatment?

Pseudoaneurysm of the Pancreatic Duodenal Artery

1. A large pear-shaped contrast-filled structure is seen on CT, representing a gastroduodenal artery pseudoaneurysm.

2. Chronic alcoholism.

3. Can be seen in up to 5% of cases of chronic pancreatitis.

4. Current treatment is usually nonsurgical, angioembolization.

Cross-Reference

Gastrointestinal Imaging: THE REQUISITES, ed 3, p 165.

Comments

Pseudoaneurysm of vessels in the pancreatic bed associated with chronic pancreatitis is not common, but can be seen in a small percentage of patients (usually < 5%). By far the most common vascular structure involved is the splenic artery. The gastroduodenal artery, as in this case, is the next most common vessel affected. If the abnormality is seen in the region of the head of the pancreas, it is usually the gastroduodenal artery. If it is in the body of the pancreas, it is the splenic artery. Apart from the expected symptoms of chronic pancreatitis, these patients often may have other symptoms relative to this vascular abnormality. However, cases of GI bleeding have been reported if the pseudoaneurysm breaks into the lumen of the gut or pancreatic duct, bile duct, or even into the retroperitoneum itself. A small number of pancreaticoduodenal artery pseudoaneurysms have also been reported. These findings will usually go undiagnosed without the use of CT or Doppler ultrasound. The differential consideration that has to be excluded is a pancreatic pseuodocyst. With the use of intravenous contrast material CT scanning can be definitive in most cases. Blood flow in the pseudoaneurysm can be detected with Doppler ultrasound in most cases. Physical examination is usually not productive, although pulsations detected in the pancreatic bed of patients with chronic pancreatitis, during physical examination, was the method of diagnosis before widespread imaging. Much of this art is lost today. Of course GDA pseudoaneurysms can occur in settings other than chronic alcoholism. Any condition that can result in pancreatitis can theoretically result in such a complication.

Notes

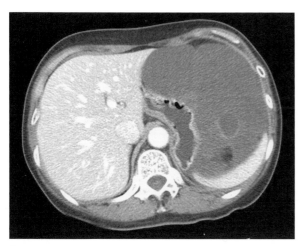

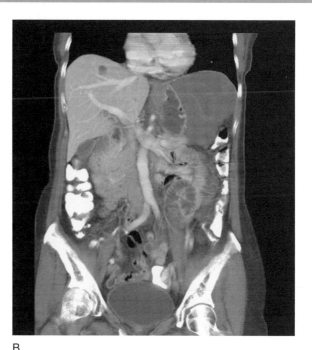

A   B

1. What is the striking feature about the CT images in this case of a women with upper abdominal discomfort?

2. What might be your differential diagnosis?

3. What is the cystic mass doing in relation to the stomach, spleen, and splenic flexure of the colon?

4. What is the site of origin for this process?

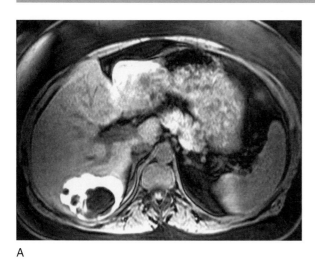

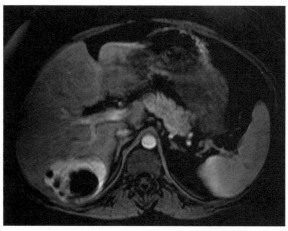

A   B

1. On these T$_1$-weighted MRI sequences, what does the mixed signal intensity of the lesion indicate?

2. Does the multilocular nature of the lesion help in diagnosis?

3. Which gender does this lesion have a predilection for?

4. What might utrasound show that is not evident in these MR images and might not be seen with CT?

Cystic Exophytic Gastrointestinal Stromal Cell Tumor of Stomach

1. A large, low-attenuation cystic mass is seen in the subphrenic left upper quadrant of the abdomen.

2. Subphrenic abscess, cystic lesions arising from the spleen stomach or pancreas.

3. The lesion is displacing all these structures.

4. The stomach. At surgery it was found to be a huge exophytic liquefied mass which was histologically a gastrointestinal stromal cell tumor (GIST).

Cross-Reference

Gastrointestinal Imaging: THE REQUISITES, ed 3, p 77.

Comments

Many of the GISTs encountered in the bowel and particularly the stomach behave in a benign fashion. They may be ulcerated and bleed if in the wall of the bowel. Most are solid tumors, although some show areas of tumor necrosis and liquefaction and resultant mixed density. By CT the GIST shown in this case is problematic, in that it does not seem to be "arising" from any particular organ and is almost entirely cystic, with the exception of some foci of density seen on the axial view. Initially GISTs were considered as mesenchymal or smooth muscle tumors, leiomyomas, or leiomyosarcoma. However, further histologic investigation began to suggest a surprising lack of smooth muscle elements in the lesion. As a result, the term gastrointestinal stromal cell tumor (GIST) was introduced to more correctly denote the spindle cell and epithelioid elements that compose these tumors. The tumor can undergo considerable necrosis and present as near-cystic lesions in some cases. However, there is also a distinctive morphologic varient of GIST characterized by myxoid content that is well encapsulated, cystic in appearance, mostly seen arising exophytically from the stomach, and mostly seen in women, and such a lesion is demonstrated in this case.

Notes

Cystadenoma of the Biliary Ducts

1. That the lesion is, in part, cystic in nature.

2. Helpful but not definitive.

3. Females, 4:1.

4. Ultrasound would probably show the septations that this cystadenoma of the bile ducts is very likely to have.

Cross-Reference

Gastrointestinal Imaging: THE REQUISITES, ed 3, p 203.

Comments

Biliary cystadenomas are a rare cystic lesion arising from the bile ducts. They are most commonly seen in middle-aged women and have some malignant potential. Often the patients present with upper abdominal discomfort; rarely jaundice or mass effect. Most of the time the finding may be incidental. The lesions are multiloculated and septated and this is usually more apparent with ultrasound than CT or MR imaging. With the lesion having malignant potential and the inability of diagnostic imaging in differentiating between a cystadenoma and a cystadenocarcinoma, needle aspiration biopsy or surgical removal is usually required for definitive histologic diagnosis. Both are slow growing and both can have similar imaging appearances. The lesions can be of varying sizes, with some as small as 3 to 5 cm and others up to 30 cm.

Alternative diagnostic considerations would be hepatic abscess and congenital biliary cysts. The latter is usually multiple and biliary cystadenomas are usually solitary. In the array of cystic lesions that may be seen in the liver, cystadenomas must be considered relatively rare, accounting for 1% to 5% of all hepatic cystic processes. In some reported cases symptomatic patients with a cystadenoma were misdiagnosed (i.e., a hydatid cyst). In general, when the finding of a multiloculated septated cyst (usually in the right lobe of the liver) is discovered in a middle-aged woman, biliary cystadenoma or cystadenocarcinoma should be considered in the differential diagnosis.

Notes